Complementary and Alternative Therapies for Epilepsy

Complementary and Alternative Therapies for Epilepsy

ORRIN DEVINSKY, MD
Professor of Neurology, Neurosurgery, and Psychiatry
NYU School of Medicine
New York, New York

STEVEN SCHACHTER, MD
Professor of Neurology
Harvard Medical School
Cambridge, Massachusetts

STEVEN PACIA, MD
Associate Professor, Department of Neurology
NYU School of Medicine
New York, New York

EDITORS

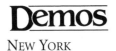

NEW YORK

Demos Medical Publishing, 386 Park Avenue South, New York, NY 10016
www.demosmedpub.com

Library of Congress Cataloging-in-Publication Data

Complementary and alternative therapies for epilepsy / Orrin Devinsky, Steven Schachter, and Steven Pacia, editors.
     p. ; cm.
 Includes bibliographical references and index.
 ISBN 1-888799-89-7 (hardcover : alk. paper)
 1. Epilepsy—Alternative treatment. [DNLM: 1. Epilepsy—therapy. 2. Complementary Therapies—methods. WL 385 C7367 2005] I. Devinsky, Orrin. II. Schachter, Steven C. III. Pacia, Steven, 1962–
 RC374.A46C66 2005
 616.8'5306—dc22

2005005690

About the cover: Portrait of Dr. Gachet, 1890, by Vincent van Gogh (1853–1890). Oil on canvas, 68.0 x 57.0 cm. Photo: Gérard Blot.

Photo credit: Réunion des Musées Nationaux/Art Resource, New York

Musee d'Orsay, Paris, France

This painting by van Gogh is of his physician, Dr. Paul-Ferdinand Gachet, holding foxglove. This plant is the source of digitalis, which was used to treat epilepsy, a disorder which van Gogh likely suffered from.

Contents

Contents

Contents

Preface

This book brings together experts in a variety of complementary and alternative medicine (CAM) disciplines who care for people with epilepsy or are working to develop new therapies for epilepsy. The group of authors is diverse in many ways—their backgrounds and geography as well as their approach to diagnosis and treatment.

Our goals are to bridge the traditional and CAM worlds. There is little doubt that most patients can benefit from both approaches. Yet the two worlds remain far apart in the United States. The vast majority of physicians are uncomfortable with CAM. The discomfort arises from a genuine distrust of therapies that lack proof of efficacy. The discomfort also arises from fear of the unknown and fear of competition. Most physicians were not taught about CAM. Unfortunately, all CAM is lumped together as "unscientific" and often spoken of pejoratively by doctors.

We provide commentary after all chapters except the introductory one. For many chapters, there is some additional information on the topic from our review of the literature. We try to provide a perspective on the content—areas we strongly support, viewpoints that we disagree with (sometimes reflecting that the quality of the data does not justify definitive or even modest support). In some cases, we are very skeptical about the data presented. When results so far exceed those for any other therapy, there should be a very healthy dose of doubt and skepticism (see Chapter 25, The Role of Carbon Dioxide in the Enhancement of Oxygen Delivery to the Brain). Such dramatic results should easily produce statistically significant benefits in controlled and blinded trials. They should be done!

We acknowledge our bias as Western physicians, trained and practicing in Western medical culture. We are academics and are all committed to the value of scientific studies—without controlled and blinded studies it is extremely hard to separate the true positive and negative effects from an intervention from the expectations, bias, hopes, and opinions that clouds everyone's vision and thinking—including Western doctors. These studies can be hard to do in the complementary and alternative medicine area. In some cases, identifying control conditions for which the patient and investigator are both blind is extremely difficult. However, this will be the only way we can move forward with confidence to identify truly effective therapies.

Finally, we thank the Finding A Cure for Epilepsy and Seizures (FACES) for the generous support in underwriting all of the expenses for a 3 day conference that brought all of the authors together at NYU Epilepsy Center and the preparation of this volume. The conference, co-sponsored by FACES, the Epilepsy Foundation, and the American

Epilepsy Society, served as a great opportunity for CAM and medical practitioners to share their experiences.

We hope that this volume helps to bring CAM and doctors caring for people with epilepsy closer, that it stimulates new research, and that it fosters a broader perspective of health for people with epilepsy.

Complementary and Alternative Therapies for Epilepsy

PART I

Complementary and Alternative Therapies: The Nature of the Evidence

Complementary and Alternative Therapies in Epilepsy: Relation to Western Medicine

Jessica Levine and Orrin Devinsky, MD

Mainstream medicine, oriented toward science-based care and prevention, is a recent advent in our species' 150,000-year history. The first effective medications for epilepsy, the bromides, were introduced 150 years ago. During the preceding 99.9% of our time, therapies we would call alternative were the *only* treatments. In their time, these treatments for epilepsy were largely considered mainstream and ranged from creating holes in the skull, exorcism of demons, bleeding and leeching, to herbs and prayer. We probably know only a small fraction of the treatments that were used to treat people with epilepsy. Some effective therapies may be lost with the cultures and healers who used them. Others may still exist but go unrecognized by our society.

Today, the paths of science-based and alternative medicine practices are largely parallel and independent—sometimes antagonistic, sometimes cooperative. Both paths have fostered many side roads. Both approaches have helped many and hurt some. A great challenge is to create a meaningful dialogue and exchange of ideas and lessons across the divide. Patients often integrate the two approaches.

The roots of modern medicine lie in *alternative medicine*, defined as those practices that are not an integral part of conventional health care. Although physicians recognize that many drugs originated as herbal folk medication, from the medical perspective, an enormous gap remains between science-based and alternative treatments.

In 1858, Sieveking, wrote that "there is not a substance in the material medica, there is scarcely a substance in the world, capable of passing through the gullet of man, that has not at one time or other enjoyed a reputation of being an anti-epileptic" (1). Although this comment focused on therapies consumed by mouth, Sieveking and other nineteenth century medical authorities recorded a spectrum of "alternative therapies," including the application of tourniquets to a seizing extremity, diets, rest, and herbal baths. The past 150 years have continued to witness an expansion in the medical and alternative therapies available to epilepsy patients.

Around the turn of the twentieth century, separating quackery from reputable therapeutic claims became a focus of the Bureau of Investigation of the American

Medical Association. From 1906 until the early 1930s, that association published a series of pamphlets on nostrums and quackery. An analysis of various tonics, renewers, remedies, syrups (Figure 1.1), and cures revealed that most contained bromides, phenobarbital, alcohol, or iodine. The majority of products were promoted by a "doctor" who was not a physician and were mislabeled if judged by the Federal Food and Drug Act guidelines. These medications were given to patients and family members with the assurance of safety and efficacy. They were also often associated with scare tactics to further stigmatize epilepsy (Figure 1.2). Quackery was not limited to individuals who peddled tonics and cures from pushcarts and pamphlets, or spiritualists who used deception. Rather, quackery extended to those with traditional medical backgrounds who used electrotherapy, surgery (e.g., removal of ovaries), and drugs (e.g., digitalis) that were ineffective and often dangerous.

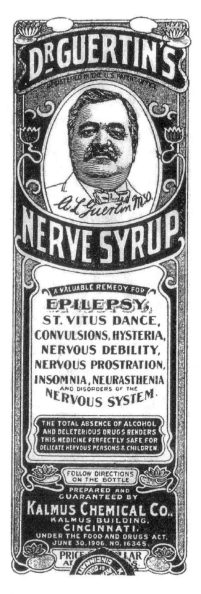

FIGURE 1.1

At the turn of the last century, a number of tonics and nostrums purported to control epilepsy were found to be ineffective or even harmful.

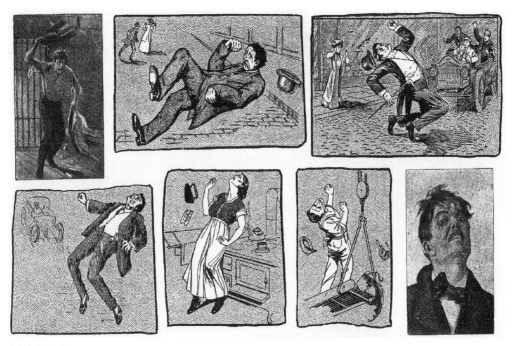

FIGURE 1.2

Many unscrupulous firms played on the fears of epilepsy patients to promote their products.

Concern about quackery persists today, despite the expectation that modern medicine should police itself. Healthcare is an enormous industry, with much of the market outside of traditional medical domains. For new medications or devices to gain the approval of regulatory boards, controlled studies must demonstrate safety, effectiveness, and tolerability. (Standards for surgical procedures may be less rigorous.) Safety data are often limited to a modest-sized sample, however. Serious, potentially life-threatening but infrequent effects may go unrecognized in premarketing studies that lead to U.S. Food and Drug Administration (FDA) approval. In 1993, this was the case with felbamate. Other important side effects may be unrecognized by the medical community despite well-documented studies. For example, the loss of bone mass from long-term treatment with antiepileptic drugs that induce the activity of certain liver enzymes (e.g., phenobarbital, carbamazepine, phenytoin, topiramate, valproate) was documented in the 1950s; however, many neurologists and most psychiatrists remain unaware of this potential effect of this commonly prescribed group of drugs. Although *quackery* is defined as the false promotion of cures, we can extend its meaning to the false promotion of a risk–benefit ratio.

Modern concerns over quackery are reflected in the existence of Quackwatch, Inc. (www.quackwatch.com), a corporation not affiliated with any commercial or industrial organization. This nonprofit corporation combats health-related fraud, myth, fad, and fallacy. Including information on both mainstream and alternative medicine, Quackwatch's primary focus is on providing information that is difficult or impossible to get elsewhere.

Modern Medical Treatment of Epilepsy

Epilepsy is a broad spectrum of disorders that affects individuals in many ways. Behind the choice of a medication or treatment for epilepsy is concern for preventing discomfort and injury from seizure, preventing brain damage, lessening social stigma, and improving outcome. The modern medications for epilepsy are acetazolamide, barbiturates, benzodiazepines [clonazepam, clobazam (not FDA-approved), clorazepate, lorazepam, valium] carbamazepine, ethosuximide, felbamate (serious risks limit its use), gabapentin, levetiracetam, lamotrigine, methsuximide, oxcarbazepine, phenytoin, primidone, tiagabine, topiramate, valproate, vigabatrin (not FDA-approved; retinal toxicity limits its use), and zonisamide.

Vagus nerve stimulation and *epilepsy surgery* are treatments for patients with epilepsy that does not respond to medication. Vagus nerve stimulation may reduce seizure frequency and intensity. The stimulating device is implanted in the chest wall and a lead (wire connection) is carefully wrapped around the left vagus nerve in the neck. The stimulator is programmed through a wand that is held to the skin or clothing over the chest wall overlying the device. The stimulator can be programmed to deliver different current strengths and different intervals of "on/off" cycles. Patients or family members can use an adjunctive external magnet to provide additional stimuli if a warning is perceived (aura) or the early part of the seizure can potentially be aborted.

Resective surgery seeks to remove the seizure focus—that area of the cerebral cortex responsible for causing the seizure. This technique is being used more frequently with increasing success and diminishing risks. Highest success rates are in cases of temporal lobe epilepsy or those with a clearly identified structural lesion on the MRI scan that corresponds with the origin of seizures as recorded on EEG or video-EEG studies. *Corpus callosotomy*, disconnecting (cutting) the fibers that connect the cerebral hemispheres in the brain, is another surgical alternative. This procedure is largely palliative (few patients have complete seizure control) and is used mainly for patients with drop seizures or tonic-clonic seizures. It has a higher complication rate than resective surgery.

The *ketogenic diet* (high in fat, low in carbohydrates and protein, limited fluids) helps children with epilepsy by raising the concentration of ketones in the body. Although it has been studied most extensively in children with symptomatic generalized epilepsies, it has been used successfully in other pediatric epilepsy syndromes and in adults. The exact mechanism by which this diet works is unknown. The diet, a complementary and alternative medicine (CAM), must be supervised by a nutritionist or physician.

Scientific Methods in Medical Research

Science is the orderly arrangement of knowledge, and *scientific methods* are the careful, systematic ways in which this knowledge increases. The scientist suggests a theory and then carefully performs tests over and over to confirm the hypothesis. The tests may include laboratory work, other observations, and clinical trials. The results of basic medical science give evidence of basic mechanisms of action that occur *in vitro* in cell culture and intracellularly, and *in vivo* in living organisms or cells. In vivo animal testing uses healthy, diseased, or genetically modified animals. Scientists know that animals and humans differ metabolically, physiologically, and hormonally, and make allowance for this fact.

Ideally, the assessment of the safety and efficacy of a CAM for epilepsy should be based on evidence from scientific research. If possible, we want to know the basic as well as the advanced research that has been performed on a CAM that is a natural product, and if possible, we want to know what the active ingredient is and if the active ingredient is always the same. Different batches of the product may not be the same. We also want to know if the product may produce allergic reactions and if any mainstream medication the patient may take will interact with the natural product.

Our motivation is to help the patient, do no harm, respect cultural differences that may incorporate CAM, and encourage the patient to safely continue receiving necessary medical treatment.

Observational Studies

Physicians decide on the treatment for patients with epilepsy based on many kinds of information, including published reports on laboratory and clinical trial research. This research is often based on studies of a large population and the synthesis of many different studies (a *meta-analysis*). The meta-analysis must account for study differences in design, patients, and statistical methods.

Physicians may also decide on treatments by using *observational studies*—careful observations (practice audits) based on the results of various treatments. What was the patient's condition? What effects (*outcome*), good and bad, did a treatment have on a patient? Is the patient happy with the treatment? It is not easy to decide if the treatment will be beneficial for one particular patient, or if the treatment will be the most effective one for that patient. Observational studies are appropriate for CAM.

Qualitative Research

Qualitative research, based on the patient's perceived *quality of care* and sometimes reported in case studies, focuses on a patient's comments. These comments may reflect a particular sociocultural context. Like the results of clinical research, this information, if distributed or published, should not reveal who the patient is.

Case Studies

Case studies, formally published as case reports or compiled informally, give details about the symptoms, treatment, and outcome of a particular patient's illness. The patient interview (and often a family interview) is an important part of the case study; it includes statements about medical history, symptoms, responses to treatment, and *quality of life*—the patient's ability to enjoy life.

Randomized Clinical Trials

Using scientific methods, *clinical trials* study the safety and effectiveness of a new medication or medical procedure. Clinical science involves the direct observation of patients, for example, how much improvement occurred and the side effects of the treatment. *Randomization* in a clinical trial is the chance assignment of a patient to active treatment or to a nontreatment control group. The control group receives a *placebo*, which is an inactive substance. The patients in the two treatment groups have similar traits, such as the extent of disease. Only authorized physicians may administer the study, and either the National Institutes of Health, a pharmaceutical company, or a private institution may sponsor them.

The trial must follow a detailed written set of rules called a *protocol*, which includes the goals of the study, the number of patients to be treated, inclusion and exclusion criteria, and how the patients will be evaluated. The research staff regularly checks the health of the participants in the trial.

A Phase 1 trial of a new medication ascertains the pharmacological activity of a new treatment and what quantity of the treatment can be prescribed. It is the first time the new medication is taken by humans. Phase 2 determines effectiveness and appropriate dosage; Phase 3, the efficacy of the treatment and the adverse experiences that occur; and Phase 4 (after approval by the FDA), the unusual and infrequent adverse experiences.

In a *blinded study*, the patient does not know whether the medication he receives is the experimental medication or the placebo. In a double-blind study, neither the patients nor the investigators know who receives the medication and who receives the inactive substance. The purpose of blinding is to eliminate bias such as the expectation of cure or of side effects.

Epidemiological research studies the incidence, distribution, and control of illness in populations, and how various influences (diet, lifestyle, environment, medication) prevent or cure the disease.

Clinical trials performed to discover new, perhaps alternative ways to treat epilepsy are especially difficult to design. Seizures occur at irregular intervals. How can we ethically assign a patient with epilepsy to a control group receiving no active treatment? Can the patient having a seizure remember and describe the effects of the intervention? Because epilepsy is a chronic illness, treatment may be required for many years. How long can a response last? What are its long-term and rare side effects?

Limits of Western Medicine and Research

Epilepsy is a difficult illness to control. The frequency of epilepsy and of seizures increases in the elderly, whose numbers are also growing. Up to 35% of patients with epilepsy do not respond fully to science-based medical treatments, which in the developed countries include at least 20 drugs (2–4). More than half of patients surveyed in the community report at least occasional seizures, and the majority report medication side effects (5). Those patients with medically refractory epilepsy suffer the greatest from the physical, mental, and psychosocial effects of epilepsy. They often take high doses of antiepileptic drugs or multiple drugs, thus leading to a greater burden of disabling side effects. Medication side effects are often underappreciated by physicians (3). People with refractory epilepsy are the greatest financial burden to the health care system (6). They often undergo extensive testing, require emergency room or inpatient care, and may undergo procedures such as epilepsy surgery. In our experience, they are also the group most likely to utilize CAM therapies. Indeed, in some cases, they may simultaneously or sequentially work with many types of CAM practitioners.

A chronic illness that does not respond to standard medical therapy, or in which those therapies have significant adverse effects, leads many individuals to explore other options. For many, the tenets of evidence-based medicine become secondary to "getting well." Modern medicine fails to effectively control or cure the symptoms of patients with many diseases, including diabetes, cancer, heart and lung diseases, and mental illness. Compounding those treatment failures are the limited economic and public health resources devoted to medical care, the growing demand for health services, and the growing number of elderly persons and chronic illnesses of old age.

For children and adults with epilepsy, approaches outside the traditional boundaries may improve seizure control. For example, stress is reported to be a factor that can provoke seizures in a large number of epilepsy patients. Stress can be reduced through a variety of approaches. Many complementary and alternative therapies reviewed in this book specifically address stress reduction. Further, relaxation techniques can provide some sense of control over the disorder. Traditional medicine should consider nonmedical healing and work to identify places where it may be helpful. Although benefits likely extend beyond stress reduction, this is one area that is worthy of further study in the near future.

Many patients achieve a balance of both medical care and alternative therapies. For example, some Navajo receive health care both from the Indian Health Service and native healers. Rarely is there a perceived conflict between the two. The native healers even treat "bad luck" (7). One observer of the Navajo commented, "Physicians and other healers simply remove obstacles to the body's restoration of homeostasis, or, as the Navajo say, to harmony.... An alternative model [of healing] might include emotional, social, or spiritual phenomena equally as significant to healing as are biochemical phenomena" (8). The Epilepsy Foundation recommends that "alternative treatments are acceptable as long as the patient continues with the traditional therapies and the alternative and traditional therapies do not conflict" (9).

We all recognize the tremendous value of offering kindness, caring, hope, and information for individuals with physical and emotional problems. By definition, these are alternative therapies that form an essential element of both mainstream Western and alternative approaches to health.

Overview of Complementary and Alternative Medicine

- On October 25, 2001, "PubMed," a U.S. National Library of Medicine online listing of journal articles in selected medical journals, had 46,847 different entries about "alternative medicine."

- The use of CAM medical treatments began growing at least 50 years ago. A 1997, U.S. telephone survey of 2,055 people from all walks of life revealed that more than one-third of the population currently used a CAM therapy. In fact, in that survey, 67.6% of respondents had used at least one CAM therapy in their lifetime. Lifetime use steadily increased with age across three age cohorts: Approximately 3 of every 10 respondents in the pre-Baby Boom cohort, 5 of 10 in the Baby Boom cohort, and 7 of 10 in the post-Baby Boom cohort reported using some type of CAM therapy by age 33 years (10).

This is the tip of the iceberg since many individuals who provide CAM do not publish (this is also true for >90% of medical doctors) and, if they do publish, the journals often are not referenced in Index Medicus or PubMed.

CAM therapies fall into extremely diverse categories with diverse origins, as varied as the countries and cultures they come from. Acupuncture, biofeedback, colonic washout, creative visualization, electrical stimulation, elimination of stress, herbal therapies, magnetic stimulation, muscle relaxation, music as sedation, nutritional therapies, prayer, and spirituality are a very partial list of CAMs.

When deciding about CAM and mainstream medical treatment for epilepsy and evaluating studies based on the treatment, physicians, patients, and families must ask these important questions:

- What was the purpose of the study?
- Who reviewed and approved the study from the perspectives of medical ethics, patient safety, and scientific merit?
- Who sponsored the study?
- How were the study data and patient safety checked?
- Did patients or investigators have an opportunity to bias the outcome of the study?

Our Challenge

The future of healthcare requires a partnership among all those who are devoted to preventing illness in the healthy and restoring health in the ill. No one approach, therapy, or model will work for all people or illnesses. We must work together, across philosophical and other divides, to find productive solutions.

References

1. Sieveking EH. *Epilepsy and Epileptic Seizures.* London: Churchill Livingstone, 1858:226.
2. Aiken SP, Brown WM. Treatment of epilepsy: existing therapies and future developments. *Front Biosci* 2000;5:E124–152.
3. Devinsky O, Penry JK. Quality of life in epilepsy: the clinician's perspective. *Epilepsia* 1993;34(suppl 4):S4–S7.

4. Devinsky O. Patients with refractory seizures. *N Engl J Med* 1999;304:1565–1570.
5. Living with epilepsy—report of a Roper poll of patients on quality of life. New York: Roper Organization, Inc., 1992.
6. Begley CE, Famulari M, Annegers JF, et al. The cost of epilepsy in the United States: an estimate from population-based clinical and survey data. *Epilepsia* 2000;41(3):342–351.
7. Kim C, Kwok YS. Navajo use of native healers. *Arch Intern Med* 1998;158:2245–2249.
8. Coulehan JL. Navaho Indian medicine: implications for healing. *J Fam Pract* 1980;10:55–61.
9. Hughes D. Patients with epilepsy increasingly embrace alternative and complementary medicines. *Neurology Reviews* 2002;(10)8.
10. Kessler RC, Davis RB, Foster DF, et al. Long-term trends in the use of complementary and alternative medical therapies in the United States. *Ann Intern Med* 2001;135:262–268.

CHAPTER 2

Double- and Dual-Blindness— Raising the Bar of Proof for Trials of Complementary and Alternative Therapies*

OPHER CASPI, MD, CORI MILLEN, DO, AND LEE SEECHREST, PHD

The *double-blind* is a fundamental concept in clinical research. It is considered a cornerstone of clinical trials of the efficacy and effectiveness of interventions. A true double-blind requires that both parties in a study—the subjects and the caregivers—are blind (i.e., ignorant of the true intervention or lack thereof). Blindness is used in clinical studies to control potential external or nonspecific influences, such as belief and expectation, as well as to maintain as much objectivity as possible on the part of the researchers (1). The double-blind method is most often used within the context of placebo-controlled randomized trials, which are considered by clinicians and researchers as the gold standard for clinical research. Is the double-blind methodology truly feasible in all medical disciplines? The answer is no.

Many interventions in medicine and surgery cannot be tested using the double-blind method because the caregiver cannot be blind to the treatment given—for example, surgery, psychotherapy, and several modalities falling into the diverse field of complementary and alternative medicine (CAM) therapies (e.g., acupuncture and osteopathy). It is not possible for an experienced acupuncturist or osteopath to carry out interventions without knowing whether their actions were intended as active treatments or as placebos. Nevertheless, numerous articles using the term "double-blind" in their title are published in these and other related fields, presumably because the term describes the methodology used to conduct these studies; however, conceptually it does not make any sense. What is the real meaning of double-blindness in these settings?

To determine just how the term double-blind is being used by researchers, we searched the literature on clinical trials assessing some CAM modalities. In many cases,

This chapter is derived from the article "Integrity and Research: Introducing the Concept of Dual-blindness. How Blind Are Double-blind Clinical Trials in Alternative Medicine?" *The Journal of Alternative and Complementary Medicine*, 2000;6:493-498. Mary Ann Liebert, Inc., Larchmont, NY. Modified with the permission of the publisher.

double-blind often indicates that a patient and an external evaluator were blind to the specific type of the intervention but the caregiver was not. Thus, double-blind is often used in studies in which the caregiver was aware of the intervention condition for each patient, even if the patient and the research staff assessing the patient were not.

A study is truly double-blind only if both the subjects and the caregivers are blind. The blinding of the caregiver is as critical as blinding the patient. The reason this distinction should be maintained is that caregivers who know whether the intervention they are administering is supposed to be the active condition or the placebo may behave differently—for example, in their enthusiasm, encouragement, body language, firmness of their directions, and subtle communications of expectations. This phenomenon was given the name the *experimenter effect* in 1966 (2), and it was especially important when a systematic evaluation of the literature on healing and spirituality was conducted and later published in 1990 (3). All these effects and others could bias the results of studies even if the patient and the clinical assessor were satisfactorily blinded to the study conditions.

To maintain integrity in research, it is necessary to clearly distinguish between these two methodological situations. We believe that the appellation *double-blind* should be reserved for studies in which no one associated with the delivery of treatment or assessment is aware of the treatment condition being received by the patient. In all other cases, for example, when the caregiver is not blind but the patient and an external evaluator/investigator are, a distinct term must describe that different study design. The term should reflect, as accurately as possible, what actually was done in the study. We therefore suggest the term *dual-blind study* as a label for a design in which the subject and an assessor, but not the caregiver, are blind. We present here an empirical justification for proposing an additional methodological complexity.

Methodology

A MEDLINE search between 1966 and April 1999 (Table 2.1) was conducted to better define the frequency with which dual-blind studies are misleadingly reported as double-blind in the CAM literature. MEDLINE is a well-known biomedical bibliographic database of articles about health care that is published by the United States National Library of Medicine. (*Double-blind method* was used as a key string and cross-referenced with different CAM modalities in which clinical trials using double-blind methodology were unlikely.) The scope note for double-blind method as a medical subject heading (MeSH) term in MEDLINE ("A method of studying a drug or procedure in which both the subjects and investigators are kept unaware of who is actually getting which specific treatment") uses the term *investigators* but implies the actual caregivers. Regrettably, in several studies (4–6), the description of the methodology was poor, and we could not discern the methods. These studies were excluded from our sample.

On obtaining MEDLINE results, the title and the abstract of each article was studied to learn whether the article claimed to be double-blind. If a double-blind methodol-

TABLE 2.1

Summary of the MEDLINE Literature

Search Findings Restricted to Publications in English for Double-blind Methodology in Various CAM Modalities (1966–1999)

Keyword		Number of References
1	Double-blind method	49,355
2	Acupuncture	6,785
3	1 and 2	64
4	Osteopathy	2,275
5	1 and 4	18
6	Chiropractic	1,714
7	1 and 6	11
8	Energy medicine	5
9	1 and 8	0

ogy was not claimed, the article was excluded. If the article claimed to be double-blind, the actual methodology of each trial was focused on. If the trial utilized a method in which both the patient and the caregiver were blind, the article was considered a true double-blind study; however, if the trial utilized a method in which the patient and an external evaluator were blind but the caregiver was not, it was considered a dual-blind study. For internal validity, we agreed in advance on the characteristics of each category. Table 2.2 summarizes the common scenarios regarding blindness in clinical studies, highlighting that blindness is a spectrum.

TABLE 2.2

Characterization of Common Categories of Blindness in Clinical Trials

Category	Patient	Caregiver	Evaluator	Comments
Triple-blind	Blind	Blind	Blind	Not included in this study
Double-blind	Blind	Blind	No evaluator	The main focus of this study
Dual-blind	Blind	Aware	Blind	The main focus of this study
Modified Dual-blind	Blind	Aware	The patient also serves as an evaluator	Possible when the outcome is blindness (pain, nausea, etc.)
Single-blind	Blind	Aware	Aware	Not included in this study
Open-label	Aware	Aware	Aware	Not included in this study

Results

In CAM, many articles are incorrectly classified as double-blind. We reviewed 40 articles in different CAM modalities: acupuncture (6–22), acupressure (5,23–28), osteopathy (29–31), and chiropractic manipulation (32–38), as well as other manual techniques (3,39–42). We could not find one study using these modalities that was truly double-blind, yet all claimed this methodology in their title or abstract. The initial hypothesis that true double-blind methodology was unlikely in these therapeutic modalities was supported. All these studies are more accurately classified as dual-blind.

The following quote from one of the studies that we reviewed exemplifies the difference between a true double-blind methodology and a dual-blind one (42): "Outcome measures were recorded by a researcher other than the one who applied the experimental conditions. This researcher was blind to the applied conditions, thus fulfilling the requirements of the tester in meeting the double-blind conditions." We strongly disagree. In contrast, we believe that a statement regarding the true nature of the methodology that was actually used to conduct a study, such as the following one: "...randomly ordered, subject and evaluator-blind crossover [study]" (14) really addresses the critical issue.

Patients also served as the evaluators in some of the studies we reviewed. This methodology is commonly used when the outcome or the independent variable is subjective (e.g., postoperative pain or nausea). We consider this methodology to be a modified version of dual-blind because patients are still open to suggestions by caregivers. Further, a patients' perception of the treatment or the interaction with their caregiver can interfere with their role as evaluators. Thus, it is even more difficult to control for all sorts of confounds using this method. These weaknesses make this modified version of the dual-blind method very problematic.

In several other studies (7,40), a combination of a specific CAM modality with a medication or another intervention was used. Our hypothesis was also confirmed, because the first part was dual-blind, whereas the latter was double-blind.

Discussion

The term *double-blind* is used in two different ways that impair its usefulness as a methodologic recommendation and as a descriptor. In its legitimate usage, double-blind implies that neither the patient nor the caregiver is aware of the intervention performed. In its aberrant use, however, this term is used to describe an experimental arrangement in which two parties are blind, but a critical third party is not. Most often, the patient and an external evaluator/investigator are blind but the person actually providing the care is unblinded. Confusion exists around this concept.

A research methodology that involves a blind third party is often valuable, but that tactic does not accomplish the ultimate goals of double-blindness. Understanding the importance of complete blindness, many researchers try to ensure it. A questionnaire administered at study completion assessing the perceptions of patients during the experiment can help differentiate between treatment and the control conditions, but it does not guarantee full blindness or the ability to detect the subtle influences on the unblinded party. Unless the caregiver is blind to the research condition, as can be done easily in most drug studies, this research methodology cannot control for the caregiver biases. The expectations of physicians, as well as subtle messages and indirect suggestions made by the clinician, can influence the patient–caregiver interaction and bias study results and outcomes. Expectancy effects were demonstrated in humans and were systematically related to the magnitude of the outcome (2). As a direct result, an objective testing of efficacy and effectiveness may be impossible under these circumstances because all the above confounds can threaten the construct validity of any experiment [see the thorough discussion by Cook and Campbell (43)].

Integrity is crucial in science. The fact that researchers and clinicians label some of their clinical trials as double-blind—even though they are not—calls for close attention.

Commentary

Dr. Caspi and his colleagues provide a valuable look at the vexing problem of proof. How do we determine if a "standard" or "alternative/complementary" therapy actually works and is safe? Western medicine has faced a challenging road to reach its current burden of proof. Complementary and alternative medicine (CAM) remains enormously popular among diverse segments of Western and non-Western societies. Proving the efficacy and safety of these techniques poses significant challenges. In part, the medical-scientific culture that defines mainstream medicine is different than the CAM culture that runs parallel and divergent from it; however, when it comes to proof, we are left with few alternatives that eliminate the bias inherent in patients, caregivers, and scientific researchers.

Western medicine is laden with numerous and deep faults. We are all biased—even the most scientifically gifted fall prey to their emotions and feelings, elevating opinions beyond their authority. Consider a lecture that was popular 15 to 20 years ago given by a prominent epilepsy specialist, whose medical and scientific publications focused on basic models of epilepsy, examining cellular mechanisms in the laboratory. He spoke on the topic of "rational polytherapy." The lecture addressed how clinicians combine two or more traditional antiepileptic drugs in a patient using "scientific" principles. For example, the lecturer advocated using drugs with alternative mechanisms of action and avoiding drugs with side effect profiles that are similar. It was a well conceived and articulated presentation. The remarkable feature was the certainty with which the argument was framed. It was not offered as "my clinical approach," or "in my experience," nor was it based on any published data. It went further. It criticized physicians who used certain combinations and clearly favored specific combinations for certain seizure types. It was presented as if it were based on rigorous studies and data. It was not. If someone had presented data with similar evidence at one of the scientific meetings on basic animal mechanisms, those in attendance would have laughed. Indeed, counter-arguments could be easily raised. Some of the most effective anti-cancer drug combinations rely on targeting a single pathway at different sites. Further, although we had a good idea about how the major antiepileptic drugs work to prevent or stop seizure spread 15-20 years ago, our knowledge remains incomplete today. We must always honestly assess what we do know and what we do not know. Medical doctors often fail to meet this challenge.

This scientist's error came from generalizing his value system and raising the height of the bar for carefully designed scientific studies to clinical medicine's lowest echelon of proof: "In my experience" or "I think." Based on these very humble origins of anecdotal observation in a few patients or interesting ideas, wonderful things have followed. Many were subsequently proven by well designed and well executed double-blind studies. In other cases, the opinions have been proven false. Darwin, in the closing chapter of *The Descent of Man*, admonished us with prophetic wisdom:

> "False facts are highly injurious to the progress of science, for they often endure long; but false views, if supported by some evidence, do little harm, for everyone takes a salutary pleasure in proving their falseness: and when this is done, one path towards error is closed and the road to truth is often at the same time opened."

Studies on traditional medical and surgical therapies can also suffer from a number of other problems. In many cases, companies that manufacture a drug or device fund the studies. The potential conflict here is enormous—study design, outcome measure, choice of investigators, control of data, statistical tests that are chosen (and possibly those that are tried and never reported), and the interpretation and "spin" on the results. For double-blind studies, much of the potential bias should be eliminated by the study design. The most notorious place for abuse is in post-marketing studies. In some cases, companies provide direct grants to investigators to study a specific question about their drug or device by reviewing patient charts. In some cases, they assist in obtaining the data and writing the manuscript. The cracks in the medical system are perhaps deepest here, and attempts are underway to fix these problems. Similar, but also different problems plague the CAM study literature.

Table 2.2 provides a nice overview of the types of studies that are used to support the effectiveness of safety of both traditional and CAM therapies. Single case reports and observations of small numbers of patients, an even more basic and less formal level of study than the "open-label" study, is often the starting ground for therapeutic advances. The use of amantadine to treat influenza led to the observation that some patients with Parkinson's disease showed improvements in energy level and motor function, leading to more formal studies and wider use of this medication in Parkinson's disease. Observations in individual cases are powerful incentives and stimulants towards new ideas, but they are also the places where the greatest errors of relating cause and effect can occur. As one moves up the ladder from open-label to single-blind to dual-blind to double-blind studies, the value of the data increases; however, many other factors can limit the value of the data and its use in drawing conclusions. If the measures are not carefully designed, if outcome measures are not defined before the study begins, if the wrong statistics are used, and if too many subgroups or too few patients are studied, the results may lack meaning.

This chapter provides an important perspective on the critical nature of proof in scientific studies, whether those studies address traditional or CAM therapies. We hope that it promotes more accurate descriptions of studies and their designs, and further raises the bar on proving the efficacy and safety of all therapies.

Several factors might contribute to the misuse of the label "double-blind studies" with interventions in which double-blind testing is difficult, if not impossible. These factors include nondiscriminating research terminology, desire for academic respectability, and competition to publish and seek funding.

Medicine is practiced under societal forces that greatly influence practitioners. Data are the only dependable currency in the scientific world. The better the source of the data, the more valuable the currency. In the perceived hierarchy of evidence, double-blind trials produce methodologically superior, higher quality data than non–double-blinded studies. The value of the label "double-blind study" contributes to the strong preference to use this potent label for clinical studies that involve a methodology with blinded parties, even if the design is not truly double-blind. Categorizing a dual-blind study as a double-blind one may be considered a "white lie," but it is a dangerous one. Are these clinical trials incorrectly described as double-blind with the possible intent that they will be regarded as somehow better and, therefore, increase the chances that they will be published or funded; or, on the other hand, is the fault merely one of an inadequate methodologic vocabulary? We believe that adopting a specific descriptor for the blinded, but less than double-blinded, study design will help foster greater truth in advertising and research reporting.

The problem of mislabeled studies is probably not unique to CAM, and it is likely that examples occur in other medical areas, especially those in which double-blind testing is very difficult. The distinction proposed herein could be generally applied; however, the field of CAM would benefit from preserving an important scientific distinction and more accurately characterizing the quality of the data that are presented.

Conclusion

Although the use of CAM remains very prevalent, recent considerable growth in research trials, improved research methodologies, and acceptance of CAM articles in mainstream medical journals provides an opportunity to better define the efficacy and safety of CAM. Moving forward, CAM must avoid spurious claims of double-blind methodologies. Standards and terminologies must avoid misleading information. A proposed new term in research methodology, *dual-blind*, can be used to describe a method in which the caregiver is not blind but the patient and an external evaluator are blind. The term *double-blind* can only accurately describe a methodology in which both the patient and the caregiver are blind. Making the distinction between these two terms will enhance both the reliability of clinical trial interpretation and research integrity.

References

1. Kazdin AE. *Research Design in Clinical Psychology*, 3rd ed. Needham Heights, MA: Allyn & Bacon, 1998.
2. Rosenthal R. *Experimenter Effects in Behavioral Research*. New York: Appelton-Century-Crofts, 1966.
3. Benor DJ. Surgery of spiritual healing research. *Complement Med Res* 1990; 4:9–33.
4. Waylonis GW, Wilke S, O'Toole D, et al. Chronic myofascial pain: management by low-output helium-neon laser therapy. *Arch Phys Med Rehabil* 1988;69:1017–1020.
5. de Aloysio D, Penacchioni P. Morning sickness control in early pregnancy by Neiguan point acupressure. *Obstet Gynecol* 1992;80:852–854.
6. Vilholm OJ, Moller K, Jorgensen K. Effect of traditional Chinese acupuncture on severe tinnitus: a double-blind, placebo-controlled, clinical investigation with open therapeutic control. *Br J Audiol* 1998;32:197–204.
7. Chapman CR, Benedetti C, Colpitts YH, et al. Naloxone fails to reverse pain thresholds elevated by acupuncture: acupuncture analgesia reconsidered. *Pain* 1983;16:13–31.
8. Lenhard L, Waite PM. Acupuncture in the prophylactic treatment of migraine headaches: pilot study. *N Z Med J* 1983;96:663–666.
9. Christensen PA, Laursen LC, Taudorf E, et al. Acupuncture and bronchial asthma. *Allergy* 1984;39:379–385.
10. Marks NJ, Emery P, Onishiphorou C. A controlled trial of acupuncture in tinnitus. *J Laryngol Otol* 1984;98:1103–1109.
11. Haas M, Peterson D, Rothman EH, et al. Responsiveness of leg alignment changes associated with articular pressure testing to spinal manipulation: the use of a randomized clinical trial design to evaluate a diagnostic test with a dichotomous outcome. *J Manip Physiol Ther* 1993;16:306–311.
12. Hackett GI, Seddon D, Kaminski D. Electroacupuncture compared with paracetamol for acute low back pain. *Practitioner* 1988;232:163–164.
13. Tandon MK, Soh PF. Comparison of real and placebo acupuncture in histamine-induced asthma. A double-blind crossover study. *Chest* 1989;96:102–105.
14. Haker E, Lundeberg T. Laser treatment applied to acupuncture points in lateral humeral epicondylalgia. A double-blind study. *Pain* 1990;43:243–247.
15. Tandon MK, Soh PF, Wood AT. Acupuncture for bronchial asthma? A double-blind crossover study. *Med J Aust* 1991;154:409–412.

16. Tavola T, Gala C, Conte G, et al. Traditional Chinese acupuncture in tension-type headache: a controlled study. *Pain* 1992;48:325–329.

17. Takeda W, Wessel J. Acupuncture for the treatment of pain of osteoarthritic knees. *Arthritis Care Res* 1994;7:118–122.

18. Schwager KL, Baines DB, Meyer RJ. Acupuncture and postoperative vomiting in day-stay paediatric patients. *Anaesth Intens Care* 1996;24:674–677.

19. Al-Sadi M, Newman B, Julious SA. Acupuncture in the prevention of postoperative nausea and vomiting. *Anaesthesia* 1997;52;658–661.

20. Biemacki W, Peake MD. Acupuncture in treatment of stable asthma. *Respiratory Med* 1998;92:1143–1145.

21. Schlager A, Offer T, Baldissera I. Laser stimulation of acupuncture point P6 reduces postoperative vomiting in children undergoing strabismus surgery. *Br J Anaesthesia* 1998;81:529–532.

22. Shlay JC, Chaloner K, Max MB, et al. Acupuncture and amitriptyline for pain due to HIV-related peripheral neuropathy: a randomized controlled trial. *JAMA* 1998;280: 1590–1595.

23. Lewis IH, Pryn SJ, Reynolds PI, et al. Effect of P6 acupressure on postoperative vomiting in children undergoing outpatient strabismus correction. *Br J Anaesth* 1991;67:73–78.

24. Stein DJ, Bimbach DJ, Danzer BI, et al. Acupressure versus intravenous metoclopramide to prevent nausea and vomiting during spinal anesthesia for cesarean section. *Anesth Analg* 1997;84:342–345.

25. Warwick-Evans LA, Masters IJ, Redstone SB. A double-blind placebo controlled evaluation of acupressure in the treatment of motion sickness. *Aviation Space Environ Med* 1991;62:776–778.

26. Belluomini J, Litt RC, Lee KA, et al. Acupressure for nausea and vomiting of pregnancy: a randomized, blind study. *Obstet Gynecol* 1994;82:245–248.

27. Ho CM, Hseu SS, Tsai SK, et al. Effect of P-6 acupressure on prevention of nausea and vomiting after epidural morphine for post-cesarean section pain relief. *Acta Anaesthesiol Scand* 1996;40:372–375.

28. Fan CF, Tanhui E, Joshi S, et al. Acupressure treatment for prevention of postoperative nausea and vomiting. *Anesth Analg* 1997;84:821–825.

29. Kelso AF, Larson NJ, Kappler RE. A clinical investigation of the osteopathic examination. *J Am Osteopathic Assoc* 1980;79:460–467.

30. Belcastro MR, Backes CR, Chila AG. Bronchiolitis: a pilot study of osteopathic manipulative treatment, bronchodilators, and other therapy. *J Am Osteopathic Assoc* 1984;83:672–676.

31. Gibson T, Grahame R, Harkness J, et al. Controlled comparison of short-wave diathermy treatment with osteopathic treatment in nonspecific low back pain. *Lancet* 1985;1: 1258–1261.

32. Sloop PR, Smith DS, Goldenberg E, et al. Manipulation for chronic neck pain. A double-blind controlled study. *Spine* 1982;7:532–535.

33. Vicenzino B, Collins D, Benson H, et al. An investigation of the interrelationship between manipulative therapy-induced hypoalgesia and sympathoexcitation. *J Manip Physiol Ther* 1998;21:448–453.

34. Haas M, Peterson D, Hoyer D, et al. Muscle testing response to provocative vertebral challenge in spinal manipulation: a randomized controlled trial of construct validity. *J Manip Physiol Ther* 1994;17:141–148.

35. Fritz-Ritson D. Phasic exercises for cervical rehabilitation after "whiplash" trauma. *J Manip Physiol Ther* 1995;18:21–24.

36. Nielsen NH, Bronfort G, Bendix T, et al. Chronic asthma and chiropractic spinal manipulation: a randomized clinical trial. *Clin Exp Allergy* 1995;25:80–88.

37. Carrick FR. Changes in brain function after manipulation of the cervical spine [published erratum appears in *J Manip Physiol Ther* 1998;21:304]. *J Manip Physiol Ther* 1997;20: 529–545.

38. Peterson KB. The effects of spinal manipulation on the intensity of emotional arousal in phobic subjects exposed to a threat stimulus: a randomized, controlled, double-blind clinical trial. *J Manip Physiol Ther* 1997;20:602–606.

39. Sims-Williams H, Jayson MI, Young SM, et al. Controlled trial of mobilisation and manipulation for patients with low back pain in general practice. *BMJ* 1978;2:1338–1340.

40. Garvey TA, Marks MR, Wiesel SW. A prospective, randomized, double-blind evaluation of trigger-point injection therapy for low-back pain. *Spine* 1989;14:962–964.

41. Melzack R, Vetere P, Finch L. Transcutaneous electrical nerve stimulation for low back pain. Comparison of TENS and massage for pain and range of motion. *Phys Ther* 1983;63: 489–493.

42. Vicenzino B, Collins D, Wright A. The initial effects of a cervical spine manipulative physiotherapy treatment on the pain and dysfunction of lateral epicondylalgia. *Pain* 1996;8: 69–74.

43. Cook TD, Campbell DT. *Quasi-Experimentation: Design and Analysis Issues for Field Settings*. Boston: Houghton Mifflin Company, 1979.

PART II

Learning to
Reduce Seizures

CHAPTER 3

Stress and Epilepsy

CAROL J. SCHRAMKE, PHD AND KEVIN M. KELLY, MD, PHD

Patients with epilepsy frequently report that stress and stressful life events influence the frequency and severity of their seizures and that epilepsy itself can cause significant stress. Despite the apparent relationship between stress and epilepsy, a relatively poor understanding exists of the specific means by which stress affects the occurrence of seizures. Clinical studies provide strong anecdotal information and evidence of stress-related seizure activity, but these studies are few and inconclusive. Basic scientific research has delineated many of the relevant anatomic pathways of the brain and the potential physiologic mechanisms that could be affected by stress, including how changing concentrations of various hormones and neurotransmitters can affect seizure threshold. Although the information from these studies is intriguing, it remains incomplete and further research is necessary.

Stress can be thought of as a diverse set of conditions, internal or external to an organism, that may disrupt physiologic balance. Categories of stressors include physiologic (sleep deprivation, hyperventilation, overexertion, dehydration, fever, illness, menstrual cycle); pharmacologic (medications, substances of abuse); environmental (extremes of temperature, noise, lighting, smells), and psychologic (situations resulting in fear, sadness, anger). These stressors, alone or in combination, can alter the normal balance of one's physical state, lower seizure threshold, and result in a seizure. The specific means by which stress precipitates a seizure is not known. How intense the stressor seems to the individual does not necessarily correlate with the likelihood of seizure occurrence. Similarly, the time that elapses between the stress and the seizure may vary; however, in many circumstances, a specific stressor can be identified, and its intensity and relationship in time to the seizure may strongly suggest a direct relationship.

Some patients with well controlled epileptic seizures experience an unexpected seizure after an unusual event has altered their typical routines and activities. Sleep deprivation is frequently the only identified change in a patient's routine associated with a breakthrough seizure. Patients report having had little or no sleep the night before a seizure. Often these circumstances include other potential stressors, such as caffeine, alcohol, and anxiety, making it more difficult to identify which stressors are the most influential in causing the breakthrough seizure. Hyperventilation, caused by an increased frequency or depth of respirations, may occasionally result in seizure and is used as a standard activating procedure in most routine electroencephalograms (EEGs). Generalized absence seizures, in particular, can easily be precipitated by hyperventilation, as can complex partial seizures, although less commonly. Vigorous physical activity may also precipitate an unexpected seizure. Seizures often occur during illness in a setting of fever and dehydration. Correspondingly, overexertion with dehydration and elevation of core body temperature is also associated with seizure.

Certain physiologic changes occur cyclically and may be related to seizure occurrence. The hormonal fluctuations of the menstrual cycle may contribute to seizure breakthrough in susceptible women at the time of ovulation, during menstruation, and throughout the luteal phase of the menstrual cycle (the time between ovulation and menstruation). Medications, prescribed or nonprescription, can stress the system and cause seizures. These seizures may be idiosyncratic or due to an interaction with the metabolism of antiepileptic or other drugs that the patient takes continuously. Cocaine, amphetamines, and similar substances may cause seizures; the withdrawal from barbiturates, benzodiazepines, or alcohol is also associated with seizures.

Environmental stressors are often difficult to identify, but in select patients specific circumstances associated with increasing levels of subjective stress may be identified. These may include extremes of temperature, persistent and offending noises, lighting that causes glare and subsequent headache, and particularly offensive smells. These situations are distinguished from "reflex epilepsy," in which seizures occur in response to specific stimuli at the time of exposure to the stimulus (e.g., exposure to a strobe light). Psychologic stressors provoking anger, fear, and mourning may result in breakthrough seizures. More chronic psychologic factors such as depression, anxiety, or hypomania fluctuate in intensity and may also increase the likelihood of seizure.

Psychologic Stress

Having epilepsy, in itself, may be a major source of stress. People with epilepsy are frequently faced with limitations in education and employment, they may be restricted or prevented from driving, and they regularly confront societal prejudices. Even well meaning friends, family members, and co-workers may interact differently with a person after witnessing a seizure or learning of this diagnosis. It is also stressful to deal with feelings centering around the loss of control, especially with uncontrolled seizures. Additionally, increased financial stress may occur due to the high cost of medical care and limited employment opportunities. Cognitive deficits, limited interpersonal skills, and psychiatric problems are also more common in some types of epilepsy, and these factors may simultaneously increase life stress and decrease the ability to cope with stress.

Although the psychological and medical literature contains many studies demonstrating that excessive stress and the inability to handle stress are harmful, both physically and mentally, unfortunately, stress is a normal part of life. Given the choice, most of us would not choose a completely stress-free existence, as that life would likely be void of challenges.

Introductory psychology textbooks often describe the relationship between stress and performance as an upside down "U." When there is no stress and no associated anxiety, we attend less to a task and reduce our effort and performance to a lower level. Yet, when stress levels are excessive, performance suffers. When trying to enhance performance, an intermediate or more moderate level of stress is best.

Both positive and negative changes in our lives may cause stress. One study describes five patients who had their first epileptic seizure or a worsening of seizures the day of or shortly before their wedding day (1).

People react differently to the same stressful situation for many reasons, some outside of their control. Studies of infants suggest that differences in temperament are apparent even at a very young age. Some of these differences seem to persist throughout life. Parents with more than one child point out that almost from birth their children are dramatically different in their ability to tolerate change and stimulation. Patients frequently tell us that being "high-strung" or "nervous" runs in their family, and it appears that both genetic (inherited) and environmental factors play a role in an individual's ability to handle stress. Growing up in a household where others handled stress and change well, versus growing up in a household where people coped with stress in less healthy ways, such as drinking to excess or blaming others, clearly has an influence on how that child handles stress in adulthood.

Convincing evidence suggests that people can learn new ways of coping with and adapting to stress. One of the most well researched forms of psychotherapy or behavioral treatment is cognitive-behavioral therapy (CBT) (2). How we think and behave strongly influences how we feel. If we approach tasks thinking they will be stressful, rather than viewing challenges in life as something to look forward to, we will probably feel apprehensive. If we think, "This will be hard but I can do it," rather than, "This is too hard for me" or "I will be so embarrassed if I make a mistake," we will probably consider this same situation as much less stressful. Patients who are depressed, anxious, and generally feel "stressed" are more likely to have ways of thinking that maintain depression, anxiety, and stressed feelings.

Learning how to put less pressure on yourself, seeing the positive as well as the negative aspects of situations, and thinking more positively would seem to be relatively simple concepts; however, many people dismiss these attitudes as trivial or too simple to be effective. It is important to remember that simple is not the same as easy, and changing how you think and behave can be difficult. People become accustomed to thinking and reacting in particular ways, and increasing awareness and altering cognition and behaviors may require considerable effort.

Psychologic Stress and Epilepsy

Too much stress or poorly managed stress can be particularly problematic for people with epilepsy. In fact, one study found that 34% of people with epilepsy reported psychologic stress as the most frequent precipitant of their seizures (3). Known factors that increase the likelihood of having a seizure, such as insufficient sleep, hyperventilation, getting overtired and overexerting oneself, are all more likely to occur when feeling stressed and overwhelmed. Many people are more likely to use drugs such as alcohol, tobacco, and caffeine in larger quantities when under stress, thereby causing physiologic changes that may precipitate seizure activity. Relatively few studies specifically look at how stress causes seizures, but interested readers are directed to Lai and Trimble (4) for a summary of the physical mechanisms and clinical studies that address this issue.

It is also stressful to worry about possible injury resulting from seizures, being embarrassed about seizures in public, and having to depend more on others due to an inability to drive. Assuming a "sick role" within a family and having physical limitations alters the dynamics within the family and increases stress.

Commentary

Some studies estimate that up to 70% of patient visits to a primary care physicians are for stress-related disorders. All chronic illnesses including hypertension, diabetes, and coronary artery disease are adversely affected by excessive stress. It is widely accepted that stressful circumstances exacerbate seizures. Spector and colleagues administered a structured interview to 100 patients with epilepsy in which stress and depression were cited as the most important seizure precipitants (1). Similarly, another study of 149 adults with epilepsy identified psychologic stress as the most important factor in provoking seizures (2). Abnormal structural changes to some brain regions have even been demonstrated in animals exposed to prolonged stress (3).

Much of this book is devoted to methods of reducing stress and harmful responses to it. It is clear that there are many ways to achieve the same goal. Whether we use progressive relaxation, neurofeedback, yoga, exercise, or another method, consistency and comfort with the techniques are critical to ensure a lasting clinical response. As comprehensive epilepsy centers continue to embrace these techniques for their patients, more practitioners will become familiar with and sensitive to the special needs of people with epilepsy. Neurologists treating patients with seizures will also become more comfortable "prescribing" stress reduction therapies for their patients.

References

1. Spector S, Cull C, Goldstein LH. Seizure precipitants and perceived self-control of seizures in adults with poorly-controlled epilepsy. *Epilepsy Res* 2000 Feb;38(2-3):207–216.
2. Spatt J, Langbauer G, Mamoli B. Subjective perception of seizure precipitants: results of a questionnaire study. *Seizure* 1998 Oct;7(5):391–395.
3. Magarinos AM, Verdugo JM, McEwen BS. Chronic stress alters synaptic terminal structure in hippocampus. *Proc Natl Acad Sci USA* 1997 Dec 9;94(25): 14002–14008.

Patients with seizure disorders are also at increased risk for experiencing nonepileptic seizure-like events that may primarily be caused by stress. Patients who have these episodes frequently believe they are experiencing epileptic seizures, and the person's appearance and symptoms during the seizure may be similar to epileptic seizures, but EEG monitoring during these episodes shows no evidence of abnormal electrical activity in the brain. An experienced epilepsy specialist recognizes subtle differences in behavior during these events as more typical of nonepileptic rather than epileptic seizures. These episodes are sometimes referred to as "pseudo-seizures." This term may be misleading, however, because the problems that cause the episodes are real, although the episodes are not due to epilepsy. Panic disorder may also cause patients to have symptoms similar to epileptic seizures.

Although rarely a person may "fake" a seizure in order to achieve some benefit or avoid something unpleasant, in the majority of cases the patient is not aware of the cause and vehemently wishes that the spells would cease. An accurate diagnosis usually requires a thorough evaluation at a center experienced in diagnosing epilepsy and nonepileptic events. An inpatient admission to obtain continuous video-EEG monitoring and evaluations by mental health specialists, including psychologists and psychiatrists, may be necessary. Although little research exists on treating nonepileptic seizure-like events, one small study found that six out of thirteen patients who participated in psychotherapy became seizure-free, while none of the seven patients who failed to follow through with the recommended psychotherapy became seizure-free (5).

Coping with Stress

Most of us would benefit from better stress management. A simple and quick way to deal with psychologic symptoms is to take medication that reduces anxiety and depression; however, this may not be the best long-term solution because medications can cause unpleasant side effects, benefits may stop once the medication is discontinued, and medication may mask the underlying problems that will not change by taking a pill. A number of behavioral treatments are as effective as medication in treating depression and anxiety; they do not cause unpleasant physical side effects, and they make it less likely that a person will have a relapse of symptoms in the future, even after treatment stops. Although some people clearly require treatment with medication for depression and anxiety, and many benefit from a combination treatment of psychotherapy and medication, alternatives to medication should always be considered.

Psychotherapy

Current psychotherapy practice has become more problem-focused and time-limited. The goal of treatment often is to help manage a specific problem. CBT is frequently used to help people handle life stress and difficult situations. Interpersonal psychotherapy may also be a helpful approach if the stress is the product of a difficult relationship. This kind of therapy targets personal interactions and helps the person recognize how personal behavior and ways of relating to others influence relationships. Psychotherapists also help patients learn new skills, including how to be assertive, how to do progressive muscle relaxation, and how to cope with anger more adaptively. Making life-style modifications, such as smoking cessation, increasing exercise, and weight reduction all involve changing behaviors, and psychotherapy may help develop relevant strategies.

Despite patients frequently noting a link between life stress and their seizures, surprisingly few studies focus on psychological and behavioral techniques to help manage seizures. One study by Schmid-Schonbein (6) observed 16 patients with seizures that were not completely controlled with medication. By learning to use behavioral means to interrupt the beginning of a seizure and to "neutralize provoking factors," 80% of the patients reduced their seizures by more than 60%.

Relaxation Techniques

A number of strategies can reduce stress and help patients cope, even without psychotherapy. (Some are reviewed in other chapters of this book.) Progressive muscle relaxation—frequently credited to Edmund Jacobson, who published his book *Progressive Relaxation* in 1929 (7)—is one of the most well known and widely taught relaxation techniques. Although relaxing sounds simple and is clearly an idea that has been around for many years, being able to relax, especially when feeling stressed or pressured, is a skill. It is possible to become more proficient at relaxation and more aware of specific muscle groups that may be more tense than they should be by progressively tightening and then relaxing specific muscle groups. Relaxation can only be used to maximum advantages if the patient is able to recognize the signs of stress and tension.

Table 3.1 contains the specific muscle groups and the corresponding motor activity necessary to practice progressive relaxation. During this routine, each part of the

TABLE 3.1

Targeted Muscle Groups for Progressive Relaxation

Body Area	Motor Activity
Hands	Make a fist
Arms	Bring your hands up to your shoulders
Shoulders and neck	Raise your shoulders up toward your ears
Lower face	Clench your teeth and tighten your jaw muscles
Nose and eyes	Wrinkle your nose and squint your eyes
Forehead	Raise your eyebrows
Abdomen	Suck in your gut
Thighs	Press down on the chair
Calves	Point your toes toward your nose
Feet	Curl your feet

body is tightened and then the tension is released. The goal is to have a brief period when the patient tightens and notices the tension in a particular muscle group, followed by a more prolonged period when she gradually releases the tension in that area, noticing how much more comfortable and relaxed that body area feels during the relaxation phase. Progressive relaxation should be done twice a day for 20 minutes in a quiet, comfortable environment, free from distractions. The tension is held for 10 to 20 seconds; the relaxation phase should last for 20 to 30 seconds. After all the muscle groups have been tensed and relaxed, the patient may relax her diaphragm and focus on her breathing. Some people also benefit from imagining themselves in a peaceful place, such as a beach or forest.

Psychotherapy, stress management, and relaxation can all help people with epilepsy but should not be expected to "cure" epilepsy or replace treatment with medication. These techniques complement conventional medical therapies as adjunct treatments and can be curative in patients with nonepileptic seizure-like events.

Mental Health Resources

Although sharing personal information can be difficult, it is important for health care professionals to know if patients are having symptoms such as depression, tearfulness, unexplained sadness, irritability, nervousness, sleep problems, decreased or increased appetite, or even general feelings of being more stressed or overwhelmed. These symptoms may be signs of other medical problems, side effects of medication, and/or signs of treatable mental health problems. It may be valuable to refer patients to a licensed psychologist, social worker, or other mental health professional for behavioral strategies.

Conclusion

Despite the relatively little amount of research on stress management and epilepsy, it is clear that better management of stress is a reasonable goal for all patients and their physicians. Recognizing that stress has a negative impact on health and well-being is an important first step.

References

1. McConnell H, Valeriano J, Brillman J. Prenuptial seizures: a report of five cases. *J Neuropsychiatry Clin Neurosci* 1995;7:72–75.
2. Dobson KS. *Handbook of Cognitive-Behavior Therapies*. New York: Guilford Press, 2001.
3. Spatt J, Langbauer G, Mamoli B. Subjective perception of seizure precipitants: results of a questionnaire study. *Seizure* 1998;7:391–395.
4. Lai C-W, Trimble MR. Stress and epilepsy. *Epilepsy* 1997;10:177–186.
5. Jongsma MJ, Mommers JM, Renier WO, et al. Follow-up of psychogenic, non-epileptic seizures: a pilot study—experience in a Dutch special centre for epilepsy. *Seizure* 1999;8:146–148.
6. Schmid-Schonbein C. Improvement of seizure control by psychological methods in patients with intractable epilepsies. *Seizure* 1998;7:261–270.

7. Jacobson E. *Progressive Relaxation: A Physiologic and Clinical Investigation of Muscular States and Their Significance in Psychology and Medical Practice.* Chicago: University of Chicago Press, 1929.

Further Information

Burns DD, Beck AT. *Feeling Good: The New Mood Therapy*, Vol 1. New York: William Morrow & Company, 1999.

Davis M, McKay M, Eshelman ER. *The Relaxation and Stress Reduction Workbook.* 5th ed. Oakland, CA: New Harbinger Publications, 2000.

Epilepsy Foundation of America: www.efa.org

American Psychological Association: www.apa.org

CHAPTER 4

Comprehensive Neurobehavioral Approach

DONNA J. ANDREWS, PHD AND JOEL M. REITER, MD

Donna Andrews experienced complex partial seizures (CPS) following acute encephalitis at age 18 years. Medications did not control her seizures and resulted in severe side effects, including the life-threatening allergic reaction Stevens-Johnson syndrome. Through careful observation, she developed techniques that allowed her to completely control her seizures. Donna Andrews met neurologist Joel Reiter in 1979, when she was his student in a course at the Berkeley Biofeedback Institute. After Dr. Reiter discussed his work with epilepsy patients using biofeedback, she challenged him to go further by incorporating the techniques she had developed to control her own CPS. He accepted the challenge and invited her to prove the efficacy of her methods by working in a pilot study directly with six of his patients with uncontrolled CPS (1). This study led to excellent results that have since been repeated with many other patients in the Andrews/Reiter Epilepsy Program (2). The Andrews/Reiter (A/R) methods were duplicated in studies at the Victoria Epilepsy Center in Canada (3) and recently at the Konigin Elisabeth Herzberge Epilepsy Center in Berlin (4).

Why the Andrews/Reiter Treatment Was Developed

Many individuals with epilepsy continue to experience seizures despite the best efforts of their neurologists. Antiepileptic drugs (AEDs) either do not control their seizures, lead to side effects, or both. Even if seizures are controlled, many patients experience fear, anxiety, and feelings of hopelessness that significantly impair their quality of life. Brain surgery is an option for some with uncontrolled seizures, but many do not want to risk possible injury from surgery; others have seizures caused by bilateral or extensive unilateral brain damage that cannot be helped by brain surgery. The A/R approach was developed to help individuals with these types of seizure disorders.

The A/R treatment method differs from the standard medical model for treating epilepsy, which assumes that seizures begin suddenly and inexplicably, that the patient is unable to expend any personal effort to control his seizures, and that all treatment must be strictly medical or surgical. The A/R method believes the onset of seizures is important to discovering ways to control seizures. All aspects of the patient's history are discussed, including where the seizure occurred; what activities preceded it over a few days to months; life events preceding the seizure, including sleep pattern, travel, work, or social changes and stresses; emotional highs and lows, including excitement, fear, boredom, worry; eating habits; alcohol or drug habits; and so forth. Were there any warning symptoms before the seizure? What repetitive patterns are present with recurrent seizures? Using the A/R method, the patient can accomplish seizure control with help from a support person and professionals.

This treatment method is based on a model of self-control developed by the A/R Epilepsy Research Program (5). The consequences of having epilepsy are numerous, complex, and varied. Psychological studies indicate this is especially true for CPS (6–10). Physicians know that the quality of life for many epilepsy patients is less than optimal because of the occurrence of seizures *and* because the drugs used to treat seizures can lead to altering and often debilitating effects on personality, intellectual performance, self-image, self-confidence, and self-acceptance (9,11–13). Seizures can distort or inhibit any brain function (10), causing changes in sensation, perception, cognition, speech output and analysis, arousal, affect, memory storage and retrieval, motor activity, and behavior (7).

Seizures cause strong emotional effects. Furthermore, the strong emotions generated by external events can precipitate seizures, often serving to reduce social interactions (14). AEDs may further impair cognitive and behavioral functioning (12,13,15). Therefore, a treatment method that both reduces seizures and the need for AEDs could significantly improve the quality of life for people with epilepsy.

Contraindications

There are no known contraindications to this approach.

Basic Concepts of the A/R Approach: Seizure Aura and Pre-Seizure

The seizure aura is actually the beginning of the seizure, and the symptoms depend on the part of the brain where the seizure begins. Examples of common seizure auras are flashing lights, tingling in a specific area of the body, sudden fear, an unpleasant smell, twitching of an extremity, or the inability to speak. Seizure auras are thought to result from an excess electrical discharge in a particular region of the brain that controls, for example, sensation, vision, and motor functions.

Pre-seizure warnings are subtle states that precede either seizure auras or full seizures. They may consist of a change in mood, a feeling of remoteness or disconnection, vague changes in sensation, or feelings of loss of control or anxiety, including agitation and withdrawal. Pre-seizure warnings become associated with a patterned physiologic response known as the *fight/flight response* (16). The first part of this response is the cessation of breathing (17), which diminishes oxygen in the brain, causing lightheadedness or disoriented feelings that move quickly into full seizures (5). An essential part of the A/R treatment is to change the patient's response to pre-seizure warnings and auras by recognizing them as a reason to institute a new response that uses *diaphragmatic breathing.*

Deep Diaphragmatic Breathing

1. Lie flat on the floor to make it easier to learn the method. Close your eyes and give your attention to your breath. Keep your eyes open if you think a seizure might occur.
2. Let your hands rest lightly on the floor beside you. Bend your elbows back toward your shoulders to take the pressure off your upper back and neck. Never touch your body with your hands or cross your legs during this exercise. Now breathe in, first inhaling into your stomach and then filling your lungs. When you can hold no more air, hold your breath to the count of three. Now exhale slowly, trying to make the exhale last as long as the inhale.
3. Repeat this up to three times. Do not exceed three repetitions without normal breathing in between. If you begin to feel dizzy at any time during this process, return to normal breathing until the dizziness passes.
4. This type of breathing can also be done standing and at any time you feel a seizure coming on. Breathing is the first line of defense against seizures. Take a diaphragmatic breath any time you start to depart from your normal feeling state.

We have repeatedly observed that as patients using the A/R approach increase their conscious awareness, they become aware of subtle cues signaling the approach of a seizure. The implementation of newly learned behavioral measures at this point can restore normal brain function, thereby preventing the seizure.

Seizure Triggers

Triggers are factors that often bring about seizures. These many potential triggers for CPS; they can be isolated, multiple, or interactive, depending on the complexity and mass of brain tissue involved. Triggers can be physical (e.g., chemical imbalance, disturbed sleep, missed medication), external (people, places, or situations that cause pressure or stress), or internal (emotional reactions and stressful states of mind) (Figure 4.1).

Standard medical approaches tend to ignore the emotional life of the patient; they overlook important information that could promote seizure control if appropriately used. The episodic nature of this chronic disorder causes certain fears and concerns that affect all individuals with epilepsy to some degree (18), leading to behavioral and emotional adjustment problems regardless of the severity of seizures (19).

Situations or life issues contributing to the onset of seizures that might have been solved early in treatment tend to become elusive. These same unresolved issues and the individual's emotional response to them tend to be stimuli overloading the patient's coping mechanism (2). The overload of this coping mechanism may be a stressor that triggers the seizure state (2,5,20).

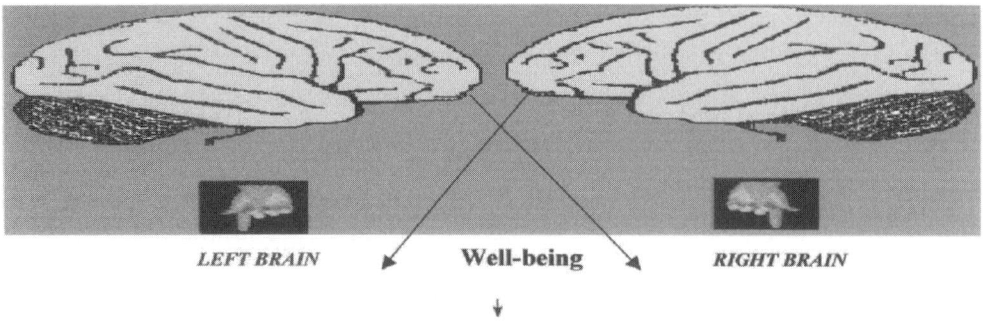

Emotion	**Emotion**
Anger	Fear
Frustration	Guilt
Excitement	Sadness
Anticipation	Joy
Mood Trap	**Mood Trap**
Depression	Anxiety Disorders
	Panic
Function	**Function**
Logic	Creativity
Reasoning	Intuition
Language	Imagination
Linear Thinking	Nonlinear Thinking

FIGURE 4.1

A comparison of right and left brain emotions, moods, and functions that trigger seizures.

Hypersensitivity to heat, the blare of sirens, and the sound of vacuum cleaners or low flying jets are common triggers (7). Dr. V. Ramani reported an unusual triggering phenomenon in the July 1991 issue of the *New England Journal of Medicine*: a 45-year-old woman was triggered into a seizure every time she heard the voice of Mary Hart, the host of *Entertainment Tonight*. Common triggers include sleep deprivation, missing medication, and strong negative or positive emotional reactions. It is commonly believed that the trigger mechanism is connected to high arousal states; however, Dahl found that low-arousal was also a trigger for seizures (21). The discovery of the triggering mechanism(s) is most important to the goal of taking control in the A/R self-control model.

Treatment with the A/R Method

The A/R treatment program includes cognitive and behavioral counseling, awareness enhancement, progressive relaxation and reinforcement, deep diaphragmatic breathing, and electroencephalographic (EEG) and electromyographic biofeedback as described in *Taking Control of Your Epilepsy: A Workbook for Patients and Professionals* (5).

A/R counseling focuses on three objectives:

- Identifying the pre-seizure warning and/or aura
- Identifying emotional, behavioral, physiologic, and/or environmental mechanisms that trigger seizure activity
- Learning to use diaphragmatic breathing as an adaptive behavior to manage the response to the trigger

The goals of this multidisciplinary approach are to:

- Discover dependable warning(s) for seizures
- Discover the elements of the triggering mechanism
- Learn diaphragmatic breathing
- Learn and improve the relaxation response
- Improve communication skills
- Set and achieve important life goals

Commentary

Since ancient times, individuals with epilepsy, their families, and physicians have been able to identify the mental, physical, and external factors (e.g., stress, sleep deprivation, premenstrual period, illness, flashing lights) that were associated with an increased likelihood of seizure occurrence, as well as premonitory symptoms that could occur hours or days before a seizure (e.g., mood changes, tiredness, mental confusion or clarity, increased frequency of urination) (1). The auras that immediately precede a seizure are actually the initial part of the seizure. Although they are commonly considered only as precursors for partial seizures, they occasionally precede generalized seizures in patients with idiopathic generalized epilepsies (e.g., juvenile myoclonic epilepsy). Auras provide only a brief warning, yet some patients can stop seizures during this short interval. For example, in some patients with tingling or jerking that rises from the foot to the hip to the arm to the head and then causes a convulsion, rubbing above where the activity is located (e.g., if the foot jerks, rub the thigh) may block the seizure from progressing.

Reflex epilepsies provide an excellent model for better understanding ways to provoke and perhaps inhibit seizure activity. Reflex epilepsy—recurrent seizures induced by specific stimuli, such as flashing lights, loud noises, reading, eating, and listening to music—is a well-described disorder that contributes to seizure provocation in many patients. How one defines *reflex* leads to different estimates of the frequency of reflex epilepsies, but estimates vary from 1 to 25%, with most authorities agreeing that traditionally defined reflex epilepsy is present in approximately 5 to 12% of patients. It is more common among patients with idiopathic generalized epilepsy, in whom light and reading are common triggers (2). Servit and colleagues reported that external factors can activate seizures in 37% of patients but could inhibit seizures in 31%.

Rarely, the induction of a seizure can prevent a subsequent seizure. For example, one woman with reading epilepsy knew that after a tonic-clonic seizure she would not have another major seizure for at least several days. Willful initiation of a seizure may be engaged to exploit a refractory period. Alajouanine and colleagues (3) reported a woman with reflex epilepsy who purposefully induced a tonic-clonic seizure on the morning of her wedding to ensure that she was seizure-free for her ceremony later that day. In her case, she would always go seizure-free for at least a day after a major seizure.

How often can children or adults with epilepsy "control" their seizures? Cull and colleagues found that in young people with epilepsy attending a specialized residential school, 63% claimed to identify seizure precipitants, 71% experienced warnings, and 51% could inhibit seizures (4). However, staff reports were much lower (56.9%, 47.2%, and 22.2%, respectively). Notably, 9% of patients and 10% of staff reported self-induction of seizures. In another study of 100 adult patients with medically refractory epilepsy, interviews and questionnaires helped separate patients into groups of low and high perceived self-control of seizures (5). The ability to identify and seek situations with low-risk for seizures, avoiding situations with high risk for seizures, and attempting to inhibit seizures discriminated high from low controllers. There were more high control subjects than low control subjects; women were over-represented in the low control group. The same investigators reported on 100 patients (many were likely in the study above), examining seizure control in adult epilepsy patients (6). Fifteen percent stated that they could induce a seizure, 52% said that they consciously try to avoid seizure precipitants, and 47% said they could sometimes stop their seizures from happening.

Approximately 50% of people with epilepsy believe that they can abort or control some seizures, thus presenting an enormous opportunity. The medical profession has failed to capitalize on this. No systematical investigations have been done of premonitory symptoms or the ability of individuals to induce or abort seizures through mental or physical activity, or sensory stimuli. Although many highly intelligent and insightful patients report similar experiences in "controlling seizures," the subject lies at the fringe or beyond the borders of traditional medicine. Furthermore, few medical models provide a mechanism to investigate this phenomenon. Articulate patients often cannot describe how they stop their seizures, they just "do it." The enormous challenge of how to turn the intriguing observation that many patients can reportedly stop seizures into a reproducible therapy is not insurmountable, as Andrews and Reiter outline in this chapter.

Andrews and Reiter provide a systematic approach to identifying pre-seizure warnings and changing the reflexive fearful and stress responses as one recognizes that a seizure is imminent into a calm response through diaphragmatic breathing. They reasonably postulate that replacing fear with calm can help inhibit seizures from progressing beyond the aura stage, because negative emotions can further enhance the development of a seizure. Their therapy goes beyond this and touches on a more careful recognition of seizure triggers and environmental factors that encourage seizures, identifying and reducing life stresses, and improving overall wellness. Their comprehensive approach and translation of theory into therapy represents an important step in the treatment of epilepsy. Identify settings that cause seizures and avoid them. Reduce life stress. Respond to an imminent seizure with calm, not fear. Common sense? Yes. But they are the first to systematically apply common sense.

A final cautionary note: Andrews and Reiter have advanced our understanding and treatment of epilepsy through the collaboration of an introspective and creative patient teaming with a professional experienced in biofeedback and relaxation techniques. This is one approach, albeit one that is broadly adaptable for many individuals. It worked extremely well for Donna Andrews and has worked well for many others; however, there are many forms of epilepsy, many environmental seizure precipitants, many stressors that are unconscious, and many ways to relax. Other approaches similar to this model, and also quite different approaches, likely exist that can help other individuals with epilepsy. Some may need to be adapted for the developmentally disabled. For some patients, inducing stress—not relaxation—may help block seizures. As we move forward and embrace the Andrews-Reiter approach, we must remain wide open to others.

References

1. Hughes J, Devinsky O, Feldmann E, et al. Premonitory symptoms in epilepsy. *Seizure* 1993;2:201–220.
2. Ritaccio A, et al., Reflex seizures. *Neuro Clinics* 1994;12:57–84.
3. Alajouanine T, Nehlil J, Gabersek V. A propos d'un cas d'epilepsie déclenché par la lecture. *Rev Neurol* 101;463–467:1959.
4. Cull CA, Fowler M, Brown SW. Perceived self-control of seizures in young people with epilepsy. *Seizure* 1996;5:131–138.
5. Spector S, Cull C, Goldstein LH. High and low perceived self-control of epileptic seizures. *Epilepsia* 2001;42:556–564.
6. Spector S, Cull C, Goldstein LH. Seizure precipitants and perceived self-control of seizures in adults with poorly-controlled epilepsy. *Epilepsy Res* 2000;38:207–216.

We found the following steps essential for the majority of patients seeking control of their epilepsy and their lives:

Step 1: Making the Decision to Begin the Process of Taking Control. To initiate treatment, patients study this approach and explore their motivating factors and the obstacles to taking control of their epilepsy. In the second session, they are asked to decide whether they want to begin this work with a counselor.

Step 2: Getting Support. Many people who begin this process lack the supportive relationships they need and often feel isolated and lonely. This step offers skills to help avoid loneliness, improve communication, and develop positive relationships with others. The patients explore their own communication style and determine how it can be improved.

Step 3: Deciding about Your Antiepileptic Drug Therapy. This step looks at the medications for epilepsy in general and specifically the effectiveness and side effects of medications the individual is taking. This provides an opportunity to report side effects and clarify any questions about AEDs. The goal is to optimize the positive effects of medication and minimize side effects. For some individuals, overmedication may interfere with the ability to participate in the A/R treatment; for others, a medication change or adjustment may enhance seizure control.

Step 4: Learning to Observe Triggers. Common examples of triggers include situations that lead to an emotional state of excitement or frustration, skipping medication, staying up late, or excessive physical exertion. In this step, individuals learn how to observe and identify their triggers.

Step 5: Channeling Negative Emotions into Productive Outlets. Some of the triggers observed in Step 4 usually lead to seizures because they first produce a negative emotion or state, such as fear, anger, or hurt. Step 5 provides skills for dealing positively with negative states, and for self-acceptance and seeing the negative state as a demand for action.

Step 6: Biofeedback: Experiencing the Sensation of the Brain Changing Itself. EEG biofeedback enables subjects to change their brainwave state at will, which usually means learning to go into an awake, relaxed state (brain waves with a frequency of 8 to 12 per second). Once this is accomplished, patients begin to be aware of the brain changing from one state of consciousness into another. This mindful state of consciousness is facilitated by biofeedback training, relaxation tapes used daily at home, and guided relaxation exercises during the training sessions. Individuals are taught to use this awareness of a possible loss of control to help them abort or stop seizures by instituting breathing or some other compensatory measure.

Step 7: Identifying the Pre-Seizure Warning. The seizure aura and pre-seizure warning consist of a symptom or sensation that precedes a seizure. Learning to identify the pre-seizure warning is an important step because it enables a person to know when a seizure is going to occur. Recognizing the pre-seizure warning may help avoid injury and embarrassment and prevent seizures by knowing when to institute a compensatory measure (breathing, focusing, interrupting a fixed gaze, and so forth). The way for patients to discover their specific aura is increased awareness, which is a by-product of an increased ability to relax and self-observe.

Step 8: Dealing with External Life Stresses. This step involves gaining awareness of the factors in one's life that are stress producing and then taking responsibility for relieving those stressors within one's control. This process can help restore self-confidence (people with uncontrolled seizures often experience low self-confidence), dramatically reduce interpersonal tension, decrease seizure frequency, and increase a sense of well-being.

Step 9: Dealing with Internal Issues and Conflicts. The feelings, conflicts, and issues that are part of a person's inner life (feelings of inadequacy, projection of blame, low levels of self-esteem, and chronic states of anxiety, anger, and depression) affect overall health as much or more than external stressors. The focus of this step is to become aware of these issues and learn to deal with them. Self-exploration with the help of a trained epilepsy counselor, the use of a personal journal, and receiving feedback from a support person can help achieve the goals of this step.

Step 10: Learning to Relax and Reduce Tension. This step is an extension of Step 6 and offers a wide variety of methods for increasing skills in reducing tension and improving relaxation. These methods offer a deeper understanding of the physical processes involved in the relaxation response, as well as exploring the benefits of regular exercise, rest and sleep, the balance between work and play, and assertive communication skills. This is an opportunity to integrate the tools of the previous nine steps and provide a chance for the counselor and patient to review those tools that are the most effective and assess progress in the goal of seizure control.

Step 11: Epilepsy's Other Symptoms. The other symptoms that occur with epilepsy include altered states, such as déjà-vu, out-of-body experiences, memory problems, and scattered thinking, as well as behavioral symptoms, such as slowing of activity or sudden outbursts of anger. The goal of this step is to recognize, accept, and cope positively with these symptoms. For example, patients with memory problems as a direct result of either their seizure disorder or their AEDs are encouraged to make a list of tasks assigned to them by a parent, teacher, or employer, and to check them off as they are completed, in order to help overcome this limitation.

Step 12: Enhancing Personal Wellness. Wellness includes all the lifestyle choices that affect bodily health. It also extends into the realm of emotion, spirit, and meaning. Step 12 encourages patients to move toward an optimum level of wellness by reviewing past successes in coping with epilepsy and assists them in making new goals for ongoing self-care. The concept of balance across a wide range of life issues (work and play, exercise and eating, and rest and productivity) is explored, while also recognizing personal limits.

References

1. Reiter JM, Lambert RD, Andrews DJ, et al. Complex-partial epilepsy: a therapeutic model of behavioral management and EEG biofeedback. *Self-Control in Epilepsy* 1990;1:27–38.
2. Andrews DJ, Schonfeld WH. Predictive factors for controlling seizures using a behavioral approach. *Seizure* 1992;1:111–116.
3. MacKinnon J. The application of behavioural and psychological methods in controlling seizures in individuals with epilepsy. Victoria Epilepsy Center 2002; Personal Communication.

4. Meencke HJ, Schmid-Schonbein C, Heinen G. Methods and results of a treatment program on self-control of epileptic seizures. Presented at the 54th Annual Meeting of the American Epilepsy Society, Los Angeles, CA. December 2000.

5. Reiter JM, Andrews DJ, Janis C. 1987. *Taking Control of Your Epilepsy: A Workbook for Patients and Professionals.* Available from Andrews/Reiter Epilepsy Research Program, 1103 Sonoma Avenue, Santa Rosa, CA 95405.

6. Fenwick P. EEG studies. In: Reynolds EH, Trimble MR (eds.) *Epilepsy and Psychiatry.* Edinburgh: Churchill Livingston, 1981.

7. Richard A, Reiter JM. *Epilepsy: A New Approach.* New York: Walker Publishing Company, 1995.

8. Neppe V, Tucker GJ. Modern perspectives in epilepsy in relation to psychiatry: classification and evaluation. *Hospital and Community Psychiatry* 1988;39:263–271.

9. Taube SL, Calman NH. The psychotherapy of patients with complex partial seizures. *Am J Orthopsychiatry* 1992;62:35–43.

10. Williams D. The structure of emotions reflected in epileptic experiences. *Brain* 1956;79:29–67.

11. Dodrill CB, Batzel LW, Queisser HR, et al. An objective method for the assessment of psychological and social problems among epileptics. *Epilepsia* 1980;21:123–135.

12. Meador K, Loring D, Huh K, et al. Comparative cognitive effects of anticonvulsants. *Neurology* 1990;40:391–394.

13. Trimble MR. Anticonvulsant drugs and cognitive function: review of the literature. *Epilepsia* 1987;28:537–545.

14. Bear DN. Temporal lobe epilepsy: a syndrome of sensory-limbic hyperconnection. *Cortex* 1979;15:357–384.

15. Andrewes DG, Bullen JG, Tomlinson L, et al. A comparative study of the cognitive effects of phenytoin and carbamazepine in new referrals with epilepsy. *Epilepsia* 1986;27:128–134.

16. Ezruel H. A psychoanalytic approach to group treatment. *J Medical Psychology* 1950;23:59–74.

17. Fried R, Rubin SR, Carlton RM. Behavioral control of intractable idiopathic seizures: self-regulation of end-tidal carbon dioxide. *Psychosom Med* 1984;46:315–329.

18. Lavender A. A behavioural approach to the treatment of epilepsy. *Behavioural Psychology* 1981;9:231–243.

19. Goldstein LH. Behavioural and cognitive-behavioural treatments for epilepsy: a progress review. *Br J Clin Psychol* 1990;29:257–269.

20. Wolf P. Psychic disorders in epilepsy. In: Canger R, Angeleri F, Penry K (eds.) *Advances in Epileptology: Eleventh International Epilepsy Symposium.* New York: Raven Press, 1979;159–160.

21. Dahl JC. The psychological treatment of epilepsy: a behavioral approach. *Acta University Uppsala.* Comprehensive Summaries of Uppsala Dissertations from the Faculty of Social Sciences. 1987;7:1–54.

CHAPTER 5

Seizure Generation

PETER FENWICK, MD

Epilepsy has been viewed as a simple medical condition for many years. This medical model of epilepsy assumes that seizures have a physiologic cause, that they arise as a result of abnormal brain discharges due either to genetic causes or to brain damage, and that the appropriate treatment is with drugs. Today, however, many recognize that this medical model is too simple and that there is another way of looking at epilepsy. As far back as 1881, Sir William Gowers said: "Of all the immediate causes of epilepsy, the most potent are physical: fright, excitement, and anxiety. To these were ascribed more than one-third in which a definite cause was given."

A recognition of the close link between brain activity, the psychic life of the individual, and the genesis of seizure activity is the foundation of the behavioral model of epilepsy. This model suggests that seizures are linked to behavior and, therefore, that by modifying behavior, a nondrug behavioral treatment of epilepsy may be possible.

What evidence do we have to support this model? Some evidence is gleaned from animal studies. Martinek and Horak (1) have shown that seizures can be triggered by emotional excitement in genetically susceptible dogs; Lockard (2) has shown that in a monkey hierarchy, seizures can be caused by exposing a subservient monkey to a dominant one. Thus, social stress is clearly a precipitating cause. Lockard went on to show that pleasant social situations (e.g., a monkey in a nonthreatening social group) produced a reduction in seizure frequency as well as a reduction in the abnormal spike discharges that often precede a seizure.

Several human studies have shown the relationship between emotional stress and the activation of the EEG. Stevens (3) gave individualized stressful interviews with criticisms and accusations to patients with temporal lobe epilepsy and found that this caused increased spiking in 66%. This was also found in other studies by Baker and Baker (4) and Small, et al. (5). Thus, the evidence points to a close relationship between mental state and the likelihood of seizure occurrence. The following case study clearly demonstrates this point.

A 22-year-old man with a strong family history of epilepsy had tonic-clonic seizures from the age of nine. There was no evidence of any brain damage either in his history or in his investigations. His seizures started with a loss of consciousness without warning, and before and after the seizures he had no focal symptoms or signs. He discovered that he could generate seizures by lying on the bed and deliberately holding his mind empty and blank for a number of minutes. This would lead to a grand mal seizure; he would then awaken in a post-ictal state—confused and disoriented—a sensation that he quite enjoyed. He would occasionally do this on weekends whenever he was bored or lonely.

Lockard's Model of Epilepsy

Lockard proposed an elegant model of seizure genesis in focal epilepsy (2). She used aluminum hydroxide paste to produce focal epileptogenic lesions on the cortex of monkeys. She then implanted this epileptogenic area with microelectrodes and defined two populations of cells that she called Group 1 and Group 2.

Group 1 neurons, situated at the center of the focus, were partially damaged and always fired in an epileptic, bursting mode. These cells were pacemaker cells that fired abnormally all the time. Their activity was not modified to any significant extent by surrounding brain activity. Group 2 cells were partially damaged neurons surrounding the focus; these could fire in both the bursting, epileptic mode and in a normal mode. Their activity could therefore be modified by surrounding brain activity. When a seizure occurred continually, discharging Group 1 cells recruited Group 2 cells into the seizure discharge. The spreading out of abnormal discharges within the Group 2 cells was a focal seizure. If Group 2 cells recruited cells in the normal brain surrounding the abnormal focus, then the focal seizure would spread throughout the brain and become secondarily generalized.

If this model is correct, the background activity of surrounding populations of cells could be of crucial importance in determining whether a seizure is likely to occur and whether it is likely to spread. If behavior can be described in terms of the excitation and inhibition of populations of neurons surrounding and influencing the focus, then it follows that behavior must be extremely important in the genesis of seizure activity. It is worth considering that the pacemaker cell in the center of the focus (e.g., those cells that are going to bring about a seizure) are firing abnormally all the time—but no one has seizures all the time. The tendency to have seizures must be influenced by other factors apart from pacemaker cells, and one of these factors is the activity in the cells surrounding the seizure focus. The Group 2 surrounding neurons must become activated and allow the seizure discharge to grow in order for a seizure to occur. Thus, modifying of the activity of these cells by making them more excited will increase the possibility of a seizure; inhibiting these cells leads to seizure reduction.

The theoretical evidence proposed by Lockard supports a behavioral model of epilepsy that ties in the patient's mental state with the likely causes of seizures. Patients often state that they seem to have learned to have seizures, because seizures occur in specific situations, such as passing a significant building or during recurring stressful events. Evidence from the animal literature suggests that seizures can be learned. The first person to test this scientifically was Forster (6), who found that seizures in cats can be conditioned. He implanted brain electrodes in a normal cat and induced a focal seizure by stimulating the electrodes. He then flashed a light at the same time as stimulation and this, too, produced a focal seizure. He then flashed the light without any electrical stimulation and found that the light alone produced no response. It produced surprised cats but no seizures.

When he carried out the same experiment in a brain-damaged cat, however, he found that he was able to produce a conditioned response in the damaged brain, so that after exposure to the light + stimulation, a focal seizure was produced in response to the light alone. This simple experiment has important implications for patients with epilepsy because it suggests that one can learn to have seizures. Conversely, one can also learn *not* to have seizures.

Changes in behavior may precipitate or inhibit seizures. The important question then is in what situations do patients believe their seizures tend to occur? To find this out, we conducted studies at the Maudsley Hospital and at a general hospital. Similar studies have also been conducted on several groups of patients in Japan. These studies have shown that although some cultural differences exist, there is a remarkable consistency in the emotional factors that are most likely to precipitate seizures (Table 5.1). This echoes the findings of Gowers (7).

TABLE 5.1

Triggers of Epileptic Seizures (In Percent)

	Maudsley Hospital Research	General Hospital Research	Japanese Studies
Tension	69	39	80
Depression	67	38	12
Tiredness	49	47	57
Anger	45	22	3
Excitement	41	36	5
Boredom	25	17	
Menstruation	19	20	
Hunger	16	14	8
Sex	10	8	1
Happiness	7	9	1

These figures suggest that tension and tiredness are the most likely precipitants of seizures, but possibly more important, happiness seems to protect against seizure occurrence.

Other groups have also looked at seizure triggers. Dahl (8) found the most common precipitants of seizures were physical activity (83%), negative stress (78%), muscle tension (71%), demanding situations (67%), and panic (64%). These figures are very close to those we found at Maudsley. Clearly, more studies are needed, but from those that we have, the message is clear. If you have epilepsy, it does matter how your life is going and what you think and feel.

Self-Induction of Seizures

Many people with epilepsy recognize the link between what they do, what is happening in their lives, and their seizure frequency. A patient who trusts her physician will often admit that she sometimes uses this knowledge to bring on a seizure. The prevalence of self-induction varies considerably from study to study. In the Maudsley clinic population, we found 23% of patients admitted to being able to self-induce seizures; however, a study in a general hospital found only 3%. The likely reason for this difference was that patients were being interviewed for the first time by a new doctor. We have found that unless you have the patient's confidence, they are unlikely to tell you that they can initiate their own seizures because they feel guilty. A further reason is that they may not be aware they are self-inducing until it is drawn to their attention and fully discussed. Studies in Sweden have found a prevalence of 16% in children and 69% in adults; a Japanese study of adults found only 8% who said they were able, on occasion, to induce a seizure. Sometimes intentional seizure generation does occur, regardless of the exact incidence of this phenomenon or physical activity.

The mechanism of self-induction varies widely and depends largely on the type of seizure. The most usual mechanisms are mimicking seizure onset, thinking stressful

Commentary

Dr. Fenwick discusses his experience with behavioral therapy in patients with uncontrolled seizures. Two cases of patients able to precipitate their own seizures for secondary gain are presented, underscoring the notion that some patients have control over the generation of seizures and therefore may also be able to prevent them. The ability of patients to induce their own seizures is generally considered rare, but the author believes it is underestimated, in part because most physicians do not inquire about it and also because patients may not divulge the information when asked.

More important, and pertinent to all patients with uncontrolled seizures, is the possibility that some seizures are preventable through an organized behavioral therapy approach. Similar to the Andrews-Reiter technique discussed in Chapter 4, Dr. Fenwick advocates an intensive investigation of seizure triggers and the circumstances that lead to seizures, followed by behavioral strategies to diminish the likelihood of a seizure occurring in a given circumstance. Admittedly, physicians treating patients with epilepsy do not always take the time to explore the psychological and environmental factors associated with a patient's seizures and spend the majority of office visit time discussing medication dosing and side effects.

Unfortunately, even when triggers are identified, they may be nonspecific or unpreventable. For instance, stress is cited as an important seizure precipitant in nearly all patients, but the causes of stress are numerous, and achieving a stress-free existence is impossible for most of us. Similarly, sleep deprivation is a common seizure precipitant, but try telling a mother with young children she must sleep through the night, every night!

A down side rarely exists to identifying and attempting to avoid seizure triggers, however, and it is certainly worth the effort. Just how many and which epilepsy patients will truly benefit from these behavioral therapy approaches is unknown. Only small clinical studies are available. Martinovic looked at behavioral therapy in 22 adolescents and young adults with juvenile myoclonic epilepsy and concluded that structured counseling resulted in complete seizure control for eight patients and was of psychotherapeutic benefit for all subjects (1). Reiter and Andrews reported similar results in a retrospective study of their behavioral approach for 11 patients with complex partial seizures (2).

Interestingly, Spector and colleagues interviewed 100 patients with poorly controlled seizures, and 47% believed that they were capable of stopping some of their seizures from happening (3). Unfortunately, seizures may vary in duration and extent of spread throughout the brain, so it is difficult to know whether these patients were actively inhibiting seizures or the events were destined to be auras or brief seizures. Again, as with behavioral therapy to avoid triggers, systematic studies of self-seizure termination are lacking; however, behavioral approaches are a safe and worthwhile adjunct to standard medical therapy, and we believe intuitively that they are reasonable approaches for many patients, even in the absence of large scale comprehensive studies.

References

1. Martinovic Z. Adjunctive behavioural treatment in adolescents and young adults with juvenile myoclonic epilepsy. *Seizure* 2001 Jan;10(1):42–47.
2. Reiter JM, Andrews DJ. A neurobehavioral approach for treatment of complex partial epilepsy: efficacy. *Seizure* 2000 Apr;9(3):198–203.
3. Spector S, Cull C, Goldstein LH. Seizure precipitants and perceived self-control of seizures in adults with poorly-controlled epilepsy. *Epilepsy Res* 2000 Feb;38(2–3):207–216.

thoughts, manipulation of attention, blanking the mind, allowing seizure-prone situations to develop, becoming angry or sad, or the like. One 34-year-old patient who experienced complex partial seizures arising bitemporally was able to induce seizures by thinking sad thoughts. His father had died during his adolescence, and he found at that time that his unhappy thoughts induced complex partial seizures. He continued to use this mechanism to deal with unhappiness in his life. He was very distressed when a relationship broke up and, as a result, he lay on his bed and deliberately thought about the sadness of the break-up. He had recurrent complex partial seizures, which he encouraged, until they developed into complex partial status. He was found by a neighbor and admitted to the hospital. I saw him 3 days later, once his epilepsy had been controlled, and we spent the session acknowledging his sadness and disappointment at the break-up of his relationship. We also discussed other ways of dealing with sad feelings that didn't involve seizure precipitation.

Behavioral Treatment

Behavioral therapy recognizes patients as individuals and presumes that seizures arise from interactions of the patient with himself, his family, his friends, and his surroundings. Behavioral treatment is based on the association between seizures and behavior, and lifestyle and relationships. Behavioral strategies are employed that may help control seizures.

Self-Control Strategies

The aim of self-control strategies is to allow the patient to gain more control over his seizures. Most patients with epilepsy have cognitive strategies that they use to inhibit seizures, both by avoiding circumstances that they know are likely to cause seizures and by trying to abort seizures once they have begun. Patients may use a wide range of self-control strategies to avoid having seizures. This phenomenon varies from patient to patient and with the type of epilepsy. Some patients have greatly reduced seizure frequency when they are on vacation. Others say that they are unlikely to have seizures at the theatre (i.e., in situations in which their interest is held). Other patients report that positive lifestyle changes may lead to freedom from seizures.

Self-control strategies are aimed at the reinforcement of seizure inhibition and the elimination of self-induction of seizures. In a study at the Maudsley Hospital, 53% of patients said they could inhibit their seizures; 27% said that they could stop a seizure from spreading once it had begun. The figures for a general hospital were 58% and 17%, respectively, which are very similar. The figures for a similar study in Japan were 13% and 19%, respectively. It is clear from these results that patients do have some control over their seizures. How do those who are successful manage it?

Several studies have looked at this. Patients develop various strategies to stop their seizures or inhibit their spread. Dahl (8) found that the most commonly used methods were: restraint of movement (74%), stimulation of sensory area (77%), visual stimulation (22%), auditory stimulation (85%), olfactory stimulation (32%), applied relaxation (78%), and using positive statements (89%). These strategies are carried out at seizure onset to reduce the likelihood of a seizure and are known as *countermeasures*. The best way to determine the most effective countermeasure is to use the ABC chart.

ABC Charts

The basis of any behavioral program is to obtain information about the behaviors that need to be changed. It is very difficult to do this unless you have a structured way of gathering information. ABC charts form the basis of a behavioral treatment program. The aim of these charts is to gather information before the seizure, during the seizure, and after the seizure, and to use this information to modify seizure activity.

- "A" is for *antecedents*. Antecedents are those experiences that occur before and at the beginning of a seizure. Take, for example, the onset of a complex partial seizure. Where were you when the seizure started? What were you thinking? Most important, what were you feeling? It is no good simply to say "I was sitting at home with some friends having a cup of coffee when suddenly a seizure came on." A patient gave the following description that allowed us to understand more about the feelings that created his seizure: He was sitting with some friends at home look-ing at their holiday photos. They were showing him what a good time they had and what fun it was bathing in the hotel pool. He noticed that he was becoming sad that he could never, or so he thought, go abroad and enjoy the fun of swimming in a hotel pool in the south of France. His thoughts became more critical, particularly of his epilepsy, and as he started to think about how limited he was by his epilep-sy his seizure began. It was clear from his account of the "A" part of the chart that many of his feelings were the result of the limitations imposed on him by his epilepsy and his sadness resulting from this. Quite clearly, if his charts showed that he felt like this on other occasions preceding a seizure, then we might be able to design a strategy to help him cope with them and possibly prevent the seizure.
- "B" is for *behavior*. That is, the behavior that occurs during the seizure. Many strategies can be used to stop a seizure from spreading if the beginning is well noted. A patient of mine told me that when a seizure started, it would slowly engulf him so that he lost control of his feelings and, if it went further, he would lose knowledge of who he was before blacking out. To help him with his loss of control and self-identity, I gave him a rubber band to put on his wrist. I instructed him to pull the rubber band and let it go with a snap when a seizure started. This is, of course, painful but one of the effects of the pain was to help him regain control. He found that the seizure would not progress any further if he used the rubber band early enough.

    Another patient who was a car mechanic told me that he would experience myoclonic jerks when he tried to fit a part onto a car and thought about the way that it would have to go in order to engage with the screw holes. The more he thought about the part he was trying to fit, the worse the myoclonic jerks would become until eventually they would run together and he would have a generalized seizure. His EEG confirmed that he had an epileptogenic focus in his parietal area, the part of the brain that deals with integrating sensory input. His seizures started when he thought about shapes, and continuing to think about shapes made the seizures spread to the point where he would have a generalized tonic-clonic seizure. I suggested that when thinking about shapes produced jerking in his arms, he should immediately stop what he was doing and not try to work through it. He reported this to be extremely effective and his seizures decreased significantly. He learned, when trying to fit a part on a car, not to think about the way it ought to go together but just do it by feel. He also never again tried to carry on working once his jerks had started.

- "C" is for the *consequences* of the seizure. It is important to know what happens after a seizure. A mother was discussing the ABC charts of her 8-year-old son with me in the clinic. It became apparent when looking at the charts that many of his seizures occurred at school, about an hour to an hour and a half after class had started. He only had small complex partial seizures that did not really inconvenience him. The teacher, however, was very worried when he had a seizure and immediately took him out of class and sent him to the school sickroom, where he would lie down and have warm milk and biscuits. He was allowed to stay there until school had ended for the morning, and sometimes he was given his lunch and did not return to the classroom in the afternoon. It was quite clear that he dealt with his anxieties about the lessons by having a seizure, and he enjoyed being rewarded with warm milk and biscuits. After talking with his teacher and the school matron, it was decided that his seizures should not be rewarded this way. We initiated a policy to first reduce his anxiety in class and then remove the positive reinforcement of the seizures. We taught him that he should tell the teacher when he was anxious and didn't understand something, and we showed him how to do this. Next we told him that it was permissible to have a seizure in class and that he didn't need to go to the school sickroom, but he should simply rest for 5 minutes and then go on with the class. When he had a small complex partial seizure, his teacher would put him at the back of the classroom for 5 minutes, bring him back into class, and immediately discuss with him any difficulties he may have been experiencing with the work. This change led to a significant reduction in seizures and a consequent reduction in medication. He also began to perform better in school.

The ABC chart is very powerful if used correctly. It requires good observational skills on the part of the patient and a close relationship between the patient and the physician. Most strategies are self-evident if the chart is filled in correctly. Here are some further examples of the use of the chart.

A patient's seizure diary showed a large increase in seizures. She was compliant with her medication and there had been no recent changes in therapy. She told me she had recently come back from vacation and that she had very much enjoyed herself; however, on her return, the vicar asked her if she had done the typing she usually did for the parish magazine. She had forgotten all about this; she was immediately overcome by guilt and had a series of complex partial seizures. She told me that when thinking about it, she realized that she tended to have a seizure whenever she was feeling guilty. The behavioral strategy I gave her was very simple—whenever she was stricken by feelings of guilt over something she had or had not done, she was instructed to say to herself: "Will it really matter in a hundred years' time?" She described this technique as the best anti-convulsant she had ever been given, and her seizure frequency dramatically fell.

The main points about an ABC chart are that, if it is filled out accurately and analyzed carefully, it should enable a precise countermeasure to be devised.

The treatment and care of a patient with epilepsy is dependent on a strong, positive working relationship between the patient and the physician. Patients should take responsibility for their epilepsy and its treatment, but they should also take advantage of the physician's specialized knowledge, help, and support.

Conclusion

In summary, the behavioral treatment of epilepsy helps patients gain an understanding of themselves and the relationship between their seizures, their life difficulties and successes, and their relationships with others. It helps them reduce seizure frequency by using countermeasures to inhibit seizure activity and by avoiding seizure-prone situations. It promotes independence and better life adjustment, and teaches that happiness and relaxation are powerful anticonvulsants.

Acknowledgments

My thanks to Dr. Masato Matsuura of the Nihon University Medical School, Tokyo; Dr. Naoto Adachi of the Adchi Medical Clinic; and Dr. Masumi Ito of the Tenshi Hospital, Sapporo for the Japanese data used in this study.

References

1. Martinek A, Horak F. Development of so-called "genuine" epileptic seizures in dogs during emotional excitement. *Physiol Bohemoslov* 1970;19:185–195.
2. Lockard JS. A primate model of clinical epilepsy: mechanism of action through quantification of therapeutic effects. In: Lockard JS, Ward AA, (eds.) *Epilepsy: A Window to Brain Mechanisms*. New York: Raven Press, 1980;11–49.
3. Stevens JR. Emotional activation of the electroencephalogram in patients with convulsive disorders. *J Nerv Ment Dis* 1959;128:339–351.
4. Baker W, Baker S. Experimental production of human convulsive brain potentials by stress-induced effects upon neural integrative function: dynamics of the convulsive reaction to stress. *Assoc Res Nerv Dis Proc* 1950;29:90–113.
5. Small JG, Stevens JR, Milstein V. Electroclinical correlates of emotional activation of the electroencephalogram. *J Nerv Ment Dis* 1954;138:146–155.
6. Forster FM. Tetanus toxoid in animals. *Intl J Neur* 1969;9:73–86.
7. Gowers W. *Epilepsy and Other Chronic Convulsive Disorders: Their Causes, Symptoms and Treatment*. London: Churchill, 1901;29.
8. Dahl J. A behaviour medicine approach to epilepsy—time for a paradigm shift? *Scand J Behav Ther* 1999;(28)3:97–114.

CHAPTER 6

Neurofeedback Therapy

M. Barry Sterman, PhD

Operant conditioning of the electroencephalogram (EEG) or brain wave recording—also known as *neurofeedback* or *neurotherapy*—is a noninvasive treatment for patients whose seizures are not adequately controlled by medication. Operant conditioning can produce meaningful functional changes that elevate the seizure threshold. Abnormal brain wave activity may be diminished and sleep normalized, but not all who respond to operant conditioning have the desired EEG changes, and even some who have the desired EEG changes do not always show actual clinical improvement.

The Technique

The first step in operant conditioning is a comprehensive mapping of the EEG over the entire head, a method called *quantitative EEG assessment* (QEEG). In early studies, however, investigators relied on a more limited assessment of the EEG, looking for abnormal sharp and slow brain wave patterns and the disturbance of normal EEG components. The EEG operant conditioning method is a learning procedure that is applied to alter recorded EEG patterns. It is based on a fundamental principle, the Law of Effect. Positive reinforcement is provided for EEG patterns that approach the desired normal EEG configuration, and negative reinforcement follows the occurrence of pathologic components in this signal. This leads to an essentially unconscious modification of these brain waves through the shaping of response patterns and, accordingly, the underlying physiology that produces these patterns. A computer processes the EEG signals, identifies the critical components, and then modifies a display on the monitor screen in front of the patient; this display provides an integrated reward for a normalized EEG pattern. This can be a simple game involving the progressive completion of a puzzle or other tasks leading to the scoring of points. With children, these points can lead to meaningful rewards, such as privileges or money. For patients with epilepsy whose EEG abnormalities have been identified, the desired response is learning how to change the underlying circuitry of the brain so that the EEG is changed and the seizure threshold is raised. Usually, the patient becomes more relaxed, but the conditioning is not a relaxation technique. It is similar to a workout in a gym, with the muscles being the brain. When the patient is a child, often psychotherapy and consultation with the parents are part of the neurotherapy treatment session.

Relevant Studies

We published the first results of the successful use of EEG biofeedback for epilepsy in 1972 (1). Work with the subject was based on biofeedback findings in animal studies that documented increased seizure thresholds in response to convulsive drugs. The patient, who had a 7-year history of generalized tonic-clonic seizures of unknown origin, became free of seizures after 3 months of training, a result that was startling given the seizure history. With a more prolonged period of treatment, this patient brought the seizures under control and stopped taking medications.

Early animal studies identified the *sensorimotor rhythm* (SMR), a rhythmic EEG pattern seen over the somatosensory cortex (or central region) of the brain. Increasing the SMR rhythm in animals through operant conditioning training eliminated or significantly reduced those seizures induced by certain chemical compounds (2). Further, sleep studies showed that animals with SMR training had an increase in SMR-like sleep EEG activity (or spindles), improved sleep organization, and less sleep-fragmenting awakenings (3). Brain wave spindles are a short series of waves with a frequency of 14 per second. In humans, sleep spindle activity increases when seizures are reduced (4,5). Other animal studies clarified more about EEG activity in epilepsy and showed evidence that EEG operant conditioning of the SMR changes the physiologic regulation of the brain (3,6–14).

Even though patients with epilepsy have different kinds of seizures, different histories, and take different medications, many controlled human studies on operant conditioning for seizure disorders were published in peer-reviewed medical journals between 1972 and 1996. These studies have consistently shown the benefits of operant conditioning (they are reviewed within Reference 15). Eighteen studies showed significant seizure reduction (over 50%) and reductions in the severity of seizures. Investigations that included sampling the blood of patients to determine anticonvulsant medication levels did not show a relationship between drug levels and the outcome of the conditioning (4,5,16–18). Additionally, studies using sham feedback, relaxation training, or alternate EEG criteria for reward showed no significant effect on seizure incidence or severity. Research using neurofeedback for seizure control is more expensive, difficult, and complex than drug studies, so the number of patients who have been studied is relatively small.

Financial Considerations

Neurofeedback treatment is administered in 1-hour sessions, 1 to 3 times per week for periods ranging from 3 months to more than 1 year, depending on the nature of the seizure disorder. The cost of treatment varies, but it is usually about $100 per session and is often covered by health insurance under the "outpatient mental health" benefit of the insurance, especially if the patient suffers from symptoms such as anxiety. Outpatient mental health benefits may have a deductible amount separate from that of the medical benefit. After the patient meets the deductible, the insurance covers from 50% to 80% of the "usual and customary" fees. The practitioner may charge an initial QEEG and intake consultation fee.

Choosing a Practitioner

The Biofeedback Certification Institute of America (www.bcia.org) oversees standards, certifies practitioners, and has information about finding and interviewing a practitioner. Although the field is rapidly evolving, unfortunately, many practitioners have not kept

---

Commentary

Just as biofeedback can train us to slow our heart rates, neurofeedback can teach us to exert some control over our brain waves. Neurofeedback is being explored not only for its potential use in epilepsy but also to enhance cognitive and memory performance (1). While any safe method of cognitive enhancement is especially exciting for our patients with memory and attentional difficulties, these claims require validation through independent, well-controlled neuropsychological studies. Other reported uses of neurofeedback include the treatment of attention deficit hyperactivity disorder (ADHD) (2), tinnitus (3), and chronic fatigue (4).

Because neurofeedback appears to be free of significant risk and because the electrophysiologic changes induced in the brain are quantifiable, there is growing interest in its use as an adjunctive epilepsy treatment. Enhancing the sensorimotor rhythm (SMR) is thought to correlate with the antiepileptic effect of neurofeedback; however, although neurofeedback may enhance this localized brain electrical rhythm, it is not clear how these changes exert an effect on epileptic activity, especially when seizures may arise in brain regions remote from the central brain regions where the SMR rhythm is located. Additional claims are being made that neurofeedback may be able to reduce the amount of slow EEG activity that corresponds to an area of brain injury, also potentially reducing its ability to produce seizures. This claim remains speculative but is worthy of further study.

In summary, neurofeedback is an intriguing therapy that is aimed at the source of seizures (i.e., the electrical activity of the brain). It has no known ill effects, as far as we know; however, prolonged therapy can become quite expensive and definitive data verifying its efficacy are lacking.

References

1. Vernon D, Egner T, Cooper N, et al. The effect of training distinct neurofeedback protocols on aspects of cognitive performance. *Int J Psychophysiol* 2003;47(1): 75–85.
2. Egner T, Gruzelier JH. Learned self-regulation of EEG frequency components affects attention and event-related brain potentials in humans. *Neuroreport* 2001;12(18):4155–159.
3. Gosepath K, Nafe B, Ziegler E, et al. Neurofeedback in therapy of tinnitus [German] *HNO* 2001;49(1):29–35.
4. James LC, Folen RA. EEG biofeedback as a treatment for chronic fatigue syndrome: a controlled case report. *Behav Med* 1996;22(2):77–81.

abreast of advances in concept and methodology. Clients should assure themselves that a provider has good credentials and is current in relevant knowledge and technology.

References

1. Sterman MB, Friar L. Suppression of seizures in an epileptic following sensorimotor EEG feedback training. *Electroencephalogr Clin Neurophysiol* 1972;33:89–95.
2. Sterman MB. Studies of EEG biofeedback training in man and cats. In: *Highlights of the 17th Annual Conference. VA Cooperative Studies in Mental Health and Behavioral Sciences.* 1972;50–60.
3. Sterman MB, Howe RD, Macdonald LR. Facilitation of spindle-burst sleep by conditioning of electroencephalographic activity while awake. *Science* 1970;167:1146–1148.
4. Sterman MB, Shouse MN. Quantitative analysis of training, sleep EEG and clinical response to EEG operant conditioning in epileptics. *Electroencephalogr Clin Neurophysiol* 1980;49:558–576.
5. Sterman MB. EEG feedback in the treatment of epilepsy: an overview circa 1980. In: White L, Tursky B, (eds.) *Clinical Biofeedback: Efficacy and Mechanisms.* New York: Guilford Press, 1982;311–330.
6. Wywricka W, Sterman MB. Instrumental conditioning of sensorimotor cortex EEG spindles in the waking cat. *Physiol Behav* 1968;3:703–707.
7. Chase MH, Harper RM. Somatomotor and visceromotor correlates of operantly conditioned 12-14 c/s sensorimotor activity. *Electroencephalogr Clin Neurophysiol* 1971;31:85–92.
8. Babb MI, Chase MH. Masseteric and digastric reflex activity during conditioned sensorimotor rhythm. *Electroencephalogr Clin Neurophysiol* 1974;36:357–365.
9. Harper RM, Sterman MB. Subcortical unit activity during a conditioned 12-14 Hz sensorimotor EEG rhythm in the cat. *Fed Proc* 1972;31:404.
10. Sterman MB. Neurophysiologic and clinical studies of sensorimotor EEG biofeedback training: some effects on epilepsy. *Semin Psychiatry* 1973;5:507–525.
11. Steriade M, Llinas R. The functional states of the thalamus and the associated neuronal interplay. *Physiol Rev* 1988;68:649–742.
12. Howe RC, Sterman MB. Somatosensory system evoked potentials during waking behavior and sleep in the cat. *Electroencephalogr Clin Neurophysiol* 1973;34:605–618.
13. Warren RA, Jones EG. Glutamate activation of cat thalamic reticular nucleus: effects on response properties of ventroposterior neurons. *Exp Brain Res* 1994;100:215–226.
14. Buchwald JS, Eldred E. Relations between gamma-efferent discharge and cortical activity. *Electroencephalogr Clin Neurophysiol* 1961;13:243–247.
15. Sterman MB. Basic concepts and clinical findings in the treatment of seizure disorders with EEG operant conditioning. *Clin Electroencephalogr* 2000;31:45–55.
16. Lantz D, Sterman MB. Neuropsychological assessment of subjects with uncontrolled epilepsy: effects of EEG biofeedback training. *Epilepsia* 1988;29:163–171.
17. Sterman MB, Macdonald LR. Effects of central cortical EEG feedback training on incidence of poorly controlled seizures. *Epilepsia* 1978;19:207–222.
18. Wyler AR, Lockard JS, Ward AA. Conditioned EEG desynchronization and seizure occurrence in patients. *Electroencephalogr Clin Neurophysiol* 1976;41:501–512.

Further Information

Jim Robbins. *A Symphony in the Brain.* Atlantic Monthly Press; 2000. (This book provides a useful, personalized history of neurofeedback.)

CHAPTER 7

Autogenic Training

NOELLE BERGER, PHD

Autogenic training (AT) is a relaxation method developed in 1924 by Johann Heinrich Schultz, a German neurologist. It is widely used in many countries, including Germany, Japan, France, Russia, England, and Canada, but it has not been popular in the United States, perhaps largely because much of the research from other countries has not been translated into English. Following the development of AT by Dr. Schultz, it was not widely used to treat epilepsy because of the belief that it might increase the frequency of seizures in some people.

We studied AT therapy in people with epilepsy and found no increase in seizure frequency in the small sample. In contrast, several patients experienced a significant reduction in the frequency of seizures, leading us to take a second look at AT and its potential use to treat people with epilepsy.

Definition

AT is a form of relaxation training, similar to self-hypnosis, that uses specific scripts. It gives some patients a high degree of physiologic and psychologic control. AT focuses on regulating body processes often thought of as uncontrollable, such as blood flow and heartbeat.

Several more complex definitions of AT have been proposed over the years. Wolfgang Luthe, a German physician and disciple of Schultz, proposed the following definition in 1963: "[AT is] … a psychophysiologic form of psychotherapy that the patient carries out himself by using passive concentration upon certain combinations of psychophysiologically adapted stimuli" (1). AT has also been described as "a psychophysiologic self-control therapy" (2). In 1990, Wolfgang Linden described AT as "a form of autonomic self-regulation therapy" (3).

The emphasis of AT is on self-control and self-administration by the patient, following training by a professional. AT differs from traditional hypnosis, which is induced by another person, usually a therapist. AT is practiced by patients themselves and promotes a feeling of self-control and independence from the therapist.

AT is based on Schultz's belief in the self-healing ability of the body and on the homeostatic model of physiologic functioning proposed by Cannon (4). The most typical application of AT is promoting relaxation by reducing *autonomic arousal* (the arousal of smooth and cardiac muscle and glandular tissues, and the arousal of involuntary actions).

History

Schultz was trained in dermatology and neurology; he became interested in hypnosis, although it was considered "unprofessional" by his peers. He began his private practice in 1924, made his first presentation on AT in 1926, and produced over 400 publications, including numerous books translated into six languages.

Schultz based his development of AT on two sources: his own experiences with clinical hypnosis and Oskar Vogt's observations on brain research. Schultz noticed that hypnotized patients usually reported two specific sensations: "a strange heaviness in the limbs" and a similarly "strange sensation of warmth." He believed hypnosis was not something the hypnotist did to patients, but instead was an experience patients allowed to happen to them. Schultz believed in a point of change, a kind of "switch" when the patient would enter into the hypnotic trance. He wanted to find a way to allow the patient to control this switch.

AT became available to English-speaking clinicians and researchers after Luthe emigrated to Canada and began publishing works on AT in English (5). Luthe later wrote a six-volume comprehensive work on AT with Schultz (6).

Relevant Research

Many studies of AT have not been properly controlled—they do not have an experimental or treatment group that receives the treatment and a control group that does not receive the treatment or receives only a placebo. No trials focus on the use of AT in people who have epilepsy. The following are reports on the use of AT with different medical conditions.

Ernst and Kanji (7) conducted a systematic review of all controlled trials of AT as a method to reduce stress and anxiety. They found that most trials were flawed because of deviations from the accepted method of AT. Eight studies were well controlled. Of these, seven reported positive effects of AT in reducing stress; one showed no benefit. Ernst and Kanji concluded that AT, properly applied, needs testing in carefully controlled trials.

Kostic and Secen (8) examined the benefits of AT in patients with adult-onset type 2 diabetes. They treated 40 patients on antidiabetic medication. They found that fasting glucose, cholesterol level, and lipid peroxidase were all significantly lower after a course of AT training. The serum level of high-density lipoprotein (HDL, the "good" cholesterol) was significantly higher after AT. The researchers concluded that in selected patients, especially those who are most responsive to stress, AT can help improve glucose control and lipid metabolism as an adjunct to conventional treatment.

Wickramasekera (9) examined the mechanism by which biofeedback (the general mechanism underlying AT) reduces clinical symptoms. He also examined whether memories and beliefs have biological consequences. He found that high and low hypnotic ability are related to dysregulation of the sympathetic ("fight or flight system") system and the parasympathetic ("rest and digest system") system. Biofeedback was most effective for reducing clinical symptoms in people of low to moderate hypnotic ability. Training in self-hypnosis, AT, or other instructional procedures produced the most rapid reduction of clinical symptoms in people with high hypnotic ability.

Mishima and associates (10) studied the psychophysiologic changes induced in subjects by standard AT. Their subjects were students studying health, who were randomly assigned either to a control group or an AT group for 3 months. In this study, AT induced significant positive changes, such as increased blood flow and relaxed mind and body, independent of breathing. (Diaphragmatic breathing may cause changes similar to those induced by AT, and it is important to differentiate the effects of each.)

Commentary

The differences between medicine as it is practiced in the United States and that of other Western countries deserves consideration. The process for approval of new medications in the United States is slower. Many countries provide over-the-counter access to medications (e.g., antibiotics) that are only available by prescription in the United States. Physicians are often more open to alternative therapies, such as AT, outside rather than inside the United States. A quick review of the medical literature since 1965 (1) shows 287 documents in English and 615 in foreign languages. Remarkably, most of the English articles come from Europe, not the United States. Why the lack of interest in study and slow adoption for use in this country? Translation into English is only part of the reason, as the 287 English documents indicate. Philosophical approaches to medical care and a lack of nonmedical champions for the therapy are also important.

What is the evidence that AT works? AT is a form of relaxation training that could be expected to help reduce stress, and to the degree that stress is a trigger for seizures, it may help improve seizure control. Evidence suggests the beneficial physiologic effects of AT (e.g., decreased resting heart rate) (2) and its effectiveness for disorders with psychological components such as atopic dermatitis (3). Positive evidence is balanced by studies showing a lack of effectiveness of AT in disorders with psychological components, such as motion sickness and asthma (4,5). The vast majority of studies are limited by inconsistent techniques of AT, small sample size, lack of blinding and controls, and other methodologic limitations.

Unfortunately, as Berger points out, Ernst and Kanji's (6) systematic review of controlled trials using AT found insufficient data to make any conclusions about its role in reducing stress or anxiety. Insufficient data is a common theme running through the complementary and alternative therapies. If we are unsure of AT's role in reducing stress and anxiety, its role in helping individuals with epilepsy remains even more uncertain. The methodology and conceptual underpinnings of AT suggest a potential role in treating epilepsy patients.

Stress may promote seizure activity by creating the physiologic milieu for seizure occurrence (lowering the seizure threshold) and by facilitating conversion of an aura (simple partial seizure) into a stronger seizure (see Chapter 4, Comprehensive Neurobehavioral Approach). AT is designed to promote relaxation and reduce stress. Its specific model, autohypnosis, combines the opportunities for self-control (often removed from individuals with epilepsy) and a personalized technique to tap the well of healing. As Gowers wrote more than a century ago, seizures may beget seizures. That is, once you have had one seizure, the second comes more easily. Once you have two, the third comes easier yet. Although good neurophysiologic evidence now supports this model in the laboratory, it is insufficient to clearly endorse its relevance in human epilepsy. AT and related relaxation therapies and mechanisms to reduce stress and enhance self-control may provide avenues to "unbeget" seizures. Time will tell, hopefully soon. We look forward to seeing the results of Berger's initial pilot study of AT in epilepsy and hope that larger and more definitive studies can be done in the not-too-distant future.

References

1. Pubmed: www.ncbi.nlm.nih.gov:80/entrez
2. Mishima N, Kubota S, Nagata S. Psychophysiologic correlates of relaxation induced by standard autogenic training. *Psychother Psychosom* 1999;68:207–213.
3. Ehlers A, Stangier U, Gieler U. Treatment of atopic dermatitis: a comparison of psychological and dermatological approaches to relapse prevention. *J Consult Clin Psychol* 1995;63:624–635.
4. Jozsvai EE, Pigeau RA. The effect of autogenic training and biofeedback on motion sickness tolerance. *Aviat Space Environ Med* 1996;67:963–968.
5. Huntley A, White AR, Ernst E. Relaxation therapies for asthma: a systematic review. *Thorax* 2002;57:127–131.
6. Ernst E, Kanji N. Autogenic training for stress and anxiety: a systematic review. *Complement Ther Med* 2000;8:106–110.

Practical Application

AT uses six standard formulas: heaviness (muscular relaxation), warmth (vascular dilation), regulation of the heart, regulation of breathing, regulation of the visceral organs, and regulation of the head. Heaviness (muscular relaxation) is the most easily influenced by conscious efforts. The effects of this formula generalize throughout the body, as do the other formulas. The practice must be consistent and always begin with the dominant arm in muscular relaxation.

The warmth formula affects blood flow in the arteries and veins, and should not be used by people with vascular disease or risk factors. The regulation of the heart formula focuses on having a quiet and strong heartbeat, not on slowing it down. Some people become so adept at AT that they can slow their heart rate. We do not advise this.

The regulation of breathing acknowledges that breathing is partly autonomous and partly intentional. The rhythm of breathing is integrated into muscular, vascular, and heart relaxation. In the case of AT, intentional modification of breathing is not desirable because it is associated with tension by way of a reflex-type mechanism. As a result, a passive formula is used: "It breathes me."

The regulation of the visceral organs focuses on the solar plexus, the area halfway between the navel and the lower end of the sternum in the upper body. The solar plexus is considered a critical nerve center for the internal organs. We sometimes use an image of the sun from which warm rays extend into other body areas.

The regulation of the head formula is based on the well-known relaxing effect of a cool cloth on the forehead. It is important not to overgeneralize by cooling the entire head with this formula. This could lead to fainting or migraine headache.

Sample Autogenic Training Exercise

The six different formulas are taught in a gradual, specific order. For the first few weeks of training, the patient concentrates on the first formula, heaviness. After this formula is learned, the others are added over a period of weeks. The training time for the complete set of exercises is 8 to 10 weeks. The following is the complete training exercise including all six formulas.

- Close your eyes and find a comfortable body position. Allow yourself to concentrate on what is going on inside you. Now concentrate on both arms and repeat this formula six times, slowly: "My arms are very heavy and warm." Use an image of warmth and heaviness that you are familiar with. Now turn your attention away from your arms and say to yourself, just once: "I am very quiet." Enjoy feeling relaxed.

- Now concentrate on the beating of your heart and repeat this formula six times, slowly: "My heartbeat is calm and strong." Now turn your attention away from your heart and say to yourself, just once: "I am very quiet." Enjoy feeling relaxed.

- Now concentrate on the rhythm of your breathing and repeat this formula six times, slowly: "It breathes me." Now direct your attention away from your breathing, and say to yourself, just once: "I am very quiet." Enjoy feeling relaxed.

- Now concentrate on your stomach area and repeat this formula six times, slowly: "Warmth is radiating over my stomach." Now turn your attention away from your stomach area and say to yourself, just once: "I am very quiet." Enjoy feeling relaxed.

- Now concentrate on your forehead and repeat this formula six times, slowly: "My forehead is cool." Now direct your attention away from your forehead and say to yourself, just once: "I am very quiet." Enjoy feeling relaxed.

- At the end of the training session, do a "take-back" exercise to maximize gains from the training and to transition back into a state of alertness. The take-back exercise consists of counting backward from 4 to 1, doing the following actions with each number:

  4 Make a couple of fists with both hands in rapid succession
  3 Bend arms inward at the elbow a few times, touching your shoulders with your hands
  2 Take a few deep breaths
  1 Open your eyes, sit up, and feel relaxed and alert

Advantages and Disadvantages of Autogenic Training

- Advantages:
  - It is cost-effective because it can be taught in a group format or individually.
  - AT gives the patient a high degree of self-control.
  - It is not time-consuming to practice, although for maximum benefit, it should be practiced two times daily.
  - AT provides lasting benefits and can be combined with other approaches.
- Disadvantages:
  - AT requires regular training to obtain and maintain its benefits.
  - It must be taught by a skilled professional, making it inaccessible to some. Powerful emotions may sometimes surface with AT that may need to be processed with a skilled psychotherapist.
  - Some patients will not benefit from AT.
  - It is not recommended for people with severe emotional or psychological disorders, or children under 5 years of age.
  - People who have diabetes, hypoglycemic conditions, or cardiac or vascular conditions need to be under a physician's supervision while undertaking AT.

Autogenic Training for Stress Management in Epilepsy

AT was integrated into a stress management program for 12 patients with epilepsy at The Epilepsy Institute in New York. The patients were taught four different methods of relaxation, including diaphragmatic breathing, progressive muscle relaxation, imagery/visualization, and AT. The effectiveness of the program was studied during its 1-year duration. The results have not yet been analyzed completely, but preliminary results indicate that some patients who practiced AT experienced a reduction in seizure frequency. More controlled research with a larger sample is needed before definitive conclusions can be made.

References

1. Luthe W. Autogenic training: method, research and application in medicine. *Am J Psychother* 1963;17:174–195.

2. Pikoff H. A critical review of autogenic training in America. *Clin Psychol Rev* 1984;4:619–639.
3. Linden W. *Autogenic Training, a Clinical Guide.* New York: Guilford Press, 1990.
4. Cannon WB. *The Wisdom of the Body.* New York: Norton, 1933.
5. Luthe W. Autogenic training: method, research and application in medicine. *Am J Psychother* 1963;17:174–195.
6. Schultz JH, Luthe W. *Autogenic Therapy,* Vol 1-6. New York: Grune & Stratton, 1969.
7. Ernst E, Kanji N. Autogenic training for stress and anxiety: a systematic review. *Complement Ther Med* 2000;8:106–110.
8. Kostic N, Secen S. Effect of autogenic training on glucose regulation and lipid status in non-insulin dependent diabetics. *Med Pregl* 2000;53:285–328.
9. Wickramasekera I. How does biofeedback reduce clinical symptoms and do memories and beliefs have biological consequences? Toward a model of mind-body healing. *Appl Psychophysiol Biofeedback* 1999;24: 91–105.
10. Mishima N, Kubota S, Nagata S. Psychophysiologic correlates of relaxation induced by standard autogenic training. *Psychother Psychosom* 1999;68:207–213.

CHAPTER 8

Massage and Seizure Control*

BERNHARD MÜLLER

This chapter outlines strategies for improving seizure control using massage. Indications, methodical components, therapeutic aims, scientific foundations, risks and contraindications, and education about massage therapy for epilepsy are covered. Massage therapy is considered as a sole therapeutic approach, as well as in combination with other psycho- and neurophysiologic approaches to seizure control. Assessing the role of massage in drug-refractory epilepsies and in patients with multiple disabilities is an important challenge that is specifically addressed. Specific types of massage, depending on symptoms and individual factors, may prevent epileptic seizures or stop them at their onset. Careful questioning by professionals and laypersons who are trusted by the patient can determine if massage therapy is helpful. Massage should not be considered as stand-alone therapy for epilepsy but as a complement to standard medical care.

Definition and Historical Background

No universal definition of massage exists. The common denominator of all described types of massage is the targeted, usually systematic manual stimulation of selected areas of the body for therapeutic purposes. Massage seeks to prevent acute or chronic disease, and—as far as possible—restore physiologic and psychological health.

Massage for alleviating pain and increasing well-being was probably known by ancient humans (1–4). Although it is one of the oldest, most commonly used treatment options for humans, the acceptance of massage within the medical-scientific community has fluctuated tremendously. Massage was included in documents on medical practice in the third millennium B.C. in ancient China, appreciated as medical art by Hippocrates and his successors, almost completely ignored or rejected in the Middle Ages, rediscovered in the sixteenth century, and used as an orthodox, first-line medical treatment in several Western countries in the late nineteenth and early twentieth centuries (2,5–9).

---

*This chapter is a condensed version of a longer, detailed study that is available on request from the author (see front matter of this book for contact information or email: bmuller@uni-mainz.de).

Types of Massage

At least four major types of massage can be used alone or in combination for the prevention and inhibition of epileptic seizures:

- Classical massage
- Acupressure, or massage of acupoints
- Synchronized massage (massage provided by two or more practitioners)
- Aroma massage with essential oils

Classical Massage

Classical massage is most often defined as one or more of five techniques that use the hands or fingers: stroking (effleurage), rubbing (friction), kneading (pétrissage), shaking (vibration), and percussion movements (tapotement), sometimes in different combinations (2,10–13). Some massage therapists use additional techniques, such as pressing (14).

The common denominator of all classical massage techniques is that they do not focus on specific points on the body, as in acupressure. Compared to massage in Asian countries, classical massage focuses on relatively few specific physiologic effects (15).

Classical massage is frequently used in healthcare, education, and emerging research in Western countries. Classical massage may be used in conjunction with other types of massage—for example, as a warm-up phase for acupressure (16,17) or to assess the usefulness and strategies of synchronized massage.

The possible use of classical massage techniques to prevent epileptic seizures gained wide support from a series of group studies, many of them conducted at the Touch Research Institute in Florida. These studies showed the largely consistent beneficial effects of simple components of classical massage techniques on anxiety levels, mood, sleep, stress hormones, and several other potentially seizure-favoring factors (18–20). The discovery of the psychophysiologic factors of massage and their possible role in behavioral and psychosomatic medicine is new and challenging (21,22).

The effects of massage on seizure inhibition or prevention may differ depending on the quality of the interaction between the therapist and the patient (23–25) and on the professional experience of the therapist. Individuals who do not respond to classical massage techniques may improve their seizure control using another type of massage.

Acupressure

The discovery of acupoints—specific points on the body that can be stimulated in order to alleviate specific ailments—is a cross-cultural phenomenon with origins dating back about 5,200 years (26–29). Variants of acupressure may be the most interesting and advanced therapies for individuals with epilepsy. An evaluation of the available literature as well as clinical observations shows that more than 40% of the 361 classical acupoints have been recommended or successfully used, often in suitable combinations, in epilepsy treatment. All twelve main, two midline, and/or six extra meridians have been involved, albeit to varying degrees. The advantages of manual stimulation (acupressure) as compared to stimulation by needles (acupuncture), are particularly important for use in epilepsy (e.g., specific stimulation during a seizure).

Synchronized Massage

Synchronized massage is provided by two or more persons whose movements mirror each other, usually at the vertical midline of the person receiving the massage. This technique was mainly developed on the Indian subcontinent for individuals with neurologic disorders (30–32). It has also been tried in other cultures (33,34).

Simultaneous treatment by more than one person has a long history. Its use in seizure control emerged from Ayurvedic traditions, which consider psychological factors in the precipitation and treatment of epilepsy (35,36). The use of synchronized massage in epilepsy control has not been scientifically studied.

The major advantages of synchronized as compared to conventional, "one-on-one" massage—both for those who receive and for those who give the massage—include: (i) the intensification or even potentiation of physiologic and psychophysiologic effects; (ii) the symmetric balancing, in some cases, of unilateral neurologic disorders; (iii) the distribution and supplementation of responsibility, observation, and continuity; (iv) the inclusion and didactically easier instruction of laypersons; and (v) the low-cost prevention of therapeutic gaps, withdrawal effects, or even traumas due to separation or long-term interruption (37). Another advantage is a decreased risk of fixation towards the therapist or other persons, that is, a decreased dependency on social patterns that favor the occurrence of both diurnal and nocturnal seizures (38,39). In some well-documented cases, bilateral stimulation appeared decisive in preventing partial seizures from generalizing.

Except for several promising studies at the beginning of the twentieth century, when massage was an established subject at the Berlin University (63), synchronized massage appears to have been forgotten by science. Randomized controlled trials (RCTs) confirmed that bilateral stimulation of an acupoint with acupressure devices is usually more effective than unilateral stimulation (64). Furthermore, manual stimulation of the same point, frequently as part of a multipoint combination in epilepsy treatment, is more effective than stimulation by technical aids (65–67). Overall, however, investigations are limited comparing synchronized versus conventional massage in epilepsy.

Synchronized massage may enhance arterial oxygen saturation more than one-on-one massage. This effect may contribute to the prevention or inhibition of seizures. Placebo-controlled research shows significant increases of cerebral blood flow velocity and slightly increased cerebral O_2 saturation upon acupoint stimulation at the head and extremities (66).

Aroma Massage

The use of aromas for stopping epileptic seizures was reported in antiquity (40). Essential oils and ointments are also mentioned in Biblical sources as both preventive and ritual treatments, although epilepsy is not specifically mentioned. This method was already differentiated from the therapeutic role of "mere" touch in Biblical times.

Seizure inhibition and the preventive applications of essential oils can be combined with massage for optimal success. True lavender (Lavandula vera) is especially useful when added to massage in the evening. (See also Chapter 9 for a discussion of aromatherapy.)

Therapeutic Self-Massage

The use of therapeutic self-massage is justified if it contributes to an individual's independence and self-control of epileptic seizures. Components of the four basic approaches can be continued if no second person is present to provide the massage. The self-control of seizures even can include the self-application of some types of bilateral stimulation.

Massage as a respectful interaction between two or more persons can be beneficial in itself, and its social value cannot be entirely replaced. Self-help should not lead to isolation, but to integration, as individuals with epilepsy teach their peers what they have learned about massage.

Scientific Foundations for the Use of Massage in Epilepsy

Scientific studies suggest or confirm the usefulness of all four types of massage in seizure control. These studies include clinical and neurophysiologic research that shows the physiologic mechanisms of action produced by massage.

Clinical Studies

Different RCTs investigating the psychologic and physiologic effects of massage to prevent seizures support the usefulness of all four massage types in helping to prevent epileptic seizures by reducing the potential factors that can provoke seizures.

Methodological challenges arise in performing a RCT to assess massage therapy to stop epileptic seizures. A comparison of different types of acupressure with or without antiepileptic medication would be most convincing (41,42).

The results of six RCTs suggest that even classical types of massage are superior to other approaches such as relaxation in reducing anxiety, sleep disturbance, or stress as potentially seizure-favoring factors. Assessments include subjective as well as objective measurements, such as measuring the levels of stress hormones (43–47).

Several studies show that acupressure combined with massage with essential oils or carrier oil can be more effective than classical massage techniques alone (48–53). The

Commentary

Massage therapy is a potentially valuable way for patients with epilepsy to reduce stress, improve emotional well-being, and possibly reduce seizure activity. Dr. Bernhard Müller provides an insightful view of massage for epilepsy based on his extensive personal experience and a thorough review of the available literature. Massage has a natural place in helping people with epilepsy relax, learn to reduce stress, and possibly through self-massage, carry these positive attributes throughout their daily life.

Reduced stress can likely help individuals with epilepsy decrease their seizure frequency or intensity. In Chapter 3, Stress and Epilepsy, Drs. Carol J. Schramke and Kevin M. Kelly provide an excellent overview of how stress reduction can improve seizure control. Self-massage offers a way to extend the window of time from a place one has to travel to receive therapy to the patient's hands and the patient's control. It extends the possible improvements temporally—so that massage could be applied by the patient or a relative—in settings where seizures occur. This might be especially helpful for those individuals with warnings before their seizures.

We suggest caution in how strongly the data support the role of massage therapy in treating seizures. Dr. Müller suggests that the documentation is clear and shows that massage can stop seizures. Massage may be effective in stopping seizures, but there are no cases of documented seizures (e.g., recorded during a video-EEG study) where massage clearly led to the termination of a seizure. Ninety-nine percent of seizures stop on their own after seconds or minutes. It is likely that any intervention can be associated with seizure offset. Many patients have nonepileptic seizures, and the criteria used to exclude this possibility is not defined in the majority of studies cited.

We remain enthusiastic about the potential role of massage and very strongly support continued development and study in this area to help people with epilepsy.

effectiveness of combined acupressure and massage with essential oils (which are both inhaled and absorbed via the skin) (54) depends on a concise knowledge of symptoms and symptom-alleviating compounds and application methods.

Neurophysiologic Studies

The development of noninvasive technology allows for improved measurement of the (dys)functions of the human body as well as mechanisms of action for manual interventions. These measurements include, for example, details (size, duration) of the release of endogenous seizure-inhibiting neurotransmitters [e.g., gamma aminobutyric acid (GABA)], or the restoration of consciousness and the stabilization of respiration following the well-defined stimulation of specific acupoints (55). Study data support electrophysiologic and electromagnetic correlates of acupoints for diagnosis and treatment, thus making acupressure a plausible therapeutic option in the short- and long-term reduction or normalization of cerebral excitability (56,57). Neuroanatomic, scintiphotographic, thermographic, functional neuroimaging, and transcranial Doppler ultrasound studies that investigate the locations of acupoints or the effects of their stimulation may further contribute to an understanding of seizure threshold regulation by means of acupressure (58–61).

The author's own preliminary investigations indicate that specific acupressure points may facilitate seizure-inhibitory reactions during the biofeedback training of slow cortical potentials.

Taking into account the pathology-dependent concepts of balancing in traditional Chinese medicine (TCM), some studies of acupressure fit well with the established model of Group 2 neurons, whose activation by manual stimulation may inhibit the spread of epileptic discharge originating from Group 1 neurons (62).

Pending and Interdisciplinary Research

The neurochemical and neurophysiologic markers of massage therapy are not well defined. Similarly, the biologic markers of relaxation and restorative sleep are incompletely defined. Understanding changes in the levels of inhibitory neurotransmitters such as GABA may help shed light on both seizure-provoking factors (e.g., sleep deprivation, stress) and seizure-relieving therapies (e.g., massage).

Based on cross-cultural RCTs of the four approaches presented here and their effects on seizure control, separately and in combination, further research is needed to evaluate the short- and long-term costs and benefits of the systematic application of massage in seizure control. Appropriate RCTs could be supplemented by meta-analyses of convincing single-case studies.

Interdisciplinary (including historical and sociological) studies may help us understand why—in contrast to antiquity and Eastern cultures—epilepsy has been excluded from the spectrum of indications in the education of classical massage therapists in Western countries.

Indication, Risks, and Contraindications

Generally, no features of epilepsy or personality discourage the use of massage. Systematic evaluations matching massage and seizure types, potential seizure precipitants, or epilepsies (68,69) underline this. In contrast, a major advantage of massage is its nonverbal nature. The application of massage in infants, for example, has yielded positive results in various cultures. Several RCTs confirm this, although the only effects on frequent seizure precipitants, such as sleep deprivation and depression, have been investigated (70). Rare negative reactions to touch can be overcome by skilled psychological treatment, thus making successful treatment possible.

Substantial differences occur with regard to the types of massage that are effective for various conditions. The choice of acupoints may depend on whether consciousness is lost during seizures, and there are points and sequences of points primarily suitable for preventing seizures or seizure-favoring factors, such as sleep deprivation. Massage can be an effective component of successful psychological approaches to control nocturnal epileptic seizures. The complexity and interactions of epilepsy, personality, and environment suggest, however, that massage must be based on individual behavioral analyses; this field is not suitable for therapeutic cookbooks.

Systematic reviews show that the number and types of contraindications to classical massage techniques varies among textbooks (71). Scientific evidence to support these contraindications is fragmentary and sometimes conflicting (72). Some conditions, such as fever, in which classical massage is considered contraindicated, are listed as explicit indications for specific acupressure treatments or essential oil massage.

Some authors consider the stimulation of several acupoints contraindicated in treating epilepsy, especially during certain stages of pregnancy (73). A careful assessment is particularly needed in this area due to the paucity of controlled studies and the disparate recommendations for both acupressure and classical massage (74–77).

Several other risks exist, such as transitory shifts of seizure activity following systematic stimulation at seizure onset, psychological dependencies (if the stimulation is provided by another person), and overly vigorous tactile stimulation that may cause injury or negative conditioning of pain to touch during a seizure with preserved consciousness, which may influence future stimulations in a negative way. Most of these issues can be addressed in a way that extends the therapeutic aims from the mere diminution of symptoms to the diminution of symptom-maintaining interaction between the individual with epilepsy and the environment. With these aims in mind, the conditions for transitory external stimulation at seizure onset can be systematized for the individual with epilepsy and for the person who stops the seizures.

Education and Costs

Although seizure inhibition through acupressure has been addressed, at least in programs specializing in this field, no school for classical massage techniques has yet been identified whose curricula include this indication (78). Occasionally, personal professional interest has surfaced, especially if inspired by observations of acupressure (79,80).

So, what can be done to initiate individually useful research and extend, quantitatively and qualitatively, offers of massage that are accessible and useful for improving the control of epileptic seizures? A critical deciding factor is an assessment of what those concerned are ready or would like to do. A survey at an epilepsy clinic in Ohio found that massage is preferred by 50% of those using alternative treatments (81). We need to define and improve the quality of epilepsy-specific manual treatments (82).

Professional Counseling

Counseling by a massage therapist who knows the patient well, especially on the issue of contraindications of preventive massage, is mandatory but not sufficient. Individuals considering massage for their epilepsy should always consult their personal physician *before* beginning therapy. Assessment by massage professionals should supplement the physician's advice.

Counseling on indications, contraindications, and measures for seizure inhibition also is desirable because individuals with epilepsy know their illness best. A compilation of systematic interviews on this issue, done between 1970 and 2000, shows that the percentage of persons who made spontaneous observations on behavioral seizure inhibition is, with few exceptions, between about 35 and 65% (83,84). The timing of a seizure does not necessarily fit in with the office hours of a professional. Therefore, the professional should carefully elicit and analyze these spontaneous observations, so that he can assist in developing new strategies for behavioral seizure inhibition (85,86).

Implementation of Treatment

Daily massage is feasible if indicated from a therapeutic view (22). A RCT on smoking in 20 subjects found less anxiety and less cigarettes smoked in the group who used daily self-massage (22). Ideally, the use of massage therapy will include "psychological parents"—persons with a history of positive interaction with the individual with epilepsy. Treatment designs utilizing laypersons as massage givers must consider that (as confirmed by video-EEGs) the quality of nonmanual interactions may also influence seizure control (22–25).

To ensure that the duration of professional counseling and treatment is determined by therapeutic needs, not economic considerations, health insurance companies should be open-minded regarding reimbursement for professional massage (87). In most countries, the addresses of massage therapists and their qualifications can be found on their organization's Web site (88). This information may be helpful in obtaining insurance reimbursement.

Treatment takes time and commitment, and is only justified if effective. Physicians should use strategies that identify those massage components that are most effective for seizure control in any individual patient. It is strongly recommended that any course of treatment chosen be individually adapted to each patient. The effectiveness of massage may be dose-dependent, often requiring daily application.

A baseline period should be long and well documented. Once a therapeutically promising measure is found, establishing the benefits of that method will be enhanced by a carefully documented baseline documentation. The following case illustrates this.

A 3-year-old, drug-resistant boy with multifocal EEG hemiparesis experienced more than 100 counted tonic seizures per day and was given the tentative diagnosis of Lennox-Gastaut syndrome. The usefulness of massage became evident because the seizure frequency dropped immediately below 100 (nearly by 50%) on the first day he received Chinese massage treatment, and it remained clearly lower as long as it was possible to implement the massage on a daily basis. It was not easy for his mother to really assess his progress, however, until her own documentation of the boy's seizures was evaluated.

Furthermore, massage treatments are not always effective on the first day of application, especially if the patient is not accustomed to the experience of touch. Thus, the time spent in documentation and planning is—as with other alternative or complementary treatments—a rewarding investment. Treatment should be identified, restricted, and focused on only those components that are effective for each individual with epilepsy.

Procedure for Preventive Massage

Preventive massage treatments in a noisy, stuffy, or cold room are not likely to be successful. Massage is always about communication and psychologic treatment as well as physical manipulation. Any negative or traumatizing experiences, especially during the first session, will negatively impact subsequent sessions, even if the technique is the most appropriate for achieving seizure control. Rather, it is advised that the therapist follow the basic rules outlined in most massage handbooks, such as working with warm hands in an agreeably temperated room (unless the weather and environment allow comparable places outside) and practicing good hygiene (10,89).

Patients and massage therapists may prefer to use additional stimulation, such as music or aromas, and also can be therapeutically relevant factors, ideally part of a larger treatment design. Patients and therapists may consider using these aids if their influence on seizure control is positive, and patients may be systematically desensitized if their influence is negative.

No hidden or manifest conflicts should exist between the person who receives and the person who gives the massage. The need to settle such conflicts—and the fact that hidden conflicts of any kind may emerge during massage—is another reason why massage is often more effective when combined with psychologic treatment. For this and a variety of other reasons, different types of psychotherapy have evolved into more comprehensive treatments that include touch. These therapies require highly skilled therapists, and results for difficult-to-treat conditions are promising, especially in group settings (38,90–92).

Long-Term Treatments

Not every patient may feel able to continuously maintain a lifestyle that includes massage (93). For patients in whom massage treatment has been limited to the improvement of seizure control, it may be useful to concentrate preventive massage on periods when seizures are more likely, such as during exams or other stressful periods (21).

It may helpful to identify the minimum duration of effective massage. This duration is usually much shorter if massage is restricted to acupressure (55). Depending on the selected point sequence and on the type of other work or activity, it is even possible that the massage therapy can be fit easily into the daily routine. Thus, the time needed for massage will not exacerbate an already time-limited day and provoke stress, but rather eliminate stress.

Conclusion

Massage increases well-being and may increase longevity and help prevent some diseases. As the ancient Chinese say: start digging a well before you are thirsty!

In summary, various types and combinations of massage can be a major component of the psychologic and neurophysiologic approaches used in the improvement of seizure control in various types of epilepsy. Massage is especially important in the individual who lacks verbal and introspective skills.

Despite examples of a more than 50% improvement in seizure control, however, and of antiepileptic and other medications becoming gradually dispensable, the successful use of massage is not always self-evident. A rational use of massage in the treatment of epilepsy takes into account the following steps:

- A careful selection of modalities (types, locations, combinations, sequences, duration, intensity, frequency, and technique) according to individual diagnoses, needs, and reactions
- A systematic examination of suitable components and strategies, as far as possible, within reasonably timed periods (seizure prevention) and/or intervention sequences (seizure inhibition)
- A replication and adaptation of the most effective and the most feasible measures
- A systematic implementation of sequences or combinations whose efficiency has been verified

In this sense, the reasonable research and investigation spent on designing a therapeutic massage program for individual patients will help contribute to the overall body of knowledge as regards massage and seizure control (94).

Despite the interactive nature of most types of massage (except therapeutic self-massage), the goal of treatment remains the self-control of epileptic seizures. Often, this requires some self-control within social surroundings as well. Although sooner or later epilepsy-specific external therapeutic support may and should become dispensable, there are many health-related reasons to maintain a lifestyle that includes massage, with or without professional assistance.

Acknowledgments

I express my gratitude to Kathie Knowles, Maria Hernandez-Reif, Heike Wicklein, Li-Chan Lin, Raymund Pothmann, Gerhard Litscher, and Michael Gach. I also wish to thank several sponsors (including the Andrews-Reiter research program), technicians, and the EEG specialists. Thanks also to Xiaoqing, Ingrid, and John for their support in overcoming several obstacles of language, and especially the many other persons with disabilities I have had the privilege of working with (and their parents) who deserve my sincere acknowledgment. Last, but not least, I thank the staff, who did a great job, especially Heidi.

References

1. Montagu A. *Körperkontakt: die Bedeutung der Haut für die Entwicklung des Menschen*, 8th ed. Stuttgart: Klett-Cotta, 1995. [Engl. original: *Touching: The Human Significance of the Skin*. New York & London: Columbia Univ Press, 1971.]
2. Kamenetz HL. History of massage. In: Basmajian JV, (ed.) *Manipulation, Traction, and Massage*, 3rd ed. Baltimore: Williams & Wilkins, 1985;211–255.
3. Hentschel HD. [On massage in their beginnings. In German.] *Physikal Therapie* 1986;7:506–509.
4. Welford M. Holistic care. Aping our ancestors. *Nursing Stand* 1992;6(20):47.
5. Veith I. *The Yellow Emperor's Classic of Internal Medicine.* 2nd ed. Los Angeles: University of California Press, 1966. [1st ed. Baltimore: Williams & Wilkins, 1949.]
6. Littré E. *Complete Works of Hippocrates* Vol 4. [In French.] Amsterdam: Hakkert, 1978. [French title: *Oevres Complètes d'Hippocrate.*]
7. Green RM. *A Translation of Galen's Hygiene (De sanitate Tuenda).* Springfield, IL: Thomas, 1951.
8. Paré A. *Complete Works.* [In French.] Geneva: Slatkine, 1970. [Reprint of Paris 1840/41.] [French title: *Oevres Complètes.*]
9. Goldstone LA. Massage as an orthodox medical treatment past and future. *Complement Ther Nurs Midwifery* 2000;6:169–175.
10. Wood EC, Becker PD. *Klassische Massagemethoden: Grundlagen—Wirkung—Technik der Ganz- und Teilmassagen.* Stuttgart: Hippokrates, 1984. [Engl. original: Beard G, Wood EC. *Massage—Principles and Techniques*, 1st ed. Philadelphia: Saunders, 1964.]
11. Hofkosh JM. Classical massage. In: Basmajian JV, (ed.) *Manipulation, Traction, and Massage*, 3rd ed. Baltimore: Williams & Wilkins, 1985;263–269.
12. Tappan FM. *Healing Massage Techniques—Holistic, Classic, and Emerging Methods*, 2nd ed. Norwalk, CT: Appleton & Lange, 1988.
13. Muschinsky B. *Massage in Theory and Practice.* [In German]. Stuttgart: Fischer, 1992. [German title: *Massagelehre in Theorie und Praxis.*]
14. Zenz G. *The Classical Therapeutic Massage.* [In German.] Heidelberg: Haug, 1993. [German title: *Die klassische Heilmassage.*]
15. Kipp Wright C. Massage by nurses in the United States and the People's Republic of China: a comparison. *J Transcult Nurs* 1995;7:24–27.
16. Chen ML, Lin LC, Wu SC, et al. The effectiveness of acupressure in improving the quality of sleep in institutionalized patients. *J Gerontol, series A: Biological sciences and medical sciences* 1999;54:M389–394.
17. Lin LC. Personal Communication, 2002.
18. Field T, Seligman S, Scafidi F, et al. Alleviating posttraumatic stress disorders in children following Hurricane Andrew. *J Appl Dev Psychol* 1996;17:37–50.
19. Field T, Ironson G, Scafidi F, et al. Massage therapy reduces anxiety and enhances EEG patterns of alertness and math computations. *Int J Neurosci* 1996;86:179–205.
20. Field T. Massage therapy effects. *Am Psychol* 1998;53:1270–1281.
21. Zeitlin D, Keller SE, Shiflett SC, et al. Immunological effects of massage therapy during acute academic stress. *Psychosom Med* 2000;62:83–84.
22. Hernandez-Reif M, Field T, Hart S. Smoking cravings are reduced by self-massage. *Prev Medicine* 1999;28:28–32.

23. Müller B. Internalization of psychosensory seizure inhibition in a severely mentally retarded adult with epilepsy, part I—a preliminary report. *Self-control in Epilepsy* 1992;3:4–28.

24. Seeck M, Mainwaring N, Yves J, et al. Differential neural activity in the neural temporal lobe evoked by faces of family members and friends. *Ann Neurol* 1993;34:369–372.

25. Müller B. Psychological approaches to seizure control in individuals with Lennox-Gastaut syndrome. Poster and lecture presented at the 24th International Epilepsy Congress. 2001 May 13-18; Buenos Aires, Argentina.

26. Dorfer L, Moser M, Bahr F, et al. A medical report from the stone age? *Lancet* 1999;354: 1023–1025.

27. Dorfer L, Moser M, Spindler K, et al. Was the man in the ice (Ötzi) acupunctured 5,200 years before? In: Litscher G, Zang HC, (eds.) *Computer-Controlled Acupuncture.* Lengerich: Pabst; 2000:176–178.

28. Agrawal AL, Marda SP. *Introduction to Acupuncture*—including a special chapter on acupressure treatment. New Delhi: Jaypee Brothers; 1985.

29. McWorther JH, Davis RB. Cherokee prescriptions for acupressure and massage. *North Carolina Med J* 1998;59:368.

30. Dash VB. *Massage Therapy in Ayurveda,* 2nd repr. New Delhi: Concept Publishing Co, 1994.

31. Devaraj TL. *The Panchakarma Treatment of Ayurveda,* 3rd ed. Bangalore: Subhas, 1996.

32. Brunner U, Wicklein H. *The Art of Ayurvedic Massage.* [In German.] München: Kösel, 1997. [German title: *Die Kunst der Ayurvedischen Massage.*]

33. Kost R. Contributions on the effects of massage on metabolism. 1st communication: the influence of massage on oxygen consumption of the rested organism. [In German.] *Zeitschrift für die gesamte physikalische Therapie* 1927;33:1–11.

34. Inkeles G. *The New Massage: Total Body Conditioning for People Who Exercise.* New York: Perigee, 1980.

35. Ramamurthi B, Gurunathan SK. Epilepsy in Ayurveda. *Neurology India* 1969;17:91–3.

36. Venkataram BS, Rangan G, David J, et al. Ayurveda and epilepsy. *Epicadec News* 1998;12: 7–9.

37. Müller B. The Ayurvedic synchronized massage—aims and implementation in healthy, chronically ill, and disabled individuals with and without epilepsy. [In German.] Manuscript including instructions for the seminar "epilepsies and other disabilities," 1999 Dec 3-4; Kleve, Germany. [German title: Die Ayurvedische Synchronmassage—Ziele und Umsetzung bei Gesunden, chronisch Kranken und Behinderten mit und ohne Epilepsie.] An English version, together with a protocol for research, is in preparation.

38. Maurer-Groeli YA. The skin as a therapeutic tool in the treatment of depressive and schizophrenic patients. [In German.] *Psychosomatische Medizin* 1975;6:67–78.

39. Groh C, Hackl S, Tatzer E, et al. Psychosocial influences on the outcome of treatment in children with seizure disorders. [In German.] *Fortschr Neurol Psychiat* 1980;48:603–611.

40. Falk F. *Galen's Teaching of the Healthy and the Ill Nervous System.* [In German.] Leipzig: Veit, 1871. [German title: *Galen's Lehre vom gesunden und kranken Nervensysteme.*]

41. Pothmann R. Emergency acupressure for epileptic seizures and fainting. [In German.] In: Bühring M, Kemper FH, (eds.) [*Naturopathic Treatment and Unconventional Medical Approaches.* In German.] Berlin, Heidelberg: Springer; 1993:1-7. [German titles: Notfall-Akupressur bei epileptischen Anfällen und Ohnmacht. In: *Naturheilverfahren und unkonventionelle medizinische Richtungen.*]

42. Pothmann R. Personal communication, 2002.

43. Field T, Grizzle N, Scafidi F, et al. Massage and relaxation therapies' effects on depressed adolescent mothers. *Adolescence* 1996;31:903–911.

44. Field T, Hernandez-Reif M, Hart S, et al. Pregnant women benefit from massage therapy. *J Psychosom Obstet Gynecol* 1999;20:31–38.

45. Hernandez-Reif M, Field T, Krasnegor J, et al. High blood pressure and associated symptoms were reduced by massage therapy. *J Bodywork Movement Therapies* 2000;4:31–38.

46. Hernandez-Reif M, Field T, Krasnegor J, et al. Lower back pain is reduced and range of motion increased after massage therapy. *Int J Neurosci* 2001;106:131–145.

47. Diego MA, Field T, Hernandez-Reif M, et al. HIV adolescents show improved immune function following massage therapy. *Int J Neurosci* 2001;106:35–45.

48. Furlan AD, Brosseau L, Imamura M, et al. Massage for low back pain: a systematic review within the framework of the Cochrane collaboration back review group. *Spine* 2002;27:1896–1910.

49. Franke A, Gebauer S, Franke K, et al. Acupuncture massage vs. Swedish massage and individal exercises vs. group exercises in low back pain sufferers— a randomized controlled clinical trial in a 2 x 2 factorial design. [In German.] *Forschende Komplementärmedizin und Klassische Naturheilkunde* 2000;7:286–293.

50. Agarwal KN, Gupta A, Pushkarna R, et al. Effects of massage and use of oil on growth, blood flow & sleep pattern in infants. *Indian J Med Res* 2000;112:212–217.

51. Field T, Schanberg S, Davalos M, et al. Massage with oil has more positive effects on normal infants. *Pre- and Perinatal Psychology J* 1996;11:75–80.

52. Dunn C, Sleep J, Collett D. Sensing an improvement: an experimental study to evaluate the use of aromatherapy, massage, and periods of rest in an intensive care unit. *J Adv Nurs* 1995;21:34–40.

53. Betts T. Further experience of the smell memory technique in the behavioral treatment of epilepsy. *Self-control in Epilepsy* 1998;9:15–19.

54. Jäger W, Buchbauer G, Jirovetz L, et al. Percutaneous absorption of lavender from a massage. *J Soc Cosmet Chem* 1992;43:49–54.

55. Omura Y. Connections found between each meridian (heart, stomach, triple burner,) & organ representation area of corresponding internal organs in each side of the cerebral cortex; release of common neurotransmitters and hormones unique to each meridian and corresponding acupuncture point & internal organ after acupuncture, electrical stimulation, mechanical stimulation (including shiatsu), soft laser stimulation or Qi Gong. *Acupunct Electrother Res* 1989;14:155–186.

56. Becker RO, Reichmanis M, Marino AA, et al. Electrophysiologic correlates of acupuncture points and meridians. *Psychoenergetic Systems* 1976;1:105–112.

57. Kail K. Clinical outcomes of a diagnostic and treatment protocol in allergy/sensitivity patients. *Altern Med Rev* 2001;6:188–202.

58. Lee MHM, Ernst M. The sympatholytic effect of acupuncture as evidenced by thermography: a preliminary report. *Orthopaed Review* 1983;12:67–72.

59. Heine H. Acupuncture therapy. Cutaneous nerve-vessel bundles passing through perforations of the superficial fascia. [In German.] *Therapeutikon* 1988;4:238–244.

60. Darras J-C, de Vernejoul P, Albarède P. Isotopical representation of acupuncture lines. [In German.] *Deutsche Zeitschrift für Akupunktur* 1992;35(1):4–15.

61. Litscher G, Zang HC, (eds.) *Computer-Controlled Acupuncture.* Lengerich: Pabst, 2000.

62. Wieser H-G. Seizure induction in reflex seizures and reflex epilepsy. In: Zifkin BG, Andermann F, Beaumanoir A, Rowan AJ, (eds.) *Reflex Epilepsies and Reflex Seizures.* Philadelphia: Lippincott-Raven, 1998;85–96 (*Advances in Neurology*, Vol 75).

63. Herxheimer H, Kost R, Wissing E. Investigations on the influence of massage, 3rd communication: The influence of massage on muscle activity and diuresis. *Zeitschrift für die gesamte physikalische Therapie* 1927;33:167–182.

64. De Aloysio D, Penachioni P. Morning sickness control in early pregnancy by neiguan point acupressure. *Obstetrics & Gynecology* 1992;80:852–854.

65. Ming J-L, Kuo BI-T, Lin J-G, et al. The efficacy of acupressure to prevent nausea and vomiting in post-operative patients. *J Adv Nurs* 2002;39:343–351.

66. Litscher G, Schwarz G, Sandner-Kiesling A. General effects of acupuncture on cerebral blood flow velocity and oxygenation of cerebral tissue. In: Litscher G, Zang HC, (eds.) *Computer-Controlled Acupuncture.* Lengerich: Pabst, 2000:11–24.

67. Wang Z-P. *Acupressure Therapy. Point Percussion of Cerebral Birth Injury, Brain Injury, and Stroke.* New York: Churchill Livingstone, 1991.

68. Müller B. Psychological approaches to the prevention and inhibition of nocturnal epileptic seizures: a meta-analysis of 70 case studies. *Seizure* 2001;10:13–33.

69. Frucht MM, Quigg M, Schwaner C, et al. Distribution of seizure precipitants among epilepsy syndromes. *Epilepsia* 2000; 41:1534-9.

70. Glover V, Onozawa K, Hodgkinson A. Benefits of infant massage for mothers with postnatal depression. *Semin Neonatol* 2002;7:495–500.

71. Westhoff S. *Massage: A Critical Analysis of Physiologic Effects and Clinical Effectiveness.* [In German.] Hannover: Diss Med, 1990. [German title: *Massage: eine kritische Analyse physiologischer Wirkungen und der klinischen Wirksamkeit.*]

72. Ernst E, Fialka V. The clinical effectiveness of massage therapy: a critical review. *Forsch Komplementärmed* 1994;1:226–232.

73. Blum JE. *Chinesische Medizin für Frauen.* Niedernhausen: Falken-Verlag; 1998. [Engl. original: *Woman Heal Thyself. An Ancient Healing System for Contemporary Women.* Boston: Tuttle, 1995.]

74. Bauer C. *Acupressure for Everybody: Gentle, Effective Relief for More Than 100 Common Ailments.* New York: Holt, 1991.

75. Wagner F. *Acupressure.* [In German.] München: Gräfe und Unzer, 1999. [German title: *Akupressur.*]

76. Schories C. *Shiatsu for an Untroubled Pregnancy.* [In German.] Stuttgart: Trias, 2000. [German title: *Shiatsu für eine unbeschwerte Schwangerschaft.*]

77. Pollmann N. *Basic Textbook Acupuncture.* [In German.] München: Urban & Fischer, 2002. [German title: *Basislehrbuch Akupunktur.*]

78. The Acupressure Institute, Berkeley, CA. See: http://www.acupressure.com/.

79. Saxe JF. Massaging clients with epilepsy. *Massage Therapy Journal* 1992;Fall:84–93.

80. Sinclair M. *Massage for Healthier Children.* Oakland: Wingbow, 1992.

81. Peebles CT, McAuley JW, Roach J, et al. Alternative medicine use by patients with epilepsy. *Epilepsy & Behavior* 2000;1:74–77.

82. Touch Research Institute. Hernandez-Reif M. Personal communication, 2002.

83. Müller B. Self-control—Can you stop your seizures from happening? Manuscript for lecture at the 4th European Epilepsy and Society Conference. Veldhoven, Holland, 1994 Sept;22–25.

84. Müller B. Behavioral approaches to seizure control in epilepsies. [In German.] Lecture series at Halle University. 2000 Dec 18; Halle, Germany. [German title: Verhaltensorientierte Ansätze der Anfallskontrolle bei Epilepsien.]

85. Müller B. Massage and seizure control. [In German.] Part 2 of the seminar "strategies of holistic epilepsy treatment" for families of the Epilepsy Association Lower Saxony; 2000 Oct 26-28; Falkenburg, Germany. [German title: *Massage und Anfallskontrolle.*]

86. Wolf P. Aura interruption: how does it become curative? In: Wolf P, (ed.) *Epileptic Seizures and Syndromes.* London: Libbey, 1994;667–673.

87. Pelletier KR, Marie A, Krasner M, et al. Current trends in the integration and reimbursement of complementary and alternative medicine by managed care, insurance carriers, and hospital providers. *Am J Health Promot* 1997;12:112–123.

88. http://www.amtamassage.org/findamassage/locator.htm and http://www.massagetoday.com/locator/

89. Lacroix N, Seager S. *Massage mit ätherischen Ölen.* Neuhausen: Urania, 1997. [Engl. original: *The Book of Aromatherapy and Massage.* London: Anness, Lorenz; 1994.]

90. Boyesen G. *Healing the Soul through the Body.* [In German.] München: Kösel, 1985. [German title: *Über den Körper die Seele heilen.*]

91. Petzold H, (ed.) *The New Body Therapies.* [In German.] Paderborn: Junfermann, 1977. [German title: *Die neuen Körpertherapien.*]

92. Mintz EE. On the rationale of touch in psychotherapy. In: Sager CJ, Kaplan HS, (eds.) *Progress in Group and Family Therapy.* New York: Brunner/Mazel, 1972:151–155.

93. Johari H. *Ancient Indian Massage: Traditional Massage Techniques Based on the Ayurveda.* New Delhi: Munshiram Manoharlal, 1984.

94. Cawley N. A critique of the methodology of research studies evaluating massage. *Eur J Cancer Care* 1997;6:23–31.

CHAPTER 9

Aromatherapy and Hypnosis

TIM BETTS, FRC PSYCH

Many patients with a genetic predisposition for epilepsy or electrically irritable lesions in the brain never have seizures. Good evidence suggests that first seizures in patients predisposed to epilepsy may occur during periods of stress or during significant life events. Once the epileptic process has been triggered, it may become self-perpetuating or, in some cases, seizures may continue to be induced by stressful circumstances.

For partial seizures (seizures originating in one brain location), the arousal state of that brain region may influence whether a seizure remains localized or spreads throughout the brain. For example, if the part of the brain surrounding a discharging focus is highly aroused (overactive), the seizure discharge is more likely to spread; an optimum level of arousal may occur that inhibits seizure spread for each individual with epilepsy (1).

Arousal can be modified and altered by life events, by stress, efforts of will and concentration, or by successfully learning to relax (2). Arousal responses can also be conditioned. Because arousal is involved in the initiation of epileptic activity and in its propagation, psychologic factors may be employed to minimize seizure spread or modify the epileptic process. This concept forms the basis of self-control techniques.

Self-control techniques for epilepsy have existed since Greco-Roman times. Despite the contemporary success of medication in controlling epilepsy, there is a developing interest in self-control techniques to complement standard medical therapies (1,3,4), both in adults and children.

Many different methods of self-control have been used, mostly involving recognizing and avoiding triggers to seizures; interposing a countermeasure when a seizure is felt to be oncoming; or, in situations where seizures are likely, by learning specific physical or psychologic mechanisms to stop them. The advantage of such methods is that people with epilepsy can take control of their own disorders. Patients who develop self awareness may be able to recognize seizure triggers or warning signs that a seizure is coming. These techniques, if successful, increase morale by giving patients some control over their epilepsy. This may be the most therapeutic factor of all.

In many of the published studies on self-control, it is difficult to determine exactly what method the person was using or what actually worked for the individual. General treatment effects may be involved, including becoming relaxed, losing the fear of seizures, cognitive changes, or a placebo effect. It does not matter to the individual how the technique works, as long as it works. When designing clinical studies on self-control techniques for epilepsy, it is often difficult to provide placebo-controlled conditions within the treatment package in order to identify which factor is really operating. Many case reports of successful behavioral treatment are of patients with unusual seizures. When reviewing the literature, the reader has to be certain that the person being treated did, in fact, have epilepsy, because nonepileptic seizures are usually of a psychologic nature and may also respond to psychologic therapy. It is possible, however, even in a single patient, to carry out a controlled study (3).

The Sense of Smell

Smell is our most primitive sense. Unlike sight, hearing, and touch, smell reception and interpretation are confined to the phylogenetically older limbic areas (5). Thus, we can only describe smell in a limited way (e.g., as pleasant or unpleasant, familiar or unfamiliar, like or unlike). We cannot describe its texture, shape, color, or rhythm, or interpret a smell as we can with sight or sound. The interpretation and reception of smell, however, occurs in those parts of the primitive brain, the limbic system, that are often the site of epileptic activity (6).

Smell is extremely important in the animal kingdom. It is used to assess the environment, pick up danger signals, and choose a mate. Although the sense of smell is not as important in humans, it remains extremely easily conditioned, often after only one trial. Such a conditioned odor memory is particularly resistant to deconditioning, and once formed, it is difficult to eradicate (7). Such a conditioned response to odor is learned best when associated with emotional experiences (8,9). Most of us know that certain odors, long forgotten, will provoke specific memories and emotions if re-encountered, often of childhood. Clear sexual differences emerge in studies of odor memory; women have more emotional and clearer odor memory than men. Women also tend to have more olfactory experiences than men (9).

Although hallucinations of smell are a common aura in human epilepsy, smell has rarely been used as a countermeasure against an oncoming seizure. In ancient medicine, physicians used unpleasant odors (such as burning hartshorn) to stop oncoming or actual seizures. This practice persisted into the Renaissance, even into Shakespeare's time (10) and was based on the idea that an unpleasant smell would drive the womb (which, in an epileptic seizure, was supposed to have wandered from its usual position into the throat) back to its normal resting place. Sometimes sweet-smelling substances were placed in the vagina to draw this errant organ back (how this technique was supposed to work in men is not clear). Even today, smelling salts are occasionally used to revive those who have fainted.

It is possible this ancient practice may have worked because smell reception often inhabits the same brain location where seizures often arise. In 1957, Efron (11) showed that an odor could be used as a conditioned countermeasure to a seizure, and could be accessed automatically without having to impose cognition (thinking) between the stimulus and the response. (This is possible because of the lack of higher brain input into the development of a smell memory.) Efron showed that within a comparatively short time of using a pleasant olfactory stimulus (jasmine) to stop a seizure, smell memory takes over. His patient no longer had to smell the jasmine oil to be able to stop a seizure, but could use just the memory of the smell. Despite interest in Efron's paper, olfactory inhibition of epileptic activity has not been employed extensively.

Definition

Aromatherapy as it is currently practiced is comparatively new, although it is rooted in older practices of massage and herbal treatments that date back to medieval times (12,13).

In the United Kingdom, the current practice of aromatherapy is largely undertaken outside the medical profession, although in France many practitioners are medically qualified. This difference may be explained by the way that the technique is used in the two countries. In the United Kingdom, the techniques used in aromatherapy are largely those of inhalation and massage; in France, aromatherapy oils are often used as external or internal medicines.

Aromatherapists use diluted aromatic oils derived by various means from various plant species. The characteristics of these oils may be markedly different, even in closely related species and even in the same species grown by different agricultural practices or in different settings. Aromatherapists try to use pure oils so that their constituents remain as constant as possible and, therefore, have predictable properties. These pure oils contain a mixture of various plant-derived compounds, many of which have a pharmacologic effect. Aromatic substances have a direct effect on the smell receptors at the end of the olfactory nerve (the first cranial nerve) at the top of the nose. This nerve sends impulses to the primitive part of the brain that receives smell. Aromatic substances are also fat soluble, and a massage with a diluted aromatic oil means that some of the active constituents of the oil will penetrate the skin easily and get into the blood stream without first being metabolized by the liver (which would break them down).

Thus, it is possible that some of these active constituents, in small amounts, may go straight to the brain. In conventional aromatherapy massage, therefore, the recipient may receive pharmacologically active compounds through the skin *and* smell the oil, which along with the massage may also be part of the therapeutic process. The oils can also be diluted in a bath or the aroma diffused into the air by a burner.

Most of the oils that aromatherapists use are relaxing and enhance feelings of well-being. A few arouse and alert (or they are said to). Some have other properties, such as diuretic action (increasing urination) or smooth muscle relaxation (potentially lowering blood pressure). In the United Kingdom, aromatherapy is mainly used for relieving tension, stress, and anxiety, and enhancing well-being. Most of the oils that aromatherapists use are safe for people with epilepsy. A few that contain a large amount of camphor, a convulsant agent, are not (see Table 9.1). One problem in recognizing whether an oil is potentially toxic is that the published information about toxicity is often not about the oil but about the plant from which the oil is derived, and, therefore, it applies only to the compound taken by mouth. Massage with small amounts of the oil, or just inhaling the fumes of the oil from a burner, is probably much safer than taking a compound by mouth (although some oils are skin irritants and must be used carefully). Trained aromatherapists know the properties of the oils they use.

TABLE 9.1

Helpful and Harmful Oils

Helpful Oils	Oils To Be Avoided
Jasmine	Rosemary
Ylang ylang	Hyssop
Lavender	Sweet fennel
Camomile	Sage
Bergamot	

Commentary

Aromatherapy with or without massage is gaining popularity in the medical community and with the public in general. Several small medical studies report benefits of aromatherapy for disorders such as anxiety in patients with brain tumors (1), pain reductions in the terminally ill (2), and even for itching associated with dialysis (3). One small double-blind, placebo-controlled study exists on the use of aromatherapy to reduce agitation in patients with dementia (4). A 35% reduction in agitated behavior was achieved using aromatherapy, while only 11% of the placebo-treated group responded. The common thread in all these studies is the use of aromatherapy to induce calm and help manage stress. Although no well controlled studies exist on the use of aromatherapy in patients with epilepsy, stress reduction is now a well-accepted strategy to reduce seizure frequency (5). Aromatherapy may be one means to accomplish this.

The olfactory system is an evolutionary old system of the brain that is highly developed in many lower animals. In humans, it has rich connections to both the memory and emotional systems of the brain within the frontal and temporal lobes. It is not difficult to imagine that the activation of the olfactory brain regions may influence function or dysfunction (as in the case of seizures) of these closely related brain regions. The authors point out that in rare cases, sensory stimuli may induce seizures. This phenomenon, known as "reflex epilepsy," may occur in different brain regions. For example, patients with a lesion in the parietal lobe (sensory cortex) hand region may have seizures when the hand that is served by that cortex is touched or stimulated. Although aromatherapy could give rise to reflex seizures, especially in patients whose seizures arise near the olfactory cortex, this is highly unlikely for the vast majority.

The author's use of hypnosis with aromatherapy is a unique approach to seizure reduction. Studies of hypnosis and epilepsy have been directed mainly at diagnosing nonepileptic or psychogenic seizure disorders. The safety of hypnosis for patients with epilepsy has not been well studied, but in the manner in which it is used by the authors, it would not seem all that different from many biofeedback protocols (see Chapter 7, Autogenic Training) and, therefore, it is unlikely to be of substantial risk.

The authors present very encouraging, albeit anecdotal, data, showing the benefits of aromatherapy in selected patients with seizures uncontrolled by conventional means. A randomized well-controlled study of this seemingly benign and even pleasant therapy could help physicians encourage the use of aromatherapy by their patients.

References

1. Hadfield N. The role of aromatherapy massage in reducing anxiety in patients with malignant brain tumors. *Int J Palliat Nurs* 2001;7(6):279–285.
2. Louis M, Kowalski SD. Use of aromatherapy with hospice patients to decrease pain, anxiety, and depression to promote an increased sense of well-being. *Am J Hosp Palliat Care* 2002;19(6):381–386.
3. Ro YJ, Ha HC, Kim CG, et al. The effects of aromatherapy on pruritus in patients undergoing hemodialysis. *Dermatol Nurs* 2002;14(4):231–234, 237–238, 256; quiz 239.
4. Ballard CG, O'Brien JT, Reichelt K, et al. Aromatherapy as a safe and effective treatment for the management of agitation in severe dementia: the results of a double-blind, placebo-controlled trial with Melissa. *J Clin Psychiatry* 2002;63(7): 553–558.
5. Wolf P. The role of nonpharmaceutic conservatic interventions in the treatment and secondary prevention of epilepsy. *Epilepsia* 2002;43(suppl 9):2–5.

Aromatherapy in Epilepsy

Interest in aromatherapy in the United Kingdom for people with epilepsy began in the Birmingham University Seizure Clinic several years ago when one of our team members was training in aromatherapy. As part of her training, she asked to try the technique on some of our patients with chronic epilepsy. The literature at that time was confused about whether aromatherapy could help people with epilepsy. Indeed, some aromatherapy authorities warned against the use of aromatherapy in epilepsy. We suspect this was related to the fear that a patient might have a seizure during a massage.

Ten patients with chronic intractable complex partial seizures, with or without secondary generalization (seizure spreading throughout the brain), agreed to take part in the study and received, during 1 month, two aromatherapy full-body massages lasting 1 hour. Most aromatherapists use a blend or mixture of different oils (diluted in a carrier oil) for massage, but we used massage with only one oil, chosen by the recipient from a variety of oils. We have continued with this monotherapy since the study.

During the treatment period itself and for about 1 month afterward, a marked reduction in seizure frequency occurred in nine of the 10 patients, although after 6 months, seizure frequency had returned to its previous baseline in all but one patient (see Table 9.2). In this patient, seizures stopped and did not return until several years later. Epilepsy is a condition that may wax and wane in frequency, so this may have been coincidence, although the patient was impressed enough to train in aromatherapy. One of the patients had an increase in seizures during the treatment period. This patient chose rosemary as the massage oil. It is a pleasant oil, but it does contain camphor.

TABLE 9.2

First Experiment Using Aromatherapy; 10 Patients with Partial Onset Epilepsy

Mean seizure frequency (range)

Month Before Treatment	During Treatment Month	Month After Treatment	Six Months After Treatment
7 (3-12)	2 (0-27)	3 (0-18)	6 (0-13)
Oils chosen	Ylang ylang (6)	Lavender (1)	Camomile (1)
	Rosemary (1)*	Rose geranium (1)	

*Seizure increase

This group of patients appeared to have definite but transient seizure reduction related to the aromatherapy treatments, but the mechanism remains uncertain. Was it the pharmacologic effect of the oils? (Several different oils were used.) Most likely it was a transient decrease in arousal or tension induced by the treatment. Reduction in stress can reduce seizure frequency (2). It could have been a placebo or general treatment effect (patients do not normally expect to go to a hospital and have a pleasant massage for an hour from someone who also talks and listens to them). Traditional aromatherapists would suggest that the aroma might have caused the seizure reduction and that patients intuitively know which oil will help them best.

Although the results of this preliminary study were promising, there were drawbacks to using aromatherapy in a clinical setting. It is difficult to provide an uninterrupted session for an hour in a quiet place. Massage is labor intensive, some oils are expensive, and employing an aromatherapist is also expensive. Could we simplify the technique so that more patients could use it? Could we encourage the initial beneficial effect to continue? Having read Efron's paper (11), we wondered whether the aroma of the oil could be used as a countermeasure and create a conditioned response against an oncoming seizure.

Although we have not been able to do a proper scientific study, we have audited our empirical experience to draw conclusions. We present here the results from 100 patients, followed up for at least 1 year after their initial treatment. These patients were treated in a variety of ways using aromatherapy. Different methods were developed to meet the particular needs of an individual patient and to help identify the best way of using aromatherapy. We attempted to measure whether it worked and by what means.

Initially, patients whom we thought suitable were asked to keep a diary for 2 to 3 months, recording not only seizures, but also triggers, seizure-related life events, and seizure-related feelings and emotions (pre- and post-seizure), because it is important to record something about the events that surround seizures. For many of these patients, over time, the documentation allowed them to identify reliable triggers or prodromes for seizures. In this way, patients could reliably recognize an oncoming seizure (or a situation in which one was likely to occur) in sufficient time to impose a blocking countermeasure. This is the kind of approach used by any therapist trying to teach patients a behavioral method for managing a seizure.

Rosalind MacCullum at our center previously showed that the instinctive reaction of most people with epilepsy to an oncoming seizure is to *increase* arousal (by concentrating hard on something else, for instance). This may not be the most effective strategy because it is difficult to keep arousal up. We now teach patients to *decrease* arousal. Sometimes this means going against their own instinctive reaction, but unless people are taught how, they usually cannot relax quickly. (If you say "relax" to the average person, he immediately tenses up.) Experience has taught us that we should teach people to relax, rather than increase arousal before an oncoming seizure.

We offer patients a range of relaxing aromatic oils to smell and invite them to choose an oil they particularly like. Not all patients like the same oil. Memory associations are important. (If you associate lavender with your favorite granny who was always nice to you and gave you sweets, you will have a positive response to its smell. But, instead, if you associate the smell of lavender with your other granny who was never nice, you will have a negative response.) People with epilepsy probably do not have the same kind of smell experiences as people who do not have epilepsy; smell appreciation and sensitivity possibly wax and wane with the nearness of a seizure. As we gained more experience, we offered an expanding range of oils. Some of the oils many of our patients find most useful, such as jasmine, are extremely expensive.

Patients were treated in various ways due to the availability of staff and premises and other factors. Some patients mainly had a series of massages with their chosen oil, but sometimes it was not possible because of the lack of someone who was trained, lack of available premises, or by the patient's own choice. (In the United Kingdom, massage has a somewhat negative connotation for many people, related to dubious goings on in "massage parlors.") Some do not perceive massage as a useful medical technique, or they are too body conscious to contemplate receiving it. We only treat someone who is comfortable with it.

Because we thought early on about using the smell of the oil as a countermeasure, some of our patients were not treated with massage using oil, but rather with an autohypnotic conditioning technique to help them associate the smell of the oil with swift relaxation. Some received both this conditioning process and massage.

Hypnosis Combined with Aromatherapy

Many patients with epilepsy are warned against hypnosis. One problem is that it has become associated by many with entertainment. Say to the average person, "I am going hypnotize you," and she will step back in alarm because of the fear of being taken over or losing control (a fear well known to anyone with epilepsy). One or two isolated case reports document people with epilepsy who have had seizures precipitated by a hypnotic technique, and there was one case in the United Kingdom of hypnosis possibly precipitating sudden death in an individual with epilepsy.

We consider hypnosis safe for people with epilepsy if a trained hypnotist is doing the hypnotic induction. The hypnotist must *not* remind the patient, while he is under the influence of hypnosis, of situations that might induce a seizure or induce a state of mind the patient associates with seizures. The "waking up" procedure should be carried out slowly so that the patient does not have a sudden change in arousal. It is sometimes said that people with epilepsy cannot be hypnotized, but in our experience, they are no more difficult, nor more easy, to hypnotize than anyone else.

Hypnosis is not fully understood but appears to be a high-arousal state. The hypnotic state requires an effort of intense concentration, and some studies suggest a degree of high arousal in the electroencephalographs (EEGs) of people being hypnotized. If patients have been taught to concentrate, either on a bodily sensation, a body part, or some external object, they pass into a state of dissociation and suggestibility (although they are completely aware of what is happening to them and retain control). If the state of dissociation and suggestibility is deep enough (it varies from person to person and from time to time), patients may be able to accept suggestions about their future behavior and later automatically act on them (posthypnotic suggestion). In people with epilepsy, who often take neurotoxic medication, the normal method of hypnotic induction (eye fixation) is often difficult because the patient's eyes wobble too much under the influence of medication. For people with epilepsy, we normally use the hand elevation method. The patient concentrates on one hand (we choose the hand opposite the side where the epileptic lesion is if she has partial epilepsy). The patient can lighten the hand by concentrating on it, and it will eventually rise from a resting position. This almost invariably works and begins to teach patients about forces in their brain that they may be able to mobilize.

After initial instruction, the patient practices at home and may use the technique without much more therapist intervention. When this occurs, and the patient can achieve the hypnotic state quickly and feel relaxed in it, a posthypnotic suggestion is given by getting the patient to smell the chosen oil and by suggesting an association between the state of relaxation and the smell of the oil. When this association has firmly developed, the patient carries a small bottle of the oil (or a handkerchief impregnated with it) around and practices gently inhaling the oil to induce relaxation. When this seems to work (observation of patients during the inhalation usually shows a characteristic sudden loss of facial tension), then patients begin to use the technique in situations where seizures are likely, if they feel that a seizure is coming on, or in situations during which they are especially concerned about having a seizure.

Patients who do well with this technique eventually use the *memory* of the aroma, rather than carrying the bottle around with them. This seems to create a specific smell memory that has a behavioral effect.

Results

One hundred patients were followed up for at least 1 year who had either a series of massages with their chosen oil, a series of massages plus the autohypnotic technique, or the autohypnotic technique without massage. We emphasize that this was not a formal trial. Patients were not randomly allocated to these three groups, but were allocated for other reasons, including some people who chose not to be hypnotized because of fear and some who wished to avoid massage.

The results (see Table 9.3) are impressive for a group of patients with chronic epilepsy who had not responded to conventional medication. These were patients, however, who had volunteered to be included, or whom we believed would benefit from the treatment. Therefore, we may be seeing the best results anyone could achieve with this method.

TABLE 9.3

First 100 Patients Followed for a Year after Treatment (In Percent)

	Hypnosis Only**	Massage with Oil Only	Massage with Oil Plus Hypnosis **
	(n=25)	(n=46)*	(n=29)
Seizure-free	12	35	38
At least 50% reduction	36	30	31
No or transient effect	48	31	25
Worse	4	4	6

*Many in this group spontaneously learned to use the aroma as a countermeasure.
**Autohypnotic conditioning technique to help patients associate the smell of the oil with swift relaxation.

Although there was no difference between the group that only had massage with oil and the group that had massage plus hypnotherapy, there was less improvement in the group that only had hypnotherapy. Several reasons may explain this, particularly because the groups that accepted massage may not have the same psychological make-up as the group that chose not to be massaged. The apparent difference between the massage-only group and the group that had massage and hypnosis may be explained in that some of the massage-only group developed their own association between the smell and the ability to relax quickly. Spontaneously and without the use of hypnosis, some patients may have used the aroma as a countermeasure to stop an oncoming seizure.

Not everyone undergoing this treatment finds it successful. Some, as Table 9.3 shows, have a transient effect that disappears quickly. This is possibly a placebo or general treatment effect, or possibly reluctance to practice. Some patients do not respond at all. As with any treatment, a few patients seemed to have an increase in seizures after a course of massage or hypnosis. This was caused inadvertently in two patients by getting them to associate the smell of the oil with having a seizure, rather than not having one. Luckily, neither of these patients were inhaling an oil whose aroma they might encounter elsewhere, and so this conditioned response disappeared quickly. But these two patients illustrate the importance of not entering into any treatment such as this lightly without due consideration; it must be undertaken with a therapist who can carefully monitor the effects. During the time that we have offered this treatment, apart from one patient having a simple partial seizure while on the massage couch, no patient has had a seizure during massage.

Possible Benefits

Aromatherapy may be useful to those who can recognize lengthy auras during seizures, or who have recognizable prodromes or triggers to their seizures. One of the advantages of the smell memory technique is that it does not require a great amount of cognition to use. Thus, even if people are slightly confused during an aura, they may still be able to interpose their aroma. We have found that patients with olfactory or taste auras find aromatherapy a particularly useful countermeasure.

Aromatherapy may be useful as a temporary adjunctive measure in people going through a stressful time in their lives, with a consequent increase in seizure frequency. It may also be useful in people with epilepsy who have sleep-related seizures. Finally, aromatherapy promotes more restful sleep. The case histories in the appendix to this chapter illustrate these uses.

Precautions

Aromatherapy is a complementary rather than an alternative therapy, and we encourage our patients to continue to take their medication. People with epilepsy who wish to try aromatherapy and hypnosis should:
- Always consult a professional
- Always tell their medical adviser what they are doing
- Avoid camphor-containing oils
- Never ingest the oils
- Avoid associating the aroma with *having* a seizure
- Use an oil they like that does not remind them of seizure situations

- Remember that the technique takes time and patience, and may not work for everyone

Further Information

International Federation of Aromatherapists
182 Chiswick High Road
London
W4 1PP
UK
www.ifaroma.org

American Aromatherapy Association
P.O. Box 1222
Fair Oaks, CA 95628
(916) 965-7546

Case Histories

Jane, Age 24 Years

During birth, Jane had a small hemorrhage into the part of the brain that controls the right side of her body. This left a scar that later became a small cyst. At age 14, she began to experience episodes of a warm feeling in her right hand. Several years later, while taking important school examinations, the warm feeling was followed by uncontrollable jerking and twitching of her right thumb and then her hand.

Further seizures followed; the jerking began to spread so that her entire arm was involved. Occasionally, the seizures were so severe that her leg would become involved and, on occasion, the twitching seemed to spread to her left hand and arm. During the attacks, she remained conscious and aware that she was out of control, which frightened her.

Her seizures had been treated with various anticonvulsants that either gave her a headache, made her gain weight, or made her feel drowsy. They also failed to control her seizures. Jane found that if she made her right hand into a tight fist as soon as she got the warm feeling, the attack would not progress. To keep the attack at bay, she had to grip something or keep making a fist. It was tiring to keep this up, and as soon as she let go, the seizure would resume.

A diary of Jane's attacks showed they were more common when she was stressed, partly because she feared the social consequences of the attacks and was embarrassed by them. She volunteered to try the aromatherapy technique.

Jane chose lavender oil and had some massages using it. She found them relaxing and noted in her diary that she never had a seizure within a few days of her massage. She learned the autohypnosis technique and had a hypnosis session at the end of each massage. Later, she accepted a posthypnotic suggestion that when she smelled lavender she would relax; she practiced this herself several times each week. When she felt the hot feeling develop in her hand, she immediately took out a handkerchief soaked with a few drops of lavender and gently inhaled the fragrance. *Gentle inhalation is important; drawing cold air rapidly through the nose may increase seizure activity* (15). Jane found that as soon as she inhaled the aroma of lavender, the warm feeling left and she felt "in control." Later, she did not have to use a handkerchief to inhale the aromatherapy oil. She merely had to think of the smell of lavender and the seizure stopped. In situations where she previously believed she might have a seizure, she now felt confident and in control.

She has been seizure-free for 5 years and no longer practices the technique, except on rare occasions. She stopped taking medication before she had her first child and has not resumed it.

Glynis, Age 30 Years

Glynis has juvenile myoclonic epilepsy with seizures that began in her early adolescence, including early-morning myoclonic jerks followed by tonic-clonic seizures. She was treated with sodium valproate. The jerks and seizures were well controlled, and she became a nurse. Some years later, while taking the same dosage of medication, she began to suffer early morning jerks again, especially if she worked a late shift followed by an early shift. Later, unfortunately, her tonic-clonic seizures returned and continued despite an increase in medication. Her nursing career was suspended. Further increases in her dosage of sodium valproate led to a marked increase in weight. She requested the chance to be included in our aromatherapy program.

It was clear from her diary that the early-morning jerking movements were related to improper sleep. If she then had to get up early in the morning to go to an early shift, she would begin to have myoclonic jerks. Perusal of her diary also revealed that although Glynis had no warning that a tonic-clonic seizure was coming, she could recognize the seizures were related to a particular frame of mind and emotion—often anger that occurred because of her stormy relationship with her boyfriend.

Glynis chose camomile as her oil, had some massages with it, learned the autohypnotic technique, and used the smell of the oil on a handkerchief whenever she was alone with her boyfriend and an argument seemed imminent, or when she noticed she was getting angry. Since learning the technique, Glynis has not had a daytime tonic-clonic seizure.

She returned to work and was encouraged to put a drop of the oil on her pillow when she went to sleep after a late shift. If she did this, she fell asleep instantly, awoke feeling refreshed in the morning, and no longer had the jerking movements. She was able to cut the amount of sodium valproate in half without an increase in seizures. She continued to use the technique if she had a hectic evening before going to bed.

Acknowledgment

This paper describes the development of a technique over many years by a group of helpful and enthusiastic students, professionals, and patients. We in particular thank Rosalind McCullum, Cathy Fox, Victoria Jackson, Eleanor Brown, Lynn Howes, and Caroline Burrow.

References

1. Fenwick P. Evocation and inhibition of seizures. In: Smith DB, Treiman D, Trimble M, (eds.) *Neurobehavioural Problems in Epilepsy: Advances in Neurology*. New York: Raven Press, 1991;Vol 55:163–183.

2. Betts T. Epilepsy and stress. *BMJ* 1992;305:378–379.

3. Dahl J. *A Behaviour Medicine Approach to Assessment and Treatment of Epilepsy in Children*. Seattle: Hogrefe and Huber, 1992.

4. Betts T. Neuropsychiatry. In: Laidlaw J, Richens A, Oxley J, (eds.) *A Textbook of Epilepsy*. Edinburgh: Churchill Livingstone, 1993:445–448.

5. Van Toller S. The brain and the sense of smell. In: Van Toller S, Dodd GH, (eds.) *Fragrance: the Psychology and Biology of Perfume*. London: Elsevier, 1992.

6. Carroll B, Richardson J, Thompson P. Olfactory information processing and temporal lobe epilepsy. *Brain Cogn* 1993;22:230–243.

7. Kirk-Smith M, Van Toller C, Dodd G. Unconscious odor conditioning in human subjects. *Biol Psychiatry* 1983;17:221–231.

8. Engen T, Ross B. Long-term memory of odours. *J Exp Psychol* 1973;100:221–227.

9. Hertz R, Cupchick C. An experimental characterisation of odour evoked memories in humans. *Chem Senses* 1992;17:519–528.

10. Betts T, Betts H. John Hall and his epileptic patients—epilepsy management in early 17th century England. *Seizure* 1998;7:411–414.

11. Efron R. The conditioned inhibition of uncinate fits. *Brain* 1957;80:251–261.

12. Davis P. *Aromatherapy: An A—Z*. Saffron Walden, UK: C.W. Daniel, 1999.

13. Price S. *Aromatherapy for health professionals*. Edinburgh: Churchill Livingstone, 1999.

14. Hirsch A. Aromatherapy: art, science or myth? In: Weintraub MI, (ed.) *Alternative and Complementary Treatment in Neurologic Illness*. New York: Churchill Livingstone, 2001:128–150.

15. Komarek V. Olfactory activation in epilepsy. In: Wolf P, (ed.) *Epileptic Seizures and Syndromes*. London: J. Libbey, 1994:107–114.

CHAPTER 10

Meditation

K. K. DEEPAK, MD, PHD

For thousands of years, philosophers have believed humans can attain "higher" states of consciousness through meditative techniques. Meditation is a form of religious or spiritual contemplation; it forms the basis of most Eastern religions, including Hinduism, Buddhism, and Taoism. It is comparable to prayer in the Christian, Islamic, and Jewish traditions. The difference between prayer and Eastern meditation is that prayer is a petition to, or dialogue with God; meditation is a detached observation of one's own mind and its processes. The word *meditation* is derived from the Latin *meditari*, meaning "contemplate." In the Indian context, the appropriate Sanskrit word is *dhyāna* (concentrated meditation). This became *Chan* in China, and *Zen* in Japan (1).

Meditation techniques developed extensively in the East and became a major element in religion, with a tendency to make them a way of life for maintaining physical, mental, and spiritual well-being. In the Western world, however, the practice of various meditative techniques—which were thought to bring forth a relaxation response—was limited primarily to religious traditions. Many Christian writers, including St. Augustine and Martin Luther, wrote descriptions of prayers, often called *contemplative exercises*. The meditation exercises of *Merkabolism* (an early form of mysticism in Judaism) included placing one's head between one's knees, whispering hymns, and repeating the name of a magic emblem.

Indian meditation (dhyāna) is an integral part of the Indian system known as *yoga*. Perhaps yoga and Ayurveda were practiced jointly in the beginning, but as time passed, the two became separate. The goal of yoga is to achieve a state of peacefulness, integration, and spiritual health. The aim of Ayurveda is to regain health after illness. Many different paths of yoga have emerged, but their aim remains the same. Among these paths, hatha yoga (the science of *asanas*: body postures, combined with *pranayam*: breathing techniques) has been widely studied by medical scientists. The best description of yoga is in the writings of Saga Patanjali, who describes eight steps to "superconsciousness." Meditation occupies the seventh step and is a requisite for further spiritual growth (Figure 10.1).

Meditation is an induced mental process that manipulates attention. Through modifying attention, a state of inattention (nonanalytic attending) can be achieved. The process may use passive attending to a featureless stimulus or may actively manipulate

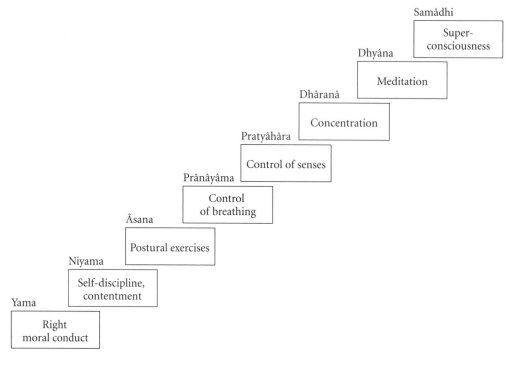

FIGURE 10.1

Eight steps of yoga. These steps are designed to achieve physical and mental control and are essential for attaining superconsciousness. The practitioner, however, may derive physiologic and psychologic benefits from following even some of the steps.

thoughts so they are not processed by the mind. Such a state of "loss of active attention" results in various psychosomatic manifestations. These effects may be beneficial. Such a definition, although limited, is adequate with reference to medical sciences for the purpose of physiologic intervention in illness.

People with religious inclinations may not agree with this narrow definition; they believe that meditation is a process that can lead to an unmeasureable superconsciousness. This limited definition is useful in a practical sense, however. It gives us the possibility of measurement at both ends: at the induction process and at the response level. Medical science can use such a limited procedure for interventional purposes in various illnesses. Such an intervention may be called the physiologic intervention of disease.

Different Types of Meditation

Many types and subtypes of meditation are possible, usually depending on the mode of induction. The author knows of no types of meditation that are defined on the basis of induced responses. Sometimes researchers define the depth of meditation on the basis of physiologic responses.

Meditation may be induced by a variety of techniques, most of which involve body immobility and repetitious mental exercises. Sometimes the exercises are based on mantras, the private repetition of a single word or phrase. Some involve inward concentration on the stream of consciousness and enhanced awareness of bodily sensation (2). Yogic meditation often involves concentration on a single point to exclude all thoughts associated with everyday life (3).

Naranjo and Ornstein (4) divided meditative techniques into two types, depending on whether the technique involves an active or passive form of concentration. This active-passive distinction is similar to the distinction in attention. In active concentration, mental effort directs the focus of attention. In passive concentration, the attention is left free to be guided by some focal object, the act of breathing, or a mantra, which is used as a point of departure (5). The mantra can be a Sanskrit word that is easy to articulate but which may have no specific meaning to the user.

Word Repetition: Meditation Using a Mantra

The most common Indian method of meditation is word repetition: the subject (i) adopts a comfortable posture; (ii) visualizes his breathing; and (iii) concentrates on repetition (silently or audibly) of a word, object, stimulus, body part, or activity. Some meditators may bypass visualization of the breath; others may visualize it throughout meditation. Often, respiratory rhythm is coupled with silent word recall. Combination and modification of these three variables determine the kind of meditation practiced.

Yoga

Yoga is a technique that often places more emphasis on the physical aspects of achieving an altered state of consciousness. Essential to this form of yoga is the adoption of an appropriate physical posture that can enhance concentration and the regulation of word repetition (6).

Buddhist Meditation

Buddhist meditation is widely practiced in Asia. One of the meditation practices of Zen Buddhism, known as *Zazen*, uses the yogic technique of coupling respiration with counting (one on inhaling, two on exhaling, and so forth). As time passes, the meditator stops counting and simply "follows the breath" in order to achieve a state of no thought, no feeling, and of complete nothingness (7,8). Many other Eastern practices, including Shintoism, Taoism, and Sufism (an Islamic mystical tradition), include similar experiences.

Vipassana Meditation

Another variant of the Buddhist tradition is *Vipassana* (mindfulness meditation), which attempts to fill the mind with several streams of thought simultaneously, focusing on everything present in the surroundings. A common technique in mindfulness meditation is the body scan, moving one's focus through the body, usually while lying down. Focusing may be comprehensive and include, for example, body parts, pain, street sounds, and other noises.

Transcendental Meditation

According to Transcendental Meditation™, which is a form of passive mantra meditation popularized by Maharishi Mahesh Yogi (9), meditators return their attention to the mantra whenever they become aware that their attention has wandered, but they do not use mental effort to maintain the mantra in conscious awareness. The result of *trying* to think of the mantra without expending effort is that TM™ meditators become increasingly aware of the effort exerted in producing thought. Wallace (9) defines TM™ as "turning attention inwards, towards subtler levels of a thought until mind transcends experience of the subtler state of the thought and arrives at the source of thought." TM™ and Buddhist meditation are common in the West because they have a minimum religious connotation.

Meditation on the Breath

At times, meditation techniques use concentration on respiration to induce and maintain the meditative state. The individual focuses her attention on the process of inhalation and exhalation passively. Some call this *breath meditation.*

Tai Chi Chuan: Moving Meditation

Tai Chi Chuan, commonly known as *moving meditation,* is a type of meditation wherein practitioners perform continuous, soft, smooth, effortless, and natural movements. Their stance always remains firmly grounded on the earth. They nonanalytically attend to the unifying sequence of movements, focusing thoughts on a series of movements in continuity. This leads to a meditative state. The participant is performing aerobic movement and that long practice renders these movements effortless. This also induces the relaxation response, but with intermittent bouts of strong contractions. The total energy required for meditation practice is less than that required in a normal state.

Effects of Meditation

In an elegant study, Telles and colleagues (10) proved a similar point by studying the effectiveness of yoga relaxation techniques. They compared oxygen consumption with respiratory and heart rates during cyclic activation by using a yoga posture alternating with *Shavasana* (the "corpse" posture), and by using Shavasana alone. To their surprise, they found more reduction in oxygen consumption during cyclic activation than during the lying down posture.

Throughout history, many similar techniques or practices have been used to achieve an altered state of consciousness. The recently documented physiologic effects of these various practices reflect the commonality of the experiences and of the relaxation response. Beary and Benson (11) point out four common elements integral to these varied practices that are necessary to evoke the relaxation response:

- Quiet environment
- Decreased muscle tone
- A mental device (a sound, word, or phrase)
- Passive attitude

Incorporating these four elements, Beary and Benson (11) developed a simple, nonreligious meditative technique:

- Sit quietly in a comfortable position and close your eyes.
- Deeply relax all your muscles, beginning at your feet and progressing up to your face.
- Breathe through your nose. Become aware of your breathing. As you breathe out, say the word one silently to yourself.
- Do not worry about whether you are successful in achieving a deep level of relaxation. Maintain a passive attitude and permit relaxation to occur at its own pace. Practice the technique once or twice daily, but not within 2 hours of a meal, because the digestive processes seem to interfere with subjective changes.

A calm and peaceful atmosphere, in conjunction with the active process by the subject, initiates meditation. Thus, holding the attention steady and ignoring events and stimulus in the environment induces tranquillity during meditation. After some time, the conditioning may take place with some nonspecific stimuli, thus facilitating subsequent meditation. Meditation can facilitate further meditation, once conditioning takes place.

Most meditation techniques, but not all, include an attempt to silence worldly thoughts and attain a state in which the mind of the meditator is focused on a single thought—or no thought at all: a state of thoughtlessness. All the different types of meditation techniques can lead to physical relaxation and mental serenity.

Physiologic Responses of Meditation

Autonomic Functions

During yogic meditation, Zen, or TM™, various physiologic experiences accompany physiologic changes (9,12–18). On two occasions, Anand (12) studied an expert yogi performing control over autonomic functions through meditation inside an airtight box—first for 8 hours and then for 10 hours. During his stay in the box, oxygen consumption and carbon dioxide output, heart rate, respiration, and body temperature were recorded,

Commentary

Dr. Deepak has written a detailed chapter on the theory and practice of meditation, as related to yoga (see Chapter 11 by Dr. Pacia). Dr. Deepak outlines the types of meditation and describes the effects of meditation on bodily functions and brain waves. He then describes a study of meditation and epilepsy that was performed in India. The results showed that patients with epilepsy who practiced meditation had a marked reduction in seizure frequency compared with patients randomized to a control group. Considering that the potential side effects of meditation are minor, and that meditation may have other general health benefits, these results are encouraging and suggest the need for further research.

One would expect that meditation would be particularly beneficial (in addition to medical therapy) for people with epilepsy who have high stress levels, are anxious, or who feel overwhelmed. People who are interested in learning to meditate should look for an instructor who is knowledgeable about epilepsy and understands what to do in the event of a seizure.

and electroencephalograms (EEGs) were taken. The yogi's average oxygen consumption dropped to about 13.3 liters per hour from a base of 19.5. His carbon dioxide output diminished proportionally. In spite of the decrease in oxygen content and increase in carbon dioxide content, the yogi did not show hyperpnea or tachycardia. The EEG results primarily showed low-voltage fast activity resembling the early stages of sleep.

Objective data support the theory that relaxation results in physiologic changes thought to characterize integrated hypothalamic function (19). Meditative practices bring about the relaxation response, as suggested by Benson (20). These physiologic changes are consistent with a generalized decrease in sympathetic nervous system activity. Uniform and significant decreases have been observed in oxygen consumption and carbon dioxide elimination with no change in respiratory quotient. In addition, heart and respiratory rates simultaneously decrease, and a marked decrease in arterial blood lactate concentration occurs. Blood flow to the muscles stabilizes (21). The physiologic changes of the relaxation response are distinctly different from those observed during quiet sitting or sleep state; they characterize a wakeful hypometabolic state that uses less energy.

An important feature of these changes in sympathetic reactivity is their carry-over effect, lasting longer than the actual period during which the mental relaxation response exercise is performed.

EEG Studies

Alpha brain waves, as recorded by EEG, represent an awake, relaxed state of unfocused attention; beta waves represent alert concentration; delta waves (the slowest) are the waves of deep sleep; theta waves occur during drowsiness.

Okuma (22) saw that the alpha waves of Zen practitioners increased remarkably with the progress of their meditation, even if their eyes were open. From EEG mapping during Zen practice, Matsuoka (15) reported specific findings. EEG changes could be classified into four states: the appearance of alpha waves, an increase of alpha amplitudes with wide distribution, a decrease of alpha waves, and the short-lived appearance of theta waves. These findings possibly indicate specific changes of consciousness.

Something more complex and more central than simple relaxation happens during meditation (23–25). The possible central mechanisms could be a cognitive manipulation of neural mechanisms. The reasons for the existence of the two central mechanisms appear to be emanating from the instructions given for induction of meditation and the subjective responses reported by long-term practitioners. In reality, meditation may use some complex mechanisms to induce the effect quickly and with more depth.

Psychophysiologic Changes during Meditation

The mental component of meditation is a mind that is concentrated, at attention, and essentially blank of distracting or disturbing thoughts. Both the physiologic and mental relaxation produced by meditation helps manifest positive change (20).

Most of the techniques used for meditation center on the concept that meditation works to gain control over the subject's attentional process. Gaining mastery over attention is difficult because of the natural tendency to constantly shift from one point of focus to another. Thus, continuous demand on attention and concentration is a prerequisite for the induction of meditation.

Van Nuys (26) measured attention in meditation and hypnotizability. He concluded that only attention measures of the meditation correlated with hypnotizability. The results also suggested that good concentration is a necessary condition for hypnotizability. Thus, it may be logically deduced that the capacity to concentrate—or the level of concentration achieved—positively correlates with better performance during meditation.

Meditation as an Intervention in Epilepsy

Numerous research papers advocate meditation to improve a variety of cardiovascular and psychologic illnesses. Stress-related disorders have been the chief target for meditation.

Epilepsy is multidimensional in origin and consequences. To a neurophysiologist, epilepsy presents an enigma of electrophysiologic changes at the neuronal level, as recorded by EEG. These changes inspire the neurophysiologist to find physiologic means of reversal using some intervention. The focus of intervention might be at various levels of disease progression, such as reduction of stress, attempts to normalize the EEG results, or avoidance of a seizure stimulus.

Current antiepileptic medications do not completely improve the clinical picture in about one-third of people with epilepsy. For more than several decades, various non-pharmacologic interventional procedures have been investigated, many of which try to reduce anxiety and stress. Excellent studies by Sterman, beginning in the 1970s (27), suggested and then proved that by modifying one's own specific EEG rhythm using *EEG biofeedback*, uneven brain wave activity in epilepsy could be enhanced and the seizure threshold raised (28). Thus, meditation and biofeedback can have a normalizing influence on EEG patterns. Later findings, however, confirmed that these EEG abnormalities could also be reduced using antiepileptic medication.

Several studies in India proved that meditation enhances alpha brain wave activity (waves occurring 8 to 13 times a second), represented by a relaxed, awake state. Also, patients with epilepsy experience a reduced occurrence of alpha waves and an increased occurrence of lower frequency waves when they are resting. The All India Institute of Medical Sciences (AIIMS) in New Delhi performed a study to examine the theory that the regular practice of meditation may lead to the reduction of frequency and duration of seizures, and a simultaneous appearance of useful changes in EEG.

AIIMS Study on Drug-Resistant Epilepsy

To observe the effect of meditation on epilepsy, during the 1990s, researchers at AIIMS used well-defined selection criteria to choose 21 patients with epilepsy. These patients had seizures that were drug-resistant, and they had no other symptomatic illness. The diagnosis was confirmed by two senior neurologists. The details of illness were collected from patients using a seizure diary/daily cards, and information about their seizures was also collected from family members. The patients were randomly divided into two groups: a treatment group of 11 that would practice meditation and a control group of nine (one dropped out). Patients in both groups visited the laboratory monthly and their baseline data were collected for 6 months to 1 year. The data included details of seizure frequency and duration, EEG details, and serum drug levels. These patients continued to receive their prescribed medications because they were drug-resistant.

We analyzed the preintervention EEG to find the presence or absence of useful frequencies, such as the intensity of alpha, beta, and other low frequencies, and of high frequencies.

Researchers told patients in the meditation intervention group that the purpose of meditation was to attain as high as possible a degree of physical relaxation and to improve their *concentration*, which was defined as "nonanalytic attending to some passive act." The method of meditation was word repetition; they were instructed to repeat a specific word while sitting in a comfortable posture. The patients practiced this for 20 minutes every day. They selected the word from a list of common words used in meditation practice and words of similar length, including both meaningful (conventionally used) and meaningless syllables (listed later on). This was done to avoid religious and cultural connotations.

We asked the subjects to repeat their chosen word in their mind only, paying continuous attention to it during these 20-minute sessions. We asked them not to change their breathing pattern during the sessions and not to speak audibly. We explained that spontaneous drift or interruption would occur and that they should avoid these drifts in concentration as much as possible and focus on bringing their attention back to their chosen mantra (6).

We gave the patients a handout describing the steps of the practice in detail to reinforce the strict methodology of meditation practice. We monitored the following in the laboratory:

- EEG parameters
- Drifts or intrusions, recorded by a microswitch connected to an event recorder (we asked them to press the microswitch when they encountered drifts or when stray thoughts intruded during meditation)
- Behavioral changes, such as body and lip movements

We recorded the EEG and analyzed it using both conventional and state-of-the-art computer equipment. The power in specific frequency bands was calculated by using Fast Fourier Transform analysis. We also studied 29 healthy subjects, including nine long-term meditators.

After 6 months of observation, we brought an additional 11 patients into the meditation training, including five with generalized tonic-clonic seizures, three with complex partial seizures, and three with simple partial seizures. We studied the effects of meditation on the parameters described above and the neuropsychologic correlates of meditation (level of relaxation, level of concentration, attention span, and intrusion rate). These patients practiced meditation for 20 minutes every day in the laboratory on the specified schedule. We asked them to report subjective responses—level of achieved relaxation and level of concentration on the Visual Analogue Scale (VAS). Their attention span and intrusion were also recorded. The other nine patients (the control group) were similarly observed.

Soon after the end of each meditation session, we assessed the levels of relaxation and concentration achieved during meditation using the VAS. Because the first response was usually difficult (lack of a reference value), we explained a hypothetical situation of maximum and minimum levels. Subsequent responses were easy to score with reference to the previous score.

We measured attention span, a subtest of clinical memory testing, by recall of digits both forward and backward. Each series began with a short list (two digits) and ended with an eight-digit list. Each had one additional set also.

Meditation Training Program

Any comfortable posture may be adopted for the practice of meditation, according to patient preference: lying down, partially lying down, or sitting. Any word may be chosen for repetition to induce meditation; however, the word should not seem disagreeable or inappropriate to the patient. We presented a long list of words to the patients and asked them to choose any one. The words included: Om, Narayan, Allah, Mohammed, Christ, Many, God, One, Yam, Two, Krishna, Sam, Jolly, Ek, Jane, Do, Shiva, Peace, Namah, and Ma.

The instructor follows these guidelines to facilitate meditation:

- Posture. Is the patient comfortable? Find the cause of discomfort, if any, and shift position to correct it.
- Clothing. Not so tight that it produces discomfort.
- Duration. 20 minutes.
- Surroundings. Avoid any distracting event. If one exists, note it.

The instructor should be able to:

- Communicate with the subject. Give time signals by saying "yes" every 5 minutes for 20 minutes; last signal marks the end of meditation. Say "stop" at the end. Monitoring of these 5-minute periods is for the initial session only.
- Provide encouragement to improve performance and achieve a high score.
- Assess the neuropsychologic status of the subject.

Successful meditation using the word-repetition model implies holding the meditative state without intrusions, finally leading to a state of physical and mental relaxation. We gave patients detailed explanations about the method of meditation and a printed sheet containing instructions for meditation (see Appendix I).

For the initial two to three sessions in the laboratory, we asked the patients to concentrate on breathing. We asked them not to increase or decrease their breathing rate for 5-minute blocks of 20 minutes, total. They practiced at home, using the instruction sheet. After three sessions in the laboratory (2 weeks), they practiced concentration using word repetition for 20 minutes. For each session in the laboratory, we interviewed the patients and entered their subjective responses on one assessment form (Appendix II).

Schedule for Meditation Practice

Practice sessions in the laboratory for training and assessment:

- Once a week for 2 weeks
- Once every 2 weeks for 1 month
- Once a month for 6 months
- Once every 2 months for 1 year

Practice session at home:

- 20-minute session once every day

Data Analysis

We collected data continuously on every visit and recorded it carefully. Several previous studies using behavior intervention have observed the effect of meditation on a short-term basis. We observed these effects in our long-term research.

We expressed seizure frequency as the total number of attacks per month. Average values for 6 months were calculated for statistical treatment because they were more stable than monthly data. We similarly treated the cumulative duration (minutes) for attacks per month.

Subjective responses to meditation were measured on every patient visit (using Appendix II) and entered into master tables from which corresponding monthly seizure data were calculated. Later (after 7 or 8 months), bimonthly data were collected. We measured attention span and intrusion rate on every visit and calculated the averages for every month. From the average values, the averages for 6 months were also calculated.

In 29 normal adults (including the nine long-term meditators), we recorded EEG frequency analysis at rest and during meditation. We compared healthy subjects and patients (before and during intervention), between patient's initial condition and condition during intervention, and between patients in the training group and controls.

Results

Complaints of seizures were the only clinical abnormalities. The patients' interictal EEGs showed low-frequency dominance in the background. Computerized frequency analysis of their EEGs showed more intensity in delta and theta waves than the comparable EEG of the healthy subjects. Normally, delta and theta waves in EEG are not present in the wakeful state. The patients with epilepsy had a low intensity of alpha waves compared to the healthy subjects. The statistical comparison of the two groups (treatment and control) revealed that both were similar for age as well as duration of illness.

The average seizure frequency before intervention in the treatment group was 68.8 attacks per month; after 6 months of meditation, 19.2 attacks per month were reported. The statistical analysis showed that the effect was significant in absolute number of attacks only after 12 months of practice. We found a significant reduction in the percentage of seizure frequency in the first 6 months that continued in the next 6-month block. We observed that meditation resulted in a significant reduction in seizure frequency when we combined the findings of percentage changes in the two time periods. The cumulative duration of seizures showed an average decline of 6.3 minutes in 6 months. This represents a highly significant reduction. In the next 6-month block, the meditation practice resulted in a continuing decline in cumulative seizure duration. We saw this effect of meditation decline in the cumulative duration of seizures in both absolute and percentage change; it was more significant than the change in seizure frequency.

We examined the changes, if any, in background frequency of EEG that resulted from meditation practice. Patients before intervention showed a slowing of background EEG, more intensity in the low-frequency arrays, and less power in the frequency range of alpha waves and sensorimotor rhythms (SMRs; rhythmic EEG patterns seen over a certain brain area).

The normal adults had an entirely different EEG profile when compared with patients with epilepsy. They had more intensity in alpha waves and higher power in the SMR band of EEG.

The percentage change between initial background frequency and background frequency during six months of meditation intervention was 4.1 hertz after meditation practice in patients, indicating a significant increment in background EEG frequency during 6 months of intervention. The next 6-month block also showed continued improvement in background EEG frequency. Thus, intervention resulted in a significant decline in the number of attacks and in cumulative duration. These declines corresponded with an increased ability to concentrate, increased ability to relax, and decreased intrusion during meditation. The EEG profile showed a tendency toward normalization during intervention. Patients in the control group did not show comparable change in their EEGs and clinical picture. These results were previously reported (29). Figure 10.2 represents the EEG data of one patient.

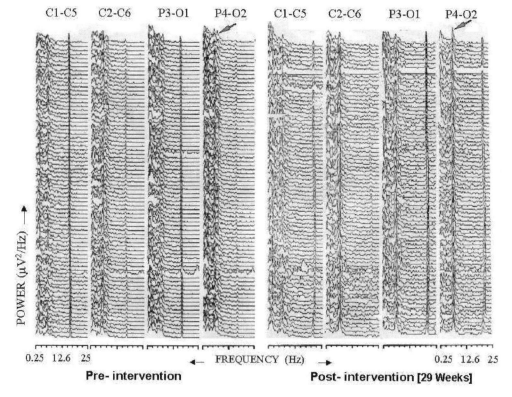

FIGURE 10.2

Electroencephalogram (EEG) comparing brain wave activity before and after the initiation of meditation therapy.

Response Variability

Meditation has been associated with variable physiologic responses. The reason for this variability may be twofold. First, the definition of meditation or the method of induction may have varied greatly. Second, the responses may have had different threshold levels of activation. The latter point was discussed by Banquet (30), who found different kinds of power spectra, which he correlated with different depths of meditation.

A literature review suggests that the views on meditation as a therapeutic modality have always been uncertain. The well-documented and important accompanying aspect of meditation is relaxation (20) and, thus, the use of meditation for stress-induced disorders is advocated. Several meta-analyses, however, suggest conflicting responses to meditation intervention for various disorders. The basic problem with meditation is identifying exactly what aspect of the meditation program the patient responds to.

Several other reasons exist for the variability observed in responses to meditation. Other problems associated with meditation are:

- Vagueness and use of mystical words in meditation instructions
- Lack of assessment method to judge whether the subject has followed the instructions
- Subject lacks prior knowledge of meditation
- Lack of knowledge of subjective response variability to meditation

We made an attempt to evolve an objective technique of meditation in the study described here. Our technique included all four components of Benson's "relaxation response" (20). Patients knew exactly what was expected of them. Consistency of responses to meditation (EEG, relaxation level, concentration level, and intrusion rate) confirmed the validity of our method.

The other component of meditation—the attentional variable—was measured directly by attention span. This method is well established and was correlated individually to one or more subjective parameters. Decline in intrusion rates was significantly correlated to sustained nonanalytic attending during meditation. The results showed a highly significant decline in the percentage of seizure frequency and cumulative duration of seizures, which correlated well with improvement in attention span. Thus, the nonanalytic attending that resulted from meditation influenced the clinical picture.

The clinical improvement was accompanied by an improved EEG background frequency. These changes were also correlated with an increase in the attention span, an increase in the level of relaxation and concentration, and a decline in intrusion rate. These had a very high level of significance.

Mechanisms of Meditation

In general, the results of the AIIMS study agree with the original theories about the relationships between intervention by meditation and alteration in seizure picture, along with its EEG correlates. The ability of patients to concentrate (nonanalytic attending) and the ability to relax, achieved through meditation, appear to bring improvement in the clinical and EEG profiles of patients with epilepsy.

The mechanism of meditation response for mediating antiepileptic response largely remains a matter of speculation. Areas in the brain that generate and modulate seizure activity have been identified. Gale (31) has done extensive studies in this direction and suggests that two brain areas, the *substantia nigra* and *area tempastas*, are connected to control of seizures. Circuits involving the thalamus and *substantia nigra* and/or limbic system and pyriform cortex may influence the activity of target areas (the seizure focus), thus modifying their activities.

Meditation induces relaxation and attentional changes. Whether attentional changes and changes in relaxation during meditation influence these areas in the brain remains to be tested. Perhaps through these changes, meditation may normalize the activity of thalamocortical circuits and produce a normal pattern of EEG frequencies. Some also propose that meditation may boost some naturally occurring endogenous antiepileptic chemical substances in the brain. Results from our study appear to be mediated through nonautonomic and nonstress mechanisms, as evidenced by specific EEG changes. Another Indian study claimed a reduction in stress after Sahaja Yoga intervention in epileptics (32).

Meditation appears to have something in common with biofeedback and autosuggestibility. It is possible to identify visceral sensation and modify it through internal cueing (33,34) that may operate on a higher nervous system level.

Precautions

Meditation is a simple and effective technique, but to use its full potential, certain steps should be assured. The basic instructions of meditation are easy, but these should be given after a good deal of explanation, preferably by an expert. If an expert teacher is not available, the teacher should be someone who has experienced the beneficial effect of meditation, either in terms of physiologic changes or psychologic manifestations. A certain receptivity is required for meditation, similar to that required for other behavioral techniques, such as hypnosis and biofeedback. Some amount of healthy skepticism is also useful, but the seeker should keep an open mind. At times, group practice, in which individuals learn to share their experiences, is more effective.

For a few, meditation can *provoke* the problems it is supposed to defeat: fear, anxiety, confusion, depression, and self-doubt. During the first 10 minutes of meditation, as one unwinds into a state of deep relaxation, it is possible for unsettling thoughts to pop up, disrupting relaxation. This problem is most common among beginners, but it occasionally happens to more experienced meditators. This may be due to anxiety over expectations. Meditation is slow to induce effects, and it demands regularity and patience.

Appendix I. Instructions for Meditation

1. Select a peaceful environment.
2. Sit comfortably. Relax the body.
3. Adopt the same posture for every session of meditation.
4. Meditate for 20 minutes daily. Remember that the duration of meditation should not be less than 20 minutes. You may use an alarm clock, watch, or timer to time it exactly, or request that someone give you an indication after 20 minutes.
5. During these 20 minutes, initially concentrate on breathing for the first 3 to 5 minutes, concentrating on the process of inhaling and exhaling. Then, repeat the selected word in your mind silently. Repeat this word quietly while exhaling. Continue this practice for 20 minutes.
6. During this practice, avoid distractions. The more you concentrate, the greater the benefit.
7. Write down your experiences and mention them in your next visit.

Appendix II. Assessment of Effects of Meditation

Name_____ Age/Sex _____ Dept. Reg. No. _____

Diagnosis_____ Treatment _____

Meditation practice started on _____ Posture _____

Word used_____ No. of sessions completed _____

No. of absences _____

Previous experience in meditation _____

Assessment Procedure:

The instructor asks each patient these questions and completes this form at the end of each session:

Questions   Score/No. of intrusions

1. Were you able to fix your attention
   on your breathing rhythm in the first 5 minutes?   _____
   If not, how many times did drifting of your
   attention occur?   _____
2. Did your attention drift during word repetition?   _____
   If it did, note the number of drifts in each period:
   1st five minutes   _____
   2nd five minutes   _____
   3rd five minutes   _____
3. Did you feel relaxed after meditation?   _____
4. Do you think you have improved your capacity
   to relax since your last visit? If so, please indicate your
   level of relaxation attained on the given scale.*   _____

Questions   Score/No. of intrusions

5.   Do you think you have improved your
     concentration or attention ability since
     the last visit? If so, please indicate this
     on a given scale.*
                                                               _____

*(Points 1 and 2 were scored from drift records from the EEG readings; Points 4 and 5
were scored from the Visual Analogue Scale.)

Acknowledgments

I thank the late Professor S.K. Manchanda, who initiated me into this study. I acknowledge the
help of Professor M.C. Maheshwari, who assisted me in acquiring patients for this study, and Dr.
Padam Singh, who assisted in statistical analysis. I express deep gratitude to the late Professor
Baldev Singh for explaining the complexities of meditation, epilepsy, and EEG. I also thank Shree
Dharmananda Jee of Adhyatma Sadhana Kendra for providing healthy people who had long-
term meditation experience for our research.

References

1. Puttick E. *Meditation.* Encarta Encyclopedia 2000.
2. Beaumont JG. *Understanding Neurophysiology.* New York: Basil Blackwell, Inc., 1988.
3. Eliade M. *Immortality and Freedom.* Trask WR (trans.) London: Routledge and Kegan Paul,
    1950.
4. Naranjo C, Ornstein RE. *On the Psychology of Meditation.* New York: Viking, 1971.
5. Cohen BH. The motor theory of voluntary thinking in consciousness and self-regulation
    advances. In: Davidson RJ, Schwartz GE, Shapiro D, (eds.) *Consciousness and Self-
    Regulation.* Vol 4. New York: Plenum Press, 1986.
6. Benson H, Beary JF, Carol MP. The relaxation response. *Psychiatry* 1974;37:37–46.
7. Johnson W. *Christian Zen.* New York: Harper and Row, 1971.
8. Ishiguro H. *The Scientific Truth of Zen.* Tokyo: Zenrigaker Society, 1964.
9. Wallace RK. Physiologic effects of Transcendental Meditation. *Science* 1970;167:1751–1754.
10. Telles S, Reddy SK, Nagendra HR. Oxygen consumption and respiration following two yoga
    relaxation techniques. *Appl Psychophysiol Biofeedback* 2000;25:221–227.
11. Beary JF, Benson H. A simple psychophysiologic technique which elicits the hypometabolic
    changes of the relaxation response. *Psychosom Med* 1974;36:115–120.
12. Anand BK, Chhina GS, Singh B. Some aspects of electroencephalographic studies in yogis.
    Electroencephalogr Clin Neurophysiol 1961;13:452–456.
13. Bagchi BK, Wenger MA. Electrophysiologic correlations of some yoga exercises.
    Electroencephalogr Clin Neurophysiol 1957;7(suppl):132–149.
14. Karambelkar PV, Vinekar SL, Bhole MV. Studies on human subjects staying in an air-tight
    pit. *Indian J Med Res* 1968;56:1282–1288.
15. Matsuoka S. Spectral EEG mapping in meditation. Proceedings of the Satellite Symposium
    on States of Consciousness. World Congress of Neurology, New Delhi. Oct. 20–21, 1989.
16. Desiraju T. Neurophysiologic assessment of brain states in meditation and yoga.
    Proceedings of the Satellite Symposium on States of Consciousness. World Congress of
    Neurology, New Delhi. Oct. 20–21, 1989.

17. Heide FJ. Psychophysiologic responsiveness to auditory stimulation during transcendental meditation. *Psychophysiology* 1986;23:71–75.
18. Davidson RJ, Goleman DJ. The role of attention in meditation and hypnosis: a psychobiological perspective on transformation of consciousness. *Int J Clin Exp Hypn* 1977;25; 291–308.
19. Wallace RK, Benson H. The physiology of meditation. *Sci Am* 1972;226:84–90.
20. Benson H: *The Relaxation Response.* New York: W.M. Morrow and Co., 1975.
21. Lavender A. A behavioral approach to the treatment of epilepsy. *Behav Psychother* 1981;9: 231–243.
22. Okuma T, Kogu E, Ikeda K, et al. The EEG of yoga and Zen practitioners. *Electroencephalogr Clin Neurophysiol* 1957;(suppl 9):51.
23. Dunn BR, Hartigan JA, Mikulas WL. Concentration and mindfulness meditations: unique forms of consciousness? *Appl Psychophysiol Biofeedback* 1999;24:147–165.
24. Lou HC, Kjaer TW, Friberg L, et al. A 15O-H2O PET study of meditation and the resting state of normal consciousness. *Hum Brain Mapp* 1999;7:98–105.
25. Lazar SW, Bush G, Gollub RL, et al. Functional brain mapping of the relaxation response and meditation. *Neuroreport* 2000;11:1581–1585.
26. Van Nuys D. Meditation, attention and hypnotic susceptibility: a correlational study. *Int J Clin Exp Hypn* 1973;21:59–69.
27. Sterman MB. Sensorimotor EEG operant conditioning: experimental and clinical effects. *Pavlovian J Bio Sci* 1977;12:63–92.
28. Sterman MB. Basic concepts and clinical findings in the treatment of seizure disorders with EEG operant conditioning. *Clin Electroencephalogr* 2000;31:45–55.
29. Deepak KK, Manchanda SK, Maheshwari MC. Meditation improves clinicoelectroencephalographic measures in drug-resistant epileptics. *Biofeedback and Self-Regulation* 1994;19:25-40 (cited in Bulletin of Breakthroughs [Los Angeles] 1995;19:9/10).
30. Banquet JP. Spectral analysis of the EEG in meditation. *EEG Clin Neurophysiol* 1973;35:143–151.
31. Gale K. Progression and generalization of seizure discharge: anatomic and neurochemical substrates. *Epilepsia* 1988;29(suppl 2):S15–34.
32. Panjwani U, Gupta, Singh SH, et al. Effect of Sahaja Yoga practice on stress management in patients of with epilepsy. *Indian J Physiol Pharmacol* 1995;39:111–116.
33. Deepak KK, Behari M. Specific muscle EMG biofeedback for hand dystonia. *Appl Psychophysiol Biofeedback* 1999;24:267–280.
34. Deepak KK, Mahapatra SC, Manchanda SK. Effect of autosuggestion on pain threshold and pain tolerance and pain induced physiologic responses. *Indian J Physiol Pharmacol* 1987;31:46.

Further Information

Goldsmith J. *The Art of Meditation.* New York: Harper Collins Publishers, 1990.
Leichtman RR, Japikse C. *Active Meditation: the Western Tradition.* Cincinnati: Ariel Press, 1990.
LeShan L. *How to Meditate: A Guide to Self-Discovery.* New York: Bantam Books, 1984.
Ozaniec N. *Basic Meditation: 101 Essential Tips.* Cheshire: Dorling Kindersley, 1997.
Rosenberg L, Guy D. *Breath by Breath: The Liberating Practice of Insight Meditation.* Boston: Shambhala Publications, 1998.
Goleman. *The Meditative Mind.* Los Angeles, CA: Jeremy P Trecher, Inc., 1988.
Borysenko J. *Minding the Body, Mending the Mind.* New York: Bantam Books, 1988.

Internet Sites

Dr. Bower's Complementry and Alternative Medicine http://galen.med.virginia.edu/~pjb3s/ Complementry_Practices.html

Yahoo provides links to over 900 health Web sites http://www.Yahoo.com/Health/ Alternative_Medicine

The Alternative Medicine Homepage http://www.pitt.edu/bw/alt.html

CHAPTER 11

Exercise and Yoga

STEVEN V. PACIA, MD

Comprehensive epilepsy centers offer the latest in medical and surgical treatments to alleviate the crippling effects of recurrent seizures; however, despite our best efforts, many patients have poorly controlled seizures or suffer from commonly associated depression or anxiety. With growing frequency, patients and their physicians are looking to complementary techniques, especially nonpharmacologic ones, to reduce the burden of seizures and to ease anxiety and depression. Exercise and yoga have well-established health benefits. Preliminary studies suggest that both may improve the quality of life for patients with epilepsy.

Patients with uncontrolled seizures cite stress as one of the most important seizure precipitants (1). Stress management may be accomplished through aerobic exercise and yoga, and some physicians are interested in these techniques as complementary therapies for patients with uncontrolled seizures (1,2). Unfortunately, many patients with seizures are counseled against exercise because of fear of seizure exacerbation and injury. Moreover, patients with epilepsy are often isolated and participate less in social and physical activities than the average individual (3). This chapter explores the potential benefits and risks of exercise and yoga for epilepsy.

Exercise and Epilepsy

The benefits of aerobic and weight-bearing exercises are well established. Exercise improves the course of many chronic illnesses and, in some cases, prevents them. The signs and symptoms of hyperlipidemia (elevated triglycerides and cholesterol), high blood pressure, obesity, coronary artery disease, osteoporosis, and diabetes are all improved by regular exercise; however, the benefits of exercise for epilepsy are less well established, and as a result, not routinely prescribed by most clinicians at comprehensive epilepsy centers.

The Relationship between Exercise and Seizures

Patients with epilepsy exercise less than the general population (4). Many physicians treating these patients are reluctant to encourage physical exercise because they fear that strenuous exercise and overheating will provoke a seizure and lead to physical injury. Several cases of exercise-induced seizures have been described in the medical literature (5–7). Patients with partial or generalized types of epilepsy are at potential risk. Unfortunately, because of the limited number of case studies, we cannot predict an individual's risk for exercise-induced seizures. Also, which exercises and how much exercise will induce seizures is unknown. A Brazilian research team, expecting exercise to increase seizures in a rat temporal lobe epilepsy model, discovered the opposite (8). Compared with controls (animals that had no physical exercise), animals that did periodic treadmill running had less seizures.

Deep breathing, or hyperventilation, is used to activate abnormal discharges (epileptiform activity) in the brain during an electroencephalogram (EEG). This provocative measure is particularly useful to diagnose absence epilepsy of childhood, a condition characterized by brief staring spells with a stereotyped, corresponding EEG abnormality (3-Hz spike and wave). The ability to activate seizures and EEG abnormalities through hyperventilation infers a potential risk of seizures from increased respirations during strenuous exercise in patients with epilepsy. Esquivel and his colleagues studied this in patients with childhood absence epilepsy and concluded that hyperventilation and strenuous exercise are not the same. Seizures and EEG abnormalities increased during hyperventilation in these children, but seizures did not occur when the children exercised (9). The authors concluded that children with this type of epilepsy should not be discouraged from exercising.

Clinical Studies

Several small clinical studies examined the effects of exercise on people with epilepsy. Denio and colleagues surveyed an epilepsy clinic population on their exercise habits and concluded that patients who exercised regularly had fewer seizures (10). After a 4-week program of exercise in 19 patients with uncontrolled seizures, Nakken found no increase in seizure frequency associated with the training program, but he did report that six of the patients had seizures while exercising (11). Whether the seizures were random events or were induced by exercise is unclear. In a follow-up study by the same group, 15 women with uncontrolled epilepsy were placed in a 15-week exercise program (12). Seizure frequency for the group decreased significantly during the program, compared with baseline seizure frequency. Additional psychological and physical benefits of exercise were documented during the training period.

In a survey of 204 Norwegian patients with epilepsy, only 10% reported that seizures occurred frequently with exercise, although nearly half of those who exercised regularly experienced at least one seizure associated with exercise (13). Of those patients able to comment on the effects of exercise on seizures, approximately one-third believed that exercise reduced seizures.

If exercise reduces seizures in some patients, is this the result of a direct effect on the brain? Some suggest that physiologic changes from daily aerobic exercise, such as general brain arousal and increased beta-endorphins (naturally occurring opiods or

Commentary

As noted throughout this book, people with epilepsy often experience high levels of stress. Exercise and yoga are excellent ways to manage stress, but people with seizures are often advised not to exercise, and they may not be told about the potential health benefits of yoga. Lack of exercise has many negative health consequences, whether or not someone has epilepsy, including obesity, cardiovascular disease, thinning of the bones, and depressed mood.

Epilepsy specialists are reconsidering whether people with epilepsy should be encouraged to exercise and participate in other forms of movement therapy, such as yoga. Dr. Pacia discusses these topics in this chapter and suggests that exercise and yoga may be beneficial for people with epilepsy, particularly for reducing stress and maintaining bone health. He reports the results of small studies and suggests the need for large-scale studies.

People who have a history of seizures induced by exercise or hyperventilation should probably proceed with caution and avoid strenuous exercise. It is also advisable that people work with exercise and yoga instructors who know what to do in the event of a seizure. For people whose seizures are not completely controlled, equipment (such as treadmills) or situations (such as swimming) that would put them at risk if a seizure occurred should probably be avoided if possible.

pain relievers present in the brain), may inhibit seizures; the effect may also be indirect. Some investigators speculate that daily aerobic exercise acts as a "stress vaccine" whereby catecholamines (including adrenaline) released in the body during stressful events seem to decrease as physical fitness increases (14). One well-controlled study in patients with congestive heart failure revealed significant improvements in stress management for patients entered into an exercise program (2). If stress is a significant provocative factor in causing seizures, then exercise may indirectly reduce seizure frequency.

Potential Benefits

In addition to the obvious general health benefits and the possibility of seizure reduction, there are more reasons for patients with epilepsy to exercise. Many patients use antiepileptic medications (AEDs) that place them at increased risk for osteoporosis and bone fractures. Medications, such as phenytoin and carbamazepine, may interfere with normal vitamin D metabolism and, therefore, with calcium deposition into bone. This effect, especially when combined with a sedentary lifestyle, is a significant risk for weak bones and possible fractures. The enhanced risk of falling from seizures, or from the gait unsteadiness that may result from certain AEDs, increases the risk of injury even more. Studies in patients with osteoporosis document a positive effect of exercise on bone strength (15,16). Thus, exercise may be an important preventive measure in patients taking AEDs.

Mood and anxiety disorders occur more often in patients with epilepsy (17). For the general population, numerous small uncontrolled studies indicate a positive effect of exercise on anxiety and depression, although no large randomized studies have been done. Similarly, no large studies confirm the benefits of exercise on mood and anxiety in epilepsy, but preliminary studies and surveys are encouraging. Roth and colleagues analyzed self-reporting measures in 114 patients with epilepsy and concluded that regular exercise reduced the incidence of depression (18). Additionally, both exercise and epilepsy studies by the Norwegian group indicated psychological benefits for those patients who exercised (11,12).

Recommendations

The benefits of regular exercise are indisputable. The use of exercise to reduce seizure frequency or alleviate anxiety and depression in epilepsy remains unproven; however, beneficial effects will be realized by most patients. At our center, we encourage regular exercise routines for all of our patients. Exercise programs should be individualized based on the relative risk of seizures and injury, because mild to moderate exercise rarely induces seizures. In the initial stages of all exercise programs, regardless of the type and intensity of exercise, we urge a gradual "ramping up" of exercise intensity in a well-supervised setting. Patients with frequent seizures that impair consciousness or motor control are encouraged to choose a safer exercise apparatus, such as a seated stationary bicycle, instead of a treadmill. In patients with seizures that cause loss of balance, padded or carpeted exercise areas and helmets are encouraged. Above all, we counsel patients not to ignore warning signs, such as auras during exercise, as these are opportunities to terminate the exercise and secure a safe position in case of a seizure.

Many patients cannot exercise for prolonged periods or participate in strenuous activities, but even modest levels of exercise may be beneficial. In a study of postmenopausal women, 41% lower risk of hip fracture occurred in women who walked at least 4 hours each week, compared with those who walked for less than 1 hour (19). For patients with epilepsy who are unwilling or unable to exercise, and for those patients whose seizures occur frequently with aerobic exercise, other forms of physical fitness, such as yoga, may be safe and effective alternatives.

Yoga and Epilepsy

Yoga has developed in India over the past 5,000 years. It has exploded in popularity as a means to maintain general health, to reduce stress, and to complement standard medical therapy. Yoga literally means "to yoke together" or to "make whole." There are several types of yoga, but the type most applicable to complementary medicine is hatha yoga or versions of it. The main components of hatha yoga are meditation, controlled breathing, and physical postures. Although elements of yoga are found in ancient Hindu spiritual texts, practicing yoga is not necessarily a religious activity for most people. Many patients need to be reassured that yoga is not at odds with their religious beliefs. Yoga is also not a competitive sport. One need not be a contortionist or gymnast to do it. Therapeutic yoga programs require instructors to be sensitive to the needs and abilities of the individual. Yoga may be practiced at many levels, and patients of all body types and abilities may derive benefits. Yoga can also be adapted for patients in wheelchairs.

For several decades, the physiologic and neurophysiologic effects of relaxation and meditation have been studied. Studies document physiologic changes in the musculoskeletal, respiratory, metabolic, and cardiovascular systems during yoga (20). These effects benefit patients with high blood pressure (21), asthma (22), and carpal tunnel syndrome (23). Additionally, yoga has measurable effects on the brain. Several studies document increased alpha waves in the EEGs of subjects performing yogic breathing and meditation (24). Alpha waves are brain waves that are abundant during calm, quiet, wakefulness. Positron emission tomography (PET) scans (studies that analyze brain blood flow and oxygen consumption) also show changes in cerebral blood flow during meditation (25). These effects on the brain may explain yoga's positive influence on stress management.

Studies of Yoga in Epilepsy

Few studies of yoga and epilepsy have been done. One study looked at yoga in three small groups of patients, all with uncontrolled seizures (26). Ten patients were prescribed a 6-month trial of yoga. Another group performed postures that only mimicked yoga. The third group did not perform yoga. Seizure frequency was reduced by 86% in the yoga group, but no change in seizure frequency occurred in the remaining two groups. Additionally, the yoga group exhibited less signs of stress after completing the yoga trial (27). This finding was based on physiologic measures of stress, such as the galvanic skin response. These results have not been replicated by other investigators.

Benefits and Precautions

At the NYU Comprehensive Epilepsy Center, we offer yoga to our patients. We hope to confirm yoga's ability to reduce seizure frequency and to improve anxiety and depression. While studies are still in progress, we receive positive feedback from nearly all participants. Instructors have tailored the program to the abilities of each patient, and even patients who have never been in exercise programs enjoy yoga. In addition to yoga, patients appreciate the camaraderie of the group.

No adverse effects of yoga for epilepsy have been reported in the medical literature. In our experience, seizures during yoga class are rare. When seizures do occur, they often happen in patients new to the program and anxious about the experience. Invariably, patients become more comfortable as they learn yoga. Controlled breathing is performed gently and slowly to avoid hyperventilation, which can cause seizures in susceptible patients. Although joint and musculoskeletal injuries may rarely result from certain yoga postures, we have not encountered them. This may be due to the gentle, therapeutic form of yoga practiced at our center. We hope to determine which routines are most beneficial to our patients as we gain more experience with yoga and epilepsy. With a flexible program tailored to the patient's individual abilities, nearly all patients can practice yoga.

References

1. Ramaratnam S, Sridharan K. Yoga for epilepsy (*Cochrane Review*). In: *The Cochrane Library*, April, 2000. Oxford: Update Software.
2. Luskin F, Reitz M, Newell K, et al. A controlled pilot study of stress management training of elderly patients with congestive heart failure. *Prev Cardiol* 2002;5(4):168–172.
3. Steinhoff BJ, Neususs K, Thegeder H, et al. Leisure time activity and physical fitness in patients with epilepsy. *Epilepsia* 1996;37(12):1221–1227.
4. Jalava M, Sillanpaa M. Physical activity, health-related fitness, and health experience in adults with childhood-onset epilepsy: a controlled study. *Epilepsia* 1997;38(4):424–429.
5. Ogunyemi AO, Gomez MR, Klass DW. Seizures induced by exercise. *Neurology* 1988;38(4): 633–634.
6. Sturm JW, Fedi M, Berkovic SF, et al. Exercise-induced temporal lobe epilepsy. *Neurology* 2002;59(8):1246–1248.
7. Schmitt B, Thun-Hohenstein L, Vontobel H, et al. Seizures induced by physical exercise: report of two cases. *Neuropediatrics* 1994;25(1):51–53.
8. Arida RM, Scorza FA, dos Santos NF, et al. Effect of physical exercise on seizure occurrence in a model of temporal lobe epilepsy in rats. *Epilepsy Res* 1999;37(1):45–52.
9. Esquivel E, Chaussain M, Plouin P, et al. Physical exercise and voluntary hyperventilation in childhood absence epilepsy. *Electrogencephalogr Clin Neurophysiol* 1991;79(2):127–132.
10. Denio LS, Drake ME Jr, Pakalnis A. The effect of exercise on seizure frequency. *J of Medicine* 1989;20(2):171–176.
11. Nakken KO, Bjorholt PG, Johannessen SI, et al. Effects of physical training on aerobic capacity, seizure occurrence, and serum level of antiepileptic drugs in adults with epilepsy. *Epilepsia* 1990;31:88–94.
12. Eriksen HR, Ellertsen B, Gronningsaeter H, et al. Physical exercise in women with intractable epilepsy. *Epilepsia* 1994;35(6):1256–1264.
13. Nakken KO, Loyning A, Loyning T, et al. Does physical exercise influence the occurrence of epileptiform EEG discharges in children? *Epilepsia* 1997;38(3):279–284.
14. Nakken KO. Physical exercise in outpatients with epilepsy. *Epilepsia* 1999;40:643–651.
15. Srivastava M, Deal C. Osteoporosis in the elderly: prevention and treatment. *Clin Geriatr Med* 2002;18(3):529–555.
16. Iuliano-Burns S, Saxon L, Naughton G, et al. Regional specificity of exercise and calcium during skeletal growth in girls: a randomized controlled trial. *J Bone Miner Res* 2003;18(1): 156–162.
17. Trimble MR, Perez MM. Quantification of psychopathology in adult patients with epilepsy. In: Kulig B, Meinardi H, Stores G, (eds.) *Epilepsy and Behavior*. Lisse: Swets and Zeitlinger, 1980;118–126.
18. Roth DL, Goode KT, Williams VL, et al. Physical exercise, stressful life experience, and depression in adults with epilepsy. *Epilepsia* 1994;35(6):1248–1255.
19. Feskanich D, Willett W, Colditz G. Walking and leisure-time activity and risk of hip fracture in postmenopausal women. *JAMA* 2002;288(18):2300–2306.

20. Vempati RP, Telles S. Yoga-based guided relaxation reduces sympathetic activity judged from baseline levels. *Psychol Rep* 2002;90(2):487–494.

21. Sundar S, Agrawal SK, Singh VP, et al. Role of yoga in management of essential hypertension. *Acta Cardiol* 1984;39(3):203–208.

22. Manocha R, Marks GB, Kenchington P, et al. Sahaja yoga in the management of moderate to severe asthma: a randomized controlled trial. *Thorax* 2002;57(2):110–115.

23. Garfinkel MS, Singhal A, Katz WA, et al. Yoga-based intervention for carpal tunnel syndrome: a randomized trial. *JAMA* 1998;280(18):1601–1603.

24. Aftanas LI, Golocheikine SA. Human anterior and frontal midline theta and lower alpha reflect emotionally positive state and internalized attention: high-resolution EEG investigation of meditation. *Neurosci Lett* 2001;310(1):57–60.

25. Lou HC, Kjaer TW, Friberg L, et al. A 15O-H2O PET study of meditation and the resting state of normal consciousness. *Hum Brain Mapp* 1999;7(2):98–105.

26. Panjwani U, Selvamurthy W, Singh SH, et al. Effect of Sahaja yoga practice on seizure control and EEG changes in patients with epilepsy. *Indian J Med Res* 1996;103:165–172.

27. Panjwani U, Gupta HL, Singh SH, et al. Effect of Sahaja yoga practice on stress management in patients of epilepsy. *Indian J Physiol Pharmacol* 1995;39(2):111–116.

PART III

Asian, Herbal, and Homeopathic Therapies

CHAPTER 12

Ayurveda: The Ancient Indian System of Medicine

Satish Jain, MD, DM

The chief source of ancient Indian Aryan culture and medicine is the four *Vedas*. The exact source and date of origin of the Vedas has always been a debatable issue, but according to Indian traditions, the Vedas were revealed to the sages by Brahma (the creator) approximately six thousand years before the Christian era. Most Western scholars believe that the oldest of the four Vedas was compiled during the second millennium B.C. The word *Ayurveda* (in Sanskrit *Ayu* means "life," and *Veda*, "to know") has traditionally been equated with the ancient Indian system of medicine. Although Ayurveda means the knowledge of life, by which the nature of life is understood and thus life is prolonged, this word does not appear in the Vedic texts. Most likely, traditional Vedic medicine flourished for several centuries before it was handed down orally from the master to the pupil. Much later, traditional Hindu medicine became synonymous with Ayurveda. Unfortunately, the text of Ayurveda is not available in its original form, but instead, most of its contents are revealed in the Samhitas, the encyclopedic works of Caraka and Susruta. These texts, originally written about 1000 B.C., are probably the most authentic and renowned representatives of the original Ayurveda (1).

In their writings, Caraka combined the role of a moralist, philosopher, and physician, and Sushruta created an atmosphere of independent thinking and investigation that later characterized Greek medicine. Caraka is credited as the oldest author in the Ayurvedic system of medicine. *Caraka Samhita* (written approximately 1000-800 B.C.) is a treatise on the ancient Indian system of medicine that was composed by Agnivesa, redacted by Caraka, and reconstructed by Drdhabla. Treatises written by later authorities borrowed heavily from this fundamental work (2–4). The *Sushruta Samhita* is acknowledged as one of the great works of its kind in Sanskrit literature, and it is especially important for its passages about surgery (1,5).

The Ayurvedic theory of *tridosha* or *tridhatu* is defined by the three elements (humors), namely *vayu* or *vata* (air), *pitta* (bile), and *kapha* (phlegm). This basis for physiology and pathology, as they were understood by the ancient Hindus, has been misunderstood by many scholars to mean literally the elements of air, bile, and phlegm. The ancients used these terms in a very broad sense, with variable meanings depending on the context in which they were used. The term *vayu* or *vata*, for example, incorporates all phenomena of motion involved in the function of life, including cell development and the functions of the central nervous system. *Pitta* does not refer to bile alone, but signifies the functions of metabolism and thermogenesis, including digestion and blood formation, and various secretions and excretions (*mala*), which are either the by-products or end products of tissue metabolism. The term *kapha* does not merely mean phlegm, but is used primarily to imply functions of cooling, preservation, and thermotaxis or heat regulation; and secondarily to denote protective fluid production of mucus, synovial fluid, and the like. The imbalance of these elements (*dhatus*) beyond normal variations causes bodily dysfunction and disturbance.

Epilepsy and Ayurveda

Abundant references to all aspects of epilepsy can be found in the Ayurvedic literature, including symptomology, etiology, diagnosis, and treatment. The eighth chapter of *Nidanasthana* (diagnosis) and tenth chapter of *Chikitsasthana* (treatment) of the *Caraka Samhita* are devoted exclusively to epilepsy (2). In Ayurvedic literature, the diseases of the head, nervous system, and mental afflictions are well classified and their treatment is given in detail. Convulsions (*akshepaka*), apoplectic fits (*apatantraka*), and hysterical fits (*daruna apatantraka*) are a few of the important nervous system disorders mentioned (1). The discussion of epilepsy in Ayurvedic literature is summarized below.

Definition and Etiology

In most Ayurvedic texts, epilepsy is mentioned as *Apasmara* (or *Apasmrti*) and classified as a mental disease. As implied by its name, it involves partial or total loss of cognition (memory and sense-perception). Epilepsy (*Apasmara*), like several psychatric illnesses (*Unmada*), is attributed to humoral derangement. The original cause of such derangement lies in wrong conduct (*mithyacara*) and improper gratification of senses. The bodily humors deranged by such conduct gradually invade the sense-carrying channels of the body, causing loss of consciousness due to the gradual accumulation of *tamas* (inertia) inside the channels. Unusual physical activity in the shape of involuntary writhing, groaning, contortions of the limbs, and uncontrolled movements of the eyes are caused by the abnormal accumulation of *rajas* (potential energy) in other channels (4).

Premonitory Symptoms

Ayurveda records many premonitory symptoms of epilepsy (2), including the contraction of eyebrows, constant irregular movement of eyes, auditory hallucination, excessive salivation and nasal secretions, anorexia and indigestion, cardiac spasm, distension of the lower abdomen with gurgling sound, weakness, pain and malaise, unconsciousness, fainting, giddiness, and frightening dreams.

Classification and Types of Epilepsy (Apasmara)

Ayurveda classifies epilepsy into four types, individually originating in the disordered states of the three *dosas* (humors): *Vatika Apasmara, Paittika Apasmara,* and *Slaismika Apasmara,* or all combined. The fourth type, the *Sannipatika* form of the disease, is caused by the simultaneous vitiation of all three dosas and is incurable; however, it is open to palliative measures. An unusual feature of all four types of epilepsy is the sudden manifestation of violent symptoms without any warning and also the sudden disappearance of symptoms without treatment (2,4).

Treatment of Epilepsy in Ayurveda

Various Ayurvedic treatment modalities that include strong elimination and alleviation therapies, depending upon specific requirements, are useful for epilepsy patients. When epilepsy is associated with extrinsic factors, then *mantras* (hymns) have been recommended. The physician is advised to first take steps to awaken the heart channels and unblock the mind blocked by the dosas through drastic emesis (*Vatika Apasmara*), enema (*Paittika Apasmara*), and purgatives (*Slaismika Apasmara*). Drug formulations are recommended only after the patient has been cleansed by all means and consoled

Commentary

Similar to traditional Chinese herbal medicine (TCHM), Ayurvedic medicine has been practiced for millennia. The practice includes not only medicinal and dietary treatments but also commonsense behavioral prescriptions such as, "Patients with epilepsy should avoid being in places where a seizure could result in injury" (1). As with TCHM, many of the compounds used are likely to be pharmacologically active agents. Fortunately, as highlighted in a review by Khan and Balick of the New York Botanical Gardens (2), the effects of many plant species used in Ayurvedic medicine have been preliminarily studied in both humans and animals. Studies now reveal the beneficial effects of several herbal remedies for ailments, including burns (3), diabetes (4), asthma, and pain (5). A study examined the antiepileptic and antianxiety effects of the common Ayurvedic epilepsy herbal medicine *Sesbania grandiflora* (6). The plant demonstrated clear antiseizure effects when evaluated using the same standard laboratory measures that assess the potential efficacy of antiepileptic medications approved in the U.S. by the FDA. Pharmacological potency will undoubtedly be found for other Ayurvedic therapies, once properly investigated.

Despite the mounting evidence that many Ayurvedic medicines do have potential benefits, most herbal treatments have never been rigorously studied, in trials like those required for the FDA approval of antiepileptic medications. Equally important, even less is known about the potential side effects and interactions of these herbs with other medications. It is impossible to advocate for the use of diets and dietary supplements without the same degree of careful testing. This applies even more strongly to invasive procedures, such as bloodletting, that have no scientific basis for the treatment of epilepsy.

The issue of safety is extremely important with regard to Ayurvedic herbs and medicines (7). Lead poisoning and other heavy metal toxicity can occur with the use of some Ayurvedic therapies (e.g., herbal tonics) (8,9). Also, although the author advocates strong cleansing regimens to purify the body, the editors only recommend the consideration of Ayurvedic medications after consultation with a neurologist: *Cleansing with emetics or purgatives can reduce antiepileptic drug levels and cause more frequent, severe, or prolonged seizures.* Their use should only be undertaken with the knowledge of the doctor prescribing antiepileptic drugs. We strongly recommend against initial treatment with Ayurvedic medications (as opposed to standard antiepileptic drugs, which have proven efficacy).

We agree with Dr. Jain that thousands of years of practical experience should not be summarily dismissed, but rather mined for its great potential. This will only occur when the most promising of these treatments are studied in an unbiased, critical manner.

References

1. Manyam BV. Epilepsy in ancient India. *Epilepsia* 1992;33(3):473–475.
2. Khan S, Balick, MJ. Therapeutic plants of Ayurveda: a review of selected clinical and other studies for 166 species. *J Altern Complement Med* 2001;7(5):389–392.
3. Priya KS, Gnanamani A, Radhakrishnan N, et al. Healing potential of *Datura alba* on burn wounds in albino rats. *J Ethnopharmacol* 2002;83(3):193–199.
4. Grover JK, Yadav S, Vats V. Medicinal plants of India with anti-diabetic potential. *J Ethnopharmacol* 2002;81(1):81–100.
5. Singh RK, Achrarya SB, Bhattacharya SK. Pharmacological activity of *Elaeocarpus sphaericus*. *Phytother Res* 2000;14(1):36–39.
6. Kasture VS, Deshmukh VK, Chopde CT. Anxiolytic and anticonvulsive activity of *Sesbania grandiflora* leaves in experimental animals. *Phytother Res* 2002;16(5):455–460.
7. Gogtay NJ, Bhatt HA, Dalvi SS, Kshirsagar NA. The use and safety of non-allopathic Indian medicines. *Drug Saf* 2002;25(14):1005–1019.
8. Dunbabin DW, Tallis GA, Popplewell PY, Lee RA. Lead poisoning from Indian herbal medicine (Ayurveda). *Med J Aust* 1992;157(11–12):835–836.
9. Parab S, Kulkarni R, Thatte U. Heavy metals in "herbal" medicines. *Indian J Gastroenterol* 2003;22(3):111–112.

well. (Note: The editors only recommend consideration of Ayurvedic medications after consultation with a neurologist; cleansing with emetics or purgatives can reduce antiepileptic drug levels and cause more frequent, severe, or prolonged seizures.)

A wide variety of *ghrtas* (purified butters) are recommended for internal use. One of the most important is *Maha Panca Gavya Ghrta*. Using mixtures of *ghrta* and *taila* (oil) cooked with drugs is also mentioned. Oils cooked with different herbal and animal products are recommended for anointing the body of the patient. *Nasyas* (nasal applications) are also used. The use of a wide variety of *anjanas* (collyriums) and *anjana vartikas* (collyriu sticks) to bring the patient to his senses is mentioned. Some unusual prescriptions are also used, such as bile of dog collected in *Pusya* constellation as collyrium and also as fumigant after mixing with *ghrta*. Another such prescription consists of a fermented liquor prepared from the half-digested contents of a pig's stomach, the pig having been previously fed with a specially prepared diet of boiled rice and the milky juice of the *bhargi* plant (*Clerodendron siphonanthus*) after a prolonged period of fasting. The contents of the pig's stomach are taken out surgically, dried, and powdered. The powder is suspended in an aqueous decoction of the *bhargi* plant. Adding sediments of wine induces fermentation, and the resulting alcoholic product is matured until it acquires a specific color and consistency. Fumigation of different types also is recommended (2,4).

The modes of drug administration for epilepsy in Ayurveda include external applications, internal use, and application in the eyes and nose. The only first-aid measure recommended in epilepsy is blood-letting (*Siravedha*) from the veins of the temples. Cauterization of both the parietal bones with needles (*Soocivedha*) has also been mentioned (2,4).

Conclusion

Abundant references to all aspects of epilepsy appear in the Ayurvedic literature dating from the second millenium B.C., including symptomatology, etiology, diagnosis, and treatment. In most texts, epilepsy is mentioned as *Apsmara* (or *Apsmari*) and classified as a mental disease. Mention has also been made of the classification of epilepsy into four subtypes and its treatment.

The Ayurvedic system of medicine made significant contributions to world civilizations. Over the years, Ayurveda has seen a progressive decline that threatens its survival; however, Ayurveda is still practiced by millions of people in India and around the world. A system that has survived through the centuries should not be summarily dismissed as being unscientific. One major reason for the decline of Ayurvedic medicine is the lack of properly conducted studies that show the effectiveness of Ayurvedic treatment for various medical disorders. Well controlled trials are necessary to assess the role of Ayurvedic treatment, either alone, or as a complementary therapy with modern medicines. Because seizures are not adequately controlled in a significant number of patients with epilepsy medications, Ayurvedic medicines may provide an alternative therapeutic modality to the management of epilepsy and other chronic disorders.

References

1. Keswani NH. Medical heritage of India. In: Keswani NH. (ed.), *The Science of Medicine and Physiologic Concepts in Ancient and Medieval India*. New Delhi, India: XXVI International Congress of Physiologic Sciences, Department of Physiology, All India Institute of Medical Sciences, New Delhi, India; 1974:1–49.

2. Tandon PN. Ayurveda and epilepsy. In: Tandon PN, (ed.), *Epilepsy in India*, Report based on a multicentric study on epidemiology of epilepsy carried out as a PL 480 funded project of the Indian Council of Medical Research, New Delhi, India; 1989:176–180.
3. Ray P, Gupta HN. *Caraka Samhita (a scientific synopsis)*, 2nd ed. New Delhi, India: Indian National Science Academy, 1980.
4. Ray P, Gupta HN, Roy M. *Susruta Samhita (a scientific synopsis)*. New Delhi, India: Indian National Science Academy, 1980.
5. Sarton G. *Introduction to the History of Science.* Carnegie Institute of Washington Publication 376 (3 volumes). Baltimore, MD: Williams and Wilkins, 1927–1948.

CHAPTER 13

Herbal Therapy in Epilepsy

JOAN A. CONRY, MD AND PHILLIP L. PEARL, MD

The use of complementary and alternative medications (CAM) in the United States has skyrocketed in the past decade. A 1998 study in the *Journal of the American Medical Association* estimated that the use of herbal medications increased from 2.5% to 12.1% in the adult population between 1990 and 1997, and that 18% of all prescription drug users were also taking herbal remedies or high-dose vitamins (1). The clinical benefit of CAM is largely unproven, because of a paucity of rigorous clinical trials evaluating safety and efficacy. Patients tend to underreport their use of alternative medicines to physicians, and physicians may discount their significance even when their use is presented. Substantial risks, however, are associated with the use of these interventions. These risks involve the direct toxicities of the alternative preparations as related to their intended ingredients, possible adulteration by other compounds, and interactions that we call "herb–drug interactions." Herb–drug interactions are related to the effects on the metabolism of standard antiepileptic drugs (AEDs) as well as factors related to AED absorption from the gastrointestinal tract and transport into the brain. This chapter presents an overview of the general principles for using alternative medicines in epilepsy and specific information on their potential effects and interactions in epilepsy patients. Data for the efficacy of these agents for use in epilepsy are also presented.

Alternative therapy may be defined in various ways. The Epilepsy Foundation (EF) recognizes different categories of alternative therapy for epilepsy:

- Excellent efficacy and excellent tolerability—example: pyridoxine (vitamin B6) in the rare neonatal syndrome of pyridoxine dependent epilepsy
- Excellent efficacy but poor tolerability—example: ACTH in West syndrome (infantile spasms)
- Promising but not proven efficacy—example: IVIG in Landau-Kleffner syndrome (acquired epileptic aphasia)
- Unproven efficacy but little evidence of side effects—examples: herbal remedies, vitamin supplements, and acupuncture

The position of the EF is that alternative therapies are *acceptable* as long as the patient also continues with traditional therapies, and the alternative and traditional therapies *do not conflict*. Although this position appears reasonable, its premise depends on evidence for efficacy of alternative therapies in the treatment of seizures and their acceptable safety without excessive toxicity. This standard applies to all therapies in medicine and should not be abrogated on behalf of alternative medicines.

Commonly Used Herbs

The top-selling herbs in the United States are: ginkgo, St. John's wort, ginseng, garlic, echinacea, saw palmetto, kava, pycnogenol, cranberry, valerian root, evening primrose, bilberry, and milk thistle. These are listed in Table 13.1, along with the indications for which they are most commonly used and the amount of annual retail sales associated with each in the United States (2). The total in U.S. sales amounts to a staggering $688.3 million, with these top 13 herbs accounting for $640.7 million of that amount.

Many herbs and supplements are recommended by herbalists to treat epilepsy. Widely accepted guidelines for these recommendations, uniformity of recommendations, and the identification of the most commonly used herbs for seizures are extremely difficult to find, either in published literature or on Internet sites. We have identified herbs described as effective, or possibly effective, for the treatment of seizures in at least two widely available and recognized reference texts (2–4). These products are listed below, with background information on each.

American Hellebore

Historically, American hellebore (*Veratrum viride*) was used as an emetic and for neuralgia, peritonitis, pneumonia, and seizures. Research is underway evaluating its use in hypertensive crises, pregnancy-induced hypertension, and myasthenia gravis. Synonyms for American hellebore are false hellebore, green hellebore, Indian poke, itchweed, and swamp hellebore. The common trade name is Cryptenamine®. This perennial herb is found in the United States. American hellebore has multiple actions. It contains ester alkaloids that are chemically similar to steroids. Variable cardiovascular effects occur, but American hellebore generally lowers blood pressure, heart rate, and possibly respiratory rate. High doses elevate blood pressure. A depolarizing action is found on cardiac tissue, nerve membranes, and muscle, increasing muscle tone. This is a highly toxic drug with a low therapeutic index.

Adverse reactions include effects on the central nervous system (CNS), heart, gastrointestinal (GI) system, lungs, and autonomic nervous system. Paresthesiae, extraocular muscle paralysis, hypertonia, weakness, and seizures may occur with CNS toxicity. Cardiac effects include syncope and bradyarrhythmias. GI symptoms include abdominal pain and distention, nausea, and vomiting. Respiratory symptoms are dyspnea and respiratory depression. Autonomic effects are increased salivation and either hypertension or hypotension. Particular caution should be taken in patients with hypertension.

Ingestion of the plant is associated with serious teratogenicity, including cyclopia and other facial deformities in animals. American hellebore is not recommended for medicinal use, particularly during pregnancy.

TABLE 13.1

Top-Selling Herbs in the United States (2)

Herb	Reported Common Uses	Retail U.S. Sales ($ Millions)
Ginkgo	Dementia Circulatory Vertigo	150.9
St. John's wort	Depression	140.4
Ginseng	Enhancement of mental and physical capacities	95.9
Garlic	Circulatory (increases blood pressure) Hyperlipidema	84.0
Echinacea/Goldenseal	Immune stimulant Antioxidant/anti-inflammatory (used for URI/flu)	69.7
Saw palmetto	Benign prostatic hypertrophy Chronic cystitis	32.1
Kava	Anxiolytic Analgesic Antiepileptic	16.6
Pycnogenol/Grape seed	Antioxidant Anti-inflammatory	12.1
Cranberry	Urinary tract infections Kidney stones	10.4
Valerian root	Mild sedative (anxiety, insomnia)	8.6
Evening primrose	Cardiovascular disease (elevated cholesterol) Rheumatoid arthritis Cough, bronchitis Multiple sclerosis Eczema PMS	8.5
Bilberry	Diarrhea Cataracts, glaucoma Diabetes mellitus	6.4
Milk thistle	Liver function	4.9

Betony

Folklore suggests many indications for the use of betony (*Stachys officinalis*), including asthma, bronchitis, diarrhea, heartburn, palpitations, renal disease, roundworm, seizures, stomachaches, toothaches, and wounds. Despite multiple claims, available evidence does not support the use of betony for any therapeutic application. Synonyms for betony are bishopswort and wood betony. Common trade names are Herb-a-Calm Formula®, Herbagessic Formula®, and HerbVal Formula®. Betony is a member of the mint family indigenous to Europe, northern Africa, and Siberia. The actions of betony are related to tannins, which constitute 15% of betony.

Adverse reactions include GI irritation (diarrhea, nausea, and anorexia), hypotension, and hepatic dysfunction. Betony should not be used in pregnancy because of the risk of uterine contractions.

Blue Cohosh

Blue cohosh (*Caulophyllum thalictroides*) is used as an anticonvulsant, to increase menstrual flow, and to induce labor. A national survey of the certified nurse-midwives who endorse herbal medicine use found that 65% used it in labor. The active agent, methylcytisine, is similar to but less potent than nicotine. Synonyms for blue cohosh are blue ginseng, caulophyllum, papoose toot, squawroot, and yellow ginseng. Common trade

Commentary

Drs. Conry and Pearl provide a careful, evidence-based review of the data to support or refute claims of effectiveness and safety for herbal therapies in epilepsy. They follow the approach of Western medicine, the culture in which the editors of this book were educated and practice. So for us, the chapter is a beacon of light and honesty. Simple questions—Does it help?, Does it harm?—but incredibly difficult to answer. That is the problem that both lay individuals face as they decide whether to "try out" one of these therapies. It is also the problem that professionals face when they try to counsel patients on the use of these therapies.

The simple answer is that none are proven to work for epilepsy. Double-blind studies find that placebos can significantly reduce seizures in up to 25% to 30% of epilepsy patients. Thus, it would be remarkable if small studies of any substance did not show some effectiveness, but what is the evidence? Drs. Conry and Pearl take a hard and close look at the evidence. Their review of the published literature reveals that the risks might actually outweigh the benefits, but that, ultimately, we are working with very limited information. The jury is out. It is leaning away from recommending any of these herbal remedies for the treatment of epilepsy. We desperately need well-controlled studies to define both safety and danger.

This chapter also highlights some of the potential dangers of using "herbal" therapies that are not produced and manufactured under any regulatory supervision. A young woman I follow was being treated with two antiepileptic drugs, but her mother had also obtained an "herbal" preparation for epilepsy from China. It was expensive, and both the mother and daughter were convinced that it helped control her seizures. One day the young woman decided to stop the Chinese herbs and shortly afterwards developed a severe cluster of seizures and symptoms suggesting withdrawal from a central nervous system depressant. Indeed, in the emergency room, a toxicology screen found that she had phenobarbital in her blood; the Chinese herb contained phenobarbital. Quite an herb! Who knows what else it contained?

Drs. Conry and Pearl take a somewhat negative voice in considering the use of various herbal preparations available in the United States and elsewhere. Their concern is justified because the negative consequences appear to outweigh the positive ones, based on the published data. In a similar way, American psychiatrists have warmly embraced the use of antiepileptic drugs for the treatment of behavioral disorders in patients without epilepsy. Mounting data suggest that many of the antiepileptic drugs do work in some psychiatric disorders, with a vast amount of positive data on patients with bipolar and pain disorders. Some drugs, however—in which well-controlled double-blind data show behavioral toxicity from epilepsy studies—are being used increasingly by psychiatrists to treat behavioral problems or counteract side effects (such as weight gain) from other psychotropic (behavioral) drugs. Medical doctors, as well as lay individuals, can easily fall into the frequent use of drugs for disorders in which the evidence is very scant. Once again, the bottom line is that we need more data. Keep in mind, once you take a plant or part of an animal, perform a series of chemical extractions, and transform it into a pill, powder, or liquid form—the end result is a drug.

names are: Blue Cohosh Low Alcohol®, Blue Cohosh Root®, Blue Cohosh Root Alcohol Free®, and Blue Cohosh Root Low Alcohol®. *Caulophyllum thalictroides* is a perennial found in the midwestern and eastern U.S. and Canada. The seeds are bright blue (as suggested by the name). Blue cohosh has some pharmacologic similarity to nicotine. Actions in animal studies include the stimulation of smooth muscle in coronary vessels, the small intestine, and uterus. Antifertility effects have been documented. Anti-inflammatory and antimicrobial actions have been reported.

Adverse reactions include chest pain, hypertension, abdominal cramps, diarrhea, hyperglycemia, and poisoning in children after ingestion of seeds. The bright blue seeds are attractive but poisonous to children. Blue cohosh is contraindicated in pregnancy because of increased uterine contractions and teratogenesis. At least two cases of severe neonatal heart failure were linked to the consumption during pregnancy. It should not be used by people with angina and other cardiac symptoms.

Kava

Kava (*Piper methysticum*) is widely used as an anxiolytic, and is commonly used in the South Pacific as a ceremonial beverage. Limited studies have identified several mechanisms of action. Kava is a strong L-type Ca^{+2} channel inhibitor and weak Na^+ channel blocker. Kava increases early K^+ outward current and GABA transmission. A serotonin 1A agonist effect has also been described (5). Limited human data exist on the use of kava in anxiety disorders. A meta-analysis of seven double-blind, randomized, placebo-controlled trials found some superiority over placebo in all trials but statistical significance in only three (6). One larger study of 101 patients with anxiety showed improvement (p<0.0001) on the Hamilton Anxiety Scale but not on the Clinical Global Impression Scale (7). Case reports suggest usefulness in "spinal seizures," epilepsy, and psychosis. Claims are made for the treatment of asthma, depression, insomnia, muscle spasms, pain, rheumatism, sexually transmitted disease, and wound healing. These are based on anecdotal reports.

Synonyms for kava are ava, awa, kava-kava, kawa, kew sakau, tonga, and yagona. Common trade names are Aigin®, Antares®, Ardeydystin®, Cekfava®, Kava Kava Liquid®, Kava Kava Root®, Kavarouse®, Kavasedon®, Kavasporal®, Kava Stress®, Kavatino®, Kavatrol®, Laitan®, Mosaro®, Nervonocton N®, Potter's Antigian Tablets®, Super 5HT with Kava®, and Viocava®. *Piper methysticum* is a member of the black pepper family, indigenous to the South Pacific islands. Clinical effects are said to include anesthetic activity, muscle relaxation, mild euphoria, and pupillary dilatation. It is also said to have fungistatic properties.

Adverse reactions include hyporeflexia, sedation, ataxia, headache, dizziness, vision changes, hypertension, diarrhea, thrombocytopenia, lymphopenia, weight loss, dyspnea, skin hypersensitivity, dopamine antagonism, red eyes, and hematuria. In the past several years, 24 cases of hepatotoxicity were reported in Germany and Switzerland, and the German government is investigating whether kava should be more closely regulated (8,9). Kava should be avoided in pregnant and lactating women, children under 12, and patients with renal disease, neutropenia, and thrombocytopenia.

Mistletoe

Despite known toxic effects, mistletoe (*Viscum* sp.) is a widely used remedy for various ailments, especially in Germany; however, this is a highly toxic substance. Mistletoe can cause cardiac, CNS, and GI toxicity. In vitro studies show antineoplastic activity, with cytotoxic effects and the release of cytokines and tumor necrosis factor (TNF-alpha). One study found increased CD3/25 lymphocyte counts in HIV patients and increased granulocyte activity. In mice, mistletoe protects against pentylenetetrazole (PTZ)-induced and bicuculline-induced seizures. No change was seen in the NMDA (tonic) seizure model (10). Claims are made for usefulness in arteriosclerosis, cancer, depression, epilepsy, hypertension, headaches, insomnia, nervousness, sterility, tachycardia, tension, ulcers, and urinary disorders. Possible improvement was reported in one patient with small cell lung cancer (11). Synonyms for mistletoe are all-heal, birdlime, devil's fuge, European mistletoe, golden bough, and viscum. Common trade names are Helixor®, Iscador®, Iscucin®, Plenosol®, and Viscum Album Quercus Frischsaft®. *Viscum* plants (leaves, branches, and berries) are native to England, Europe, and Asia. North American mistletoes are primarily used as Christmas greens. They are parasitic plants that grow on fruit trees, poplars, and oaks. Mistletoe contains amines, acetylcholine, choline, histamine, tyramine, flavonoids, lectins, alkaloids, acids, and other components that cause a number of adverse effects.

Adverse reactions include coma, sedative effects, seizures, bradycardia, cardiac arrest, cardiac depression, hypotension and hypertension, hepatitis, uterine stimulation, nausea, vomiting, diarrhea, gastritis, psychosis, miosis, and mydriasis. Mistletoe should not be used in pregnant or lactating women. The patient should be monitored for dehydration and electrolyte imbalance.

Mugwort

Mugwort (*Artemisia vulgaris*) has generated positive results in Western medicine for the correction of breech presentation (12). There is a lack of clinical data supporting mugwort's safety and efficacy, however, and its use cannot be recommended. Synonyms for mugwort are ai ye, armoise commune, artemesia, carline thistle, felon herb, gemeiner beifuss, hierba de San Juan, sailor's tobacco, St. John's plant, Summitates artemisiae, and wild wormwood. The common trade name is Phyto Surge®.

Artemisia vulgaris is a member of the daisy family, native to northern Europe, Asia, and North America. Mugwort is not the same as wormwood (*A. absinthium*). Claimed therapeutic actions are multiple: abortifacient, analgesic, antihelminthic, antibacterial, antiflatulent, antifungal, antirheumatic, antiseptic, aphrodisiac, appetite stimulant, bile stimulant, CNS depressant, diaphoretic, digestive, diuretic, emetic, expectorant, hemostatic, laxative, sedative, uterine stimulant, and uterine vasodilator. The use of mugwort is similar to that of traditional wormwood: as an antihelminthic and for amenorrhea and dysmenorrhea. Mugwort is used in moxibustion treatments at acupuncture points in Chinese traditional medicine. It has also been used for abdominal cramps, constipation, diarrhea, chills, depression, epilepsy, fever, menopausal and menstrual complaints, rheumatism, vomiting, and psychiatric symptoms, including anxiety, depression, hysteria, hypochondriasis, insomnia, irritability, restlessness, neuroasthenia, and neuroses.

Adverse reactions include significant uterine stimulant effects, contact dermatitis, allergic reactions, and anaphylaxis. Mugwort is contraindicated in pregnancy, lactation, coagulopathies, and gastroesophageal reflux. Mugwort pollen is an allergen that contributes to hay fever, with cross-sensitivity to hazelnut, tobacco, honey, or jelly.

Pipsissewa

Claims are made for efficacy of pipsissewa (*Chimaphila umbellate*) as an anticonvulsant, antispasmodic, astringent, diaphoretic, and diuretic. This herb lacks clinical evidence at safe doses and therapeutic claims, and should not be consumed. Synonyms for pipsissewa are ground holly, prince's pine, spotten wintergreen, and wintergreen. The common trade name is Pipsissew Fresh Upper Leaves®. *Chimaphila umbellate* is a creeping perennial herb of the heath family native to Eurasia and northern North America. Clinical actions include hypoglycemic action in animals, and it reportedly increases renal circulation and stimulates renal tubular function.

Adverse reactions are GI irritation, nausea, vomiting, diarrhea, and rash. Pipsissewa should be used with caution in patients with GI disorders, iron deficiency, and malabsorption disorders. It should not be used in lactating patients.

Scullcap

Virtually no clinical trial evidence exists regarding the use of scullcap (*Scutellaria laterifolia, S. baicalensis*), and insufficient evidence recommends it for any condition or disease. Some studies suggest immunogenic (13) and hematopoietic benefits (14) in cancer patients. Anti-inflammatory action is reportedly produced by inhibiting interleukin-1, prostaglandin E2, and leukotriene B4 (15). Other studies show decreased 5-FU and cyclophosphamide myelotoxicity and tumor cell viability in mice (16). In vitro studies have evaluated its effect as an antiviral agent (influenza, HIV, EBV). It may have antioxidant effects (17). Synonyms for scullcap are helmet flower and hoodwort. The source is leaves and roots of *Scutellaria laterifolia* and *S. baicalensis*, native to temperate regions of North America. Claims are made for clinical activity as an anticonvulsant, sedative, antihelminthic, and antibacterial. It is also said to have anti-inflammatory, cholesterol-lowering, and antispasticity effects.

Adverse reactions are hepatotoxicity, confusion, seizures, stupor, cardiac arrhythmias, and fasciculations. It should be used with great caution during pregnancy and lactation, and liver function studies should be monitored. Commercial forms are often adulterated with other herbs and alcohol.

Melatonin

Although melatonin is not an herb, its widespread use warrants discussion. Melatonin is a chronobiotic, a term analogous to nutribiotic when used for vitamins and herbs. Melatonin is a derivative of serotonin metabolism. It is marketed as a dietary supplement because it is found in some plants. It is neither FDA-approved nor regulated. Melatonin is normally produced by the pineal gland, and it is secreted to the hypothalamus, where it likely promotes sleep. The circadian rhythm of melatonin production reveals secretion beginning in the evening, with peak melatonin levels about 2–3 A.M., and then a rapid fall at approximately 6 A.M. Melatonin can be helpful for jet lag and disorders of delayed sleep phase. Normal sleep phase can be restored in patients with delayed sleep phase syndrome after administration of melatonin for 2 to 6 weeks.

There are reports of antiseizure effects of melatonin. Animal models suggest a link between seizures and melatonin. In animals, antimelatonin antibody can induce seizures (18). Pinealectomy may produce seizures in rats (19). Audiogenic seizures in rats produce pineal damage (20). In adult humans, no placebo-controlled trials in epilepsy have been undertaken; however, no change in melatonin rhythms were observed after daytime tonic-clonic, complex partial, or psychogenic seizures (21). A small number of pediatric patients with photosensitive epilepsy had low melatonin levels (22). Variable effects of melatonin on seizure frequency are reported, with both an increase (23) and a decrease in seizure frequency (24). Improvement in sleep may confound the assessment of improved seizures associated with the use of melatonin.

Several formulations are commercially available, including immediate release capsules (containing lactose and starch), slow release capsules (psyllium), slow release (OROS), and transdermal. It is recommended to use synthetic (crystalline/white) [not beef-derived (yellow/brown)], to avoid allergic reactions such as serum sickness. The dosing is unknown. Doses range from 0.1 to 2000 mg per day in anecdotal reports. A usual recommended dose is generally in the range of 2 to 5 mg, but no evidence supports this other than common usage. The oral bioavailability of melatonin is 10% to 15% absorption, and metabolism is via the cytochrome P450 (1A2 enzyme) system of the liver. Melatonin enters the brain rapidly; the elimination half-life is 30 to 50 minutes. Interactions with AEDs can occur. An acute oral dose of valproic acid suppressed nocturnal melatonin (25). Carbamazepine may decrease melatonin levels (26).

Melatonin affects multiple systems, including circadian rhythms, reproductive organs, thermoregulation, and immunoregulation (27). Concerns exist regarding its safety. Adverse effects reported include drowsiness, sleep disruption, nightmares, hypotension, male gynecomastia with low sperm count, and abdominal pain. Concerns also exist regarding effects on puberty, in light of delayed sexual maturation in animal studies (28). Melatonin may also cause vasoconstriction, a particular concern for patients with coronary artery disease. The effects of chronic use are unknown (29).

Important Herb–Drug Interactions

Although herbs and supplements are used commonly by patients with epilepsy, their effects on concomitant medications and on seizures themselves are seldom considered. The physician may not inquire about vitamins and supplements. If the question is asked, knowledge is sparse about the desired effects, adverse side effects, and interactions of herbs and supplements with other medications.

Three major types of interactions involving herbs and epilepsy should be considered: pharmacokinetic effects—the effects of herbs on drug metabolism; pharmacodynamic effects—herb–drug interactions that occur in the brain and other organ systems but are not predictable based on pharmacokinetic principles of absorption and metabolism; and the direct effects of herbs on the seizure threshold.

Two principal pharmacologic systems are affected by herbs: the P450 and P-glycoprotein systems. The liver enzymatic system for drug metabolism, the P450 system, may be induced (activated) or inhibited by medications, including herbs. The P-glycoprotein (Pgp) transport system, which regulates the entry of medicines and herbs into the vascular and central nervous systems, may be induced or inhibited by medications, including herbs. Many AEDs affect the P450 system of hepatic metabolism. For example, phenobarbital, phenytoin, primidone, and carbamazepine are inducers of this system. Other agents metabolized by the P450 system have accelerated metabolism and, subsequently, lower blood levels and efficacy when given together with these hepatic inducers. Other medications, such as verapamil, affect the Pgp transport system and lead to less availability of substances to remain in the central nervous system when Pgp is stimulated. Pgp has an extruder function, acting as a gateway to remove substances from compartments.

Although many AEDs affect the P450 system, nearly all available AEDs are themselves metabolized by this system (exceptions are gabapentin and levetiracetam). Carbamazepine, clonazepam, ethosuximide, felbamate, lamotrigine, oxcarbazepine, phenobarbital, phenytoin, primidone, tiagabine, topiramate, valproic acid, and zonisamide all are eliminated (to variable degrees) via the P450 system (30).

Herbs that induce or inhibit the cytochrome P450 enzyme systems will reduce or increase, respectively, the AED level. Several commonly used herbs interact with the P450 system (Table 13.2). This potentially results in unexpected (and unrecognized) subtherapeutic AED levels or toxicity. Foods also may affect the P450 system. Grapefruit juice inhibits P450, increasing many AED serum levels. Broccoli, charbroiled foods, and cigarettes are P450 inducers, lowering many AED levels.

The transport system is the other major pharmacokinetic system important when considering the effects of herbs on AEDs and seizures. Several systems are probably involved with this function; the Pgp system is the most thoroughly studied.

P-glycoprotein (Pgp) is an adenosine triphosphate-dependent pump that moves substrates out of cells. Pgp is controlled by the multidrug-resistance gene (MDR-1). Pgp is found in the choroid plexus and cerebral endothelium, where it contributes to the blood–brain barrier and limits the entry of drugs into the brain. Pgp is also found in the intestinal epithelium, where it limits absorption from the gut. MDR-1 expression, and therefore Pgp transport, is affected by many naturally occurring compounds (31). Any agent that affects Pgp transport potentially affects the intestinal absorption of AEDs as well as their regional delivery to the epileptogenic zone of brain. Herbs that affect Pgp are St. John's wort, garlic, pycnogenol, and pipsissewa. These properties are summarized in Table 13.2.

Pharmacodynamic interactions occur when herbs have clinical effects that may potentiate or reduce the actions of other drugs. For example, betony has antihypertensive properties and may exacerbate the effects of medications a patient is taking for hypertension, thus leading to low blood pressure and fainting. Blue cohosh has antidiabetic properties and may aggravate the hypoglycemic effects of medications prescribed for a patient with diabetes. Kava has increased toxicity in combination with alcohol, benzodiazepines, and barbiturates (39).

Products containing herbs are often combinations of multiple products or are adulterated with impure products. The effects of such compounds are unpredictable. An example is that of case reports supporting an antiepileptic effect of MSM, a nonprescription supplement containing methsuximide (40). Methsuximide, marketed as Celontin®, is a prescription AED used for decades in epilepsy, but practically abandoned due to moderate side effects and limited effectiveness.

TABLE 13.2

Effects of Herbs on Drug Metabolism

Herb	Effect on P450 Enzymes	Effect on Pgp-Mediated Transport
St. John's wort (32, 33)	Controversial ? Inhibits acutely ? Induces chronically	Induces
Garlic (34)	Inhibits	Minimal interaction (? Low to moderate inhibition)
Echinacea (35)	Inhibits	
Pycnogel (36)	Inhibits	Inhibits
Milk thistle	Inhibits	
American hellebore (37)		Inhibits
Mugwort (38)	Inhibits	
Pipsissewa (36)	Inhibits	Inhibits

The direct effect of herbs on seizures is a critical issue. Several herbs used to treat seizures can exacerbate seizures. These include American hellebore, mistletoe, and scullcap. Table 13.3 lists some of the known effects of herbs on seizures.

TABLE 13.3

Effects of Commonly Used Herbs on Seizures

Herb	Effect on Seizures
Ginkgo	Proconvulsant (41)
Evening primrose	Proconvulsant
Ephedra	Proconvulsant (42)
Mistletoe	Anticonvulsant Proconvulsant
American hellebore	Anticonvulsant Proconvulsant
Scullcap	Anticonvulsant Proconvulsant

Conclusion

Herbs that are commonly and consistently cited as effective treatments for epilepsy in the alternative medicine literature have been reviewed here for their efficacy and safety data. Although these herbs are used to treat seizures, a lack of clinical or laboratory data supports the antiepileptic properties for six of the eight commonly referenced products: American hellebore, betony, blue cohosh, mugwort, pipsissewa, and skullcap. Laboratory data support antiepileptic effects for kava and mistletoe, but objective data for clinical efficacy are unavailable for any herb. Safety data are lacking and, instead, significant potential toxicities are associated with each. Several of the top selling herbs paradoxically have effects that may lower the seizure threshold and, hence, provoke seizures.

Herb–drug interactions are important in managing epilepsy, and the use of herbal and alternative products by patients cannot be discounted as irrelevant to the treatment of epilepsy. Herbs or supplements may increase or decrease the metabolism, absorption, or transport of AEDs. Herbs may therefore alter the effectiveness or side effects of the medications a patient is taking for epilepsy. In addition to these pharmacokinetic factors, herbs may alter the pharmacodynamics of multiple medications, altering the effect of medications a patient is taking for epilepsy or other medical or psychiatric conditions. Commonly used herbs may also directly affect the seizure disorder.

The role of alternative medicine in epilepsy is unclear. It is difficult to adopt a position of comfort with the utilization of herbs for the treatment of seizures without evidence of human efficacy, safety, or tolerability. Patients and physicians must be increasingly aware that a complete medication history includes information on supplements and herbs, with consideration of the implications associated with the use of these products.

Sources of Information on Safety of Herbal Products

National Center for Complementary and Alternative Medicine
  http://nccam.nih.gov
Office of Dietary Supplement
  http://odp.od.nih.gov/ods/
EXTRACT database
  Centre for Complementary Health Studies, Exeter University, Exeter EX4 4RG
  Tel: 01392 264496
PhytoNet Home Page
www.exeter.ac.uk/phytonet/
  An information resource concerning development, manufacture, regulation, and surveillance of herbal medicines

Main Regulatory and Registering Bodies in Herbal Medicine

National Institute of Medical Herbalists (NIMH)
56 Longbrook St., Exeter, EX4 6AH
Tel: 01392 426022
Fax: 01392 498963
Email: nimh@ukexeter,freeserve.co.uk
URL: www.btinternet.com/~nimh/

Register of Chinese Herbal Medicine
PO Box 400, Wembley, Middlesex HA9 9NZ
Tel: 0171 470 8740
URL: www.rchm.co.uk

European Herbal Practitioners Association
Midsummer Cottage Clinic, Nether Westcote, Chipping, Norton OX7 6SD
Tel: 01993 830419
Fax: 01993 830957
URL: www.users.globalnet.co.uk/~epha/

References

1. Astin J. Why patients use alternative medicine. *JAMA* 1998;279(19):1548–1553.
2. Blumenthal M, Goldberg A, Brinckmann J, (eds.) Herbal Medicine: Expanded Commission E Monographs. Newton, NJ: *Integrative Medicine Communications*, 2000.
3. Fetrow CW, Avila JR, (eds.) *Professional's Handbook of Complementary and Alternative Medicines*, 2nd ed. Springhouse, PA: Springhouse Corp., 2001.
4. Skidmore-Roth L. *Handbook of Herbs and Natural Supplements*. St. Louis: Mosby, 2001.
5. Grunze H, Langosch J, Schirrmacher K, et al. Kava pyrones exert effects on neuronal transmission and transmembraneous cation currents similar to established mood stabilizers-a review. *Prog Neuropsychopharmacol Biol Psychiatry* 2001;25(8):1555–1570.
6. Pittler MH, Ernst E. Efficacy of kava extract for treating anxiety. Systematic review and meta-analysis. *J Clin Psychopharmacol* 2000;20:84–89.
7. Volz HP, et al. Kava-kava extract WS-1490 versus placebo in anxiety disorders—a randomized placebo-controlled 25-week outpatient trial. *Pharmacopsychiatry* 1997;30:1–5.
8. American botanical council announces new safety information on kava. Available at: http://www.herbalgram.org_site.php/122001press/. [Accessed January 10, 2002.]
9. Connor KM, Davidson JRT, Churchill LE. Adverse-effect profile of kava. *CNS Spectrums* 2001;6(10):848–853.
10. Amabeoku GJ, Leng MJ, Syce JA. Antimicrobial and anticonvulsant activities of Viscum capense. *J Ethnopharmacol* 1998;61(3):237–241.
11. Bradley GW, et al. Apparent response of small cell lung cancer to an extract of mistletoe and homeopathic treatment. *Thorax* 1989;44:1047–1048.
12. Cardini F, Weixin H. Moxibustion for correction of breech presentation: a randomized controlled trial. *JAMA* 1998;280:1580–1584.
13. Smolianinov DA, et al. Effect of S. baicalensis extract on the immunologic status of patients with lung cancer receiving antineoplastic chemotherapy. *Eksp Klin Farmakol* 1997;69:49–51.
14. Goldberg BE, et al. Dry extract of S. baicalensis as a hemostimulant in antineoplastic chemotherapy in patients with lung cancer. *Eksp Klin Farmakol* 1997;60:28–30.
15. Chung CP, et al. Pharmacological effects of methanolic extract from the root of Scutellaria baicalensis and its flavonoids on human fibroblast. *Planta Med* 1995;61:150–153.
16. Razina TG, et al. Enhancement of the selectivity of the action of the cytostatics cyclophosphane and 5-FU by using an extract of the baikal skullcap in an experiment. *Vopr Onkol* 1987;33:80–84.
17. Shaeo ZH, et al. Extract from Scutellaria baicalensis georgi attenuates oxidative stress in cardiomyocytes. *J Mol Cell Cardiol* 1999;31:1885–1895.
18. Fariello RG, Bubenik GA, Brown GM. Epileptogenic action of intraventricularly injected antimelatonin antibody. *Neurology* 1977;27:567–570.

19. Philo R, Reiter RJ. Characterization of pinealectomy induced convulsion in the Mongolian gerbil (Meriones unguiculatus). *Epilepsia* 1978;19:485–492.

20. Alves de Azevedo B, Fontana P Jr. Audiogenic seizures and the pineal gland. *Biol Psychiatry* 1988;23:734–740.

21. Rao ML, Stefan H, Bauer J. Epileptic but not psychogenic seizures are accompanied by simultaneous elevation of serum pituitary hormones and cortisone levels. *Neuroendocrinology* 1989;49:33–39.

22. Miyamoto A, Hara M, Ito M, et al. Serum melatonin kinetics in epileptic children with or without photosensitivity. *Jpn J Psychiat Neurol* 1990;44:432–433.

23. Sheldon SH. Pro-convulsant effects of oral melatonin in neurologically disabled children. *Lancet* 1998;351:1254.

24. Fauteck L, et al. Melatonin in epilepsy: first results of replacement therapy and clinical results. *Biol Signals Recept* 1999;8:105–110.

25. Monteleone P, et al. Suppression of nocturnal plasma melatonin levels by evening administration of sodium valproate in healthy humans. *Biol Psych* 1997;41:336–341.

26. Schapel GJ, et al. Melatonin response in active epilepsy. *Epilepsia* 1995;36:75–78.

27. Weaver DR. Reproductive safety of melatonin: a "wonder drug" to wonder about. *J Biol Rhythms* 1997;12:707–708.

28. Meredith S, et al. Long-term supplementation with melatonin delays reproductive senescence in rats, without an effect on number of primordial follicles. *Exp Gerontol* 2000;35:343–352.

29. Arendt J. Safety of melatonin in long-term use. *J Biol Rhythms* 1997;12:673–681.

30. Fischer JH, Patel T. Guide to antiepileptic agents 2001. *CNS News Special Edition.* December 2001;101–107.

31. Cot JM. Herb-drug interactions: focus on pharmacokinetics. *CNS Spectrums* 2001;6(10): 827–832.

32. Obach RS. Inhibition of human cytochrome P450 enzymes by constituents of St. Johns Wort, an herbal preparation used in the treatment of depression. *J Pharmacol Exp* 2000; 294(1):88–95.

33. Li Y, et al. Effect of flavinoids on cytochrome p450-dependent acetaminophen metabolism in rats and human liver microsomes. *Drug Metab Dispos* 1994;22:566–571.

34. Foster BC, et al. An in vitro evaluation of human cytochrome P450 3A4 and P-glycoprotein inhibition by garlic. *J Pharm Pharm Sci* 2001;4(2):176–184.

35. Budzinski JW, et al. An in vitro evaluation of human cytochrome P450 3A4 inhibition by selected commercial herbal extracts and tinctures. *Phytomedicine* 2000;7(4):273–282.

36. Leonessa F, et al. C-7 analogues of progesterone as potent inhibitors of the P-glycoprotein efflux pump. *J Med Chem* 2002;45(2):390–398.

37. Cox DS, et al. Influence of multidrug resistance (MDR) proteins at the blood-brain barrier on the transport and distribution of enamione anticonvulsants. *J Pharm Sci* 2001;90(10): 1540–1552.

38. Eissa FZ, et al. Effects of feeding Artemissa filifolia and Helenium flexuosum on rabbit cytochrome P450 isoenzymes. *Vet Hum Toxicol* 1996;38(1):19–23.

39. Almeida JC, et al. Coma from the health food store: interaction between kava and alprazolam. *Ann Intern Med* 1996;125:940.

40. Sigler M, et al. Effective and safe but forgotten: methsuximide in intractable epilepsies in childhood. *Seizure* 2001;10:120–124.

41. Granger AS. Ginkgo biloba precipitating epileptic seizures. *Age Ageing* 2001;30(6):523–525.

42. Haller CA, Benowitz NL. Adverse cardiovascular and central nervous system events associated with dietary supplements containing ephedra alkaloids. *N Engl J Med* 2000;343(25): 1886–1887.

CHAPTER 14

Herbal Treatment of Epilepsy: Phytotherapy

Daniel J. Luciano, MD and Marcello Spinella, PhD

Phytotherapy is a form of complementary and alternative medicine (CAM) that uses plants to treat diseases, including epilepsy. The World Health Organization (WHO) has estimated that 80% of the world population uses some form of herbal medication, and it is estimated that greater than 50% of the United States population uses herbs for medicinal purposes, at a cost greater than $3 billion annually. Herbs and other forms of alternative therapy are most commonly used for chronic disorders that may not respond ideally to conventional forms of therapy. In addition, many patients have become disillusioned with the Western model of medicine. They are concerned about the potential toxic side effects and cost of artificially produced medications and would prefer to use "natural" remedies.

Herbs have been popular in Europe for centuries and remain so today. They were also quite popular in American medicine until the twentieth century, when they were largely replaced by pharmaceuticals. In the United States and elsewhere, they remain a mainstay of treatment in the practice of homeopathy and naturopathy. They are still used extensively in many developing nations.

Recently, herbs were found in a pouch worn by a 5,200-year-old prehistoric frozen mummy ("Oetzi") found in Northern Italy; he is now on display in Bolzano, Italy. The first official compilation of herbal treatments was ordered by the King of Sumeria in 2000 B.C. and consisted of 250 substances. The ancient Greeks and Romans also produced written texts on herbal medicine, such as the Roman *De Materia Medica* from the first century A.D.

In early herbology, the principle of the *Doctrine of Signatures* was used. Under this principle, a heart-shaped leaf was used for heart disorders and red leaves were used for bleeding disorders. Of course, this involved a great deal of trial and error. Interestingly, many modern drugs were derived from plants that were used by the ancients. The word *drug* was derived from the old Dutch word *drogge*, meaning, "to dry." At least 30% of the pharmaceutical drugs currently in use may have some plant derivatives in them (1). For example, aspirin was derived from white willow bark, atropine from belladonna, digoxin from foxglove, ephedrine from ephedra, morphine from the poppy, and quinine from chinchona bark.

Commentary

Drs. Luciano and Spinella review herbal therapies for epilepsy. This review complements the previous chapter by Drs. Conry and Pearl. The two sets of authors take different approaches to this important area in complementary and alternative therapies for epilepsy. Whereas the previous chapter by Drs. Conry and Pearl takes a more scientific—What's the evidence?—viewpoint while simultaneously taking a hard look at toxicity data, in this chapter, Drs. Luciano and Spinella provide a comprehensive review of major herbal therapies, examining data for mechanisms of action based on animal or other studies, as well as efficacy in what are largely uncontrolled studies.

The result of these two chapters is a balanced view of herb use for epilepsy, given our current level of knowledge. It is both a frustrating and exciting area for epilepsy therapy. Several herbs are likely to modulate seizure activity and could, if well studied, provide help to many people with epilepsy. In some medical cultures, especially in Asia, herbs have been used continuously for millenia, and their experience could provide a valuable starting point for systematic study. The herbs that have been traditionally used or shown in animal or small human studies to have antiepileptic effects should undergo more rigorous study to examine their potential therapeutic and toxic effects. As highlighted in Chapter 17 on Traditional Chinese Medicine, Drs. Shaobai Wang and Yanmei Li give other examples of herbal preparations that show benefits in preliminary studies. Emerging research in this area will provide more definitive information on the benefits and risks of these therapies. We anxiously await the results!

Herbal Research

Limited scientific research addresses the use of herbs for the treatment of epilepsy, and the experiments primarily involve animal models, rather than human subjects. Over 100 compounds from around the world have been tested; approximately half of them show antiepileptic effects in one or more animal models of epilepsy (2). Only a small number of human studies have been undertaken, performed primarily in the Far East. The results are of questionable validity, however, because the studies involve small numbers of patients. They are not the randomized, double-blinded, placebo-controlled trials required for a sound scientific study.

The lack of human testing results from a number of factors. Herbs are considered dietary supplements rather than drugs by the FDA and, therefore, clinical trials for usefulness and toxicity are not required. Western medicine also has ignored and avoided alternative therapies until recently, and pharmaceutical companies lack interest because patents cannot be issued for naturally occurring products. In addition, Western medical and pharmaceutical research favors the study of isolated chemical compounds, as opposed to the multiple agents found in herbs and herbal mixtures. Clearly, with basic science suggesting the utility of a number of herbal compounds, and the persistence of seizures in many patients despite the use of all approved medications, more human research in this area is sorely needed.

Possible Antiepileptic Mechanisms of Action

Herbs may have antiepileptic effects in several ways. The most obvious may be via tranquilizing properties and improvement of sleep, because sleep-deprivation can precipitate seizures. Valerian, kava, and passion flower may work in this fashion. Valerian and kava may also increase brain levels and/or the binding of the nerve transmitter gamma aminobutyric acid (GABA), which quiets nerve activity (3). Passion flower may act by stimulating sites in the brain that usually receive tranquilizing benzodiazepine drugs, such as diazepam (Valium®) (3). Finally, some herbs, such as TJ-960, may act as antioxidants and prevent cell damage in the brain.

Western Herbs

Many herbs from around the world show some antiepileptic effects in cellular preparations or live animals. These herbs have not been systematically studied in humans, however, and recommendations are based almost exclusively on anecdotal data. Table 14.1 lists Western herbs that have been recommended in various sources for the treatment of epilepsy. Those that are italicized are the most commonly cited and will be discussed in greater detail. Table 14.2 lists typically recommended doses of some of the most commonly used herbs.

TABLE 14.1

Herbs for Epilepsy

Valerian root	Scullcap	European mistletoe
Black cohosh	Kava	Marijuana
Hyssop	Blue vervain	Yarrow
Geranium	Kelp	Bupleurum
Passion flower	Carline thistle	Elderberry (inner bark)
Mugwort	Lady's slipper	Aloe
Betony	European peony	Ginseng
Flax seed oil	Ginger	Linden flowers
Chrysanthemum	Forskolin	Behen
Burning bush	Calotropis	Gotu kola
Groundsel	Lily-of-the-valley	Tree of heaven
Yew		

TABLE 14.2

Recommended Doses of Western Herbs Used in Epilepsy

Valerian	150–450 mg per day at bedtime or in divided doses. Dr. Andrew Weil recommends one dropperful of tincture with water three or four times a day (4).
Scullcap	1–2 grams three times a day. Liquid extract, 2–4 mL three times a day.
European mistletoe	10 grams per day. Liquid extract 1–3 mL three times a day.
Black cohosh	800–2400 mg per day.
Kava	Capsules of root extract, 150–300 mg twice a day with food or liquid.

Valerian (Valeriana officinalis)

Valerian is a flowering herb native to Europe and Asia that has been known as a sedative for thousands of years. It has remained an extremely popular herb in Western countries, particularly in Germany and Russia. Research has shown it to improve the quality of sleep (5), and it is the active component in many of the prescribed and nonprescription preparations used for nervousness and insomnia. Although it has been perhaps the most common herb prescribed for epilepsy throughout the ages, there remains no significant animal or human proof of its usefulness in this disorder. It might work against seizures by increasing the release of and inhibiting the breakdown of the brain transmitter GABA, thereby inhibiting nerve activity in a manner similar to that of the benzodiazepine drugs, such as diazepam (5). Alternatively, valerian might have an indirect antiepileptic action because of its sedative effect and normalization of sleep. Notably, sudden discontinuation of valerian after chronic use can cause a withdrawal syndrome characterized by delirium, similar to withdrawal from benzodiazepines or alcohol (6).

Valerian has been one of the most widely prescribed herbs throughout history for the treatment of epilepsy. It was probably named after the Roman emperor Valerianus, who reigned from 253 to 260 A.D. The Roman doctor Galen called it *phu* because of its foul odor. Known as a tranquilizing agent for many centuries, it was the substance German folklore claimed that the Pied Piper used to charm the rats of Hamlin. (He used it to charm their children away, too, when the townsfolk refused to pay him.) In the sixteenth century, an Italian physician claimed that valerian cured him of epilepsy. In 1597, the herbalist John Gerard prescribed it for convulsions. Valerian was later used to treat "shell shock" during World War I and to calm civilians during bombing raids in World War II. It was in the *U.S. Pharmacopoeia* until 1946, and remains popular as a sleeping aid and tranquilizing agent in many herbal preparations in Europe.

Scullcap (Scutellaria galericulata, S. lateriflora)

Scullcap is an herb, native to North America, that has been used as a nerve tonic for the treatment of restlessness, insomnia, spasms, and delirium tremens in alcoholics. It has been used to wean addicted individuals from morphine, barbiturates, diazepam, and meprobamate. A chemical in the plant, scutellarin, has sedative and antispasmodic effects. It has been used to treat epilepsy, but no experimental data support its use. Scullcap may be used as the dried herb or liquid extract (see Table 14.2). Side effects may include giddiness, confusion, stupor, and twitching (7). This herb should not be used in conjunction with the drug disulfiram (Antabuse®) or drugs designed to suppress the immune system, because it may enhance the immune response (7). Preparations of scullcap may be contaminated with another herb, teucrium, which may cause liver damage (7). Thus, monitoring of liver function may be warranted when using scullcap, particularly if used in conjunction with antiepileptic drugs (AEDs) that are potentially toxic to the liver.

Kava (Piper methysticum)

Kava is an herb native to the South Seas, where it is valued for its calming and sedative properties. Double-blind studies in humans have shown efficacy for treating anxiety (8). Kava also appears to have analgesic, muscle-relaxing, and anticonvulsant effects, though these have not been scientifically proven in humans. The anticonvulsant potential of kava may be mediated via an enhancement of GABA within the brain, or possibly via blockade of sodium and calcium channels, similar to the actions of several standard AEDs (8). Rare instances of abnormal movements, acute hepatitis, liver failure, and rash (8) have been reported with kava. This herb is contraindicated in depressed patients because the danger of suicide may be increased (8).

Black Cohosh (Cimicifuga racemosa)

Black cohosh is a plant native to North America. Its root is used for menstrual and premenstrual symptoms. It may have an estrogenic effect (8). It has also been used as a sedative and in the treatment of epilepsy and chorea. A report documents one person experiencing a seizure when taking this herb, but the subject was also using evening primrose oil, a possible proconvulsant (1). Black cohosh is generally well tolerated at usual doses, producing occasional gastrointestinal side effects. This herb is contraindicated during pregnancy due to an increased incidence of spontaneous abortion. It also amplifies the effects of antihypertensive medications, possibly resulting in low blood pressure (8).

European Mistletoe (Viscum album)

European mistletoe is an epiphytic parasitic plant found primarily in Europe. Though unproven, the stem acts as a tranquilizer and the fruit is used to treat epilepsy and regulate blood pressure. Chemicals in the herb (lectins) are cytotoxic and immune-enhancing. Mistletoe may also improve joint problems and enhance survival time in cancer (8).

Marijuana (Cannabis sativa)

Marijuana is an herb with several potential medicinal properties, including antiepileptic effects. It was first used for the treatment of epilepsy in the nineteenth century. The plant contains approximately 60 active substances; cannabinoids, including THC (delta-9-tetrahydrocannibinol), the main chemical responsible for the mental effects of the drug; and CBD (cannabidiol). Specific receptors for cannabinoids are located throughout the brain in areas that modulate seizure activity. Several small studies have examined these chemicals in various models of epilepsy and in various animal species. THC has variable effects, being antiepileptic in some models and forms of epilepsy (e.g., partial epilepsy), but with evidence that it can provoke seizures in inherited generalized epilepsies (9). Studies using CBD—which does not cause a "high"—seem to indicate it is more purely anticonvulsant. Several small double-blind human studies of CBD in epilepsy found an insignificant reduction in seizures; however, the study populations were small, and low doses of CBD were used (9). One epidemiologic study of drug use and new onset seizures found that marijuana may be protective against first seizures in men (10). As with alcohol, withdrawal seizures may occur upon sudden discontinuation after regular use (10); the author (DL) has seen this occur in four patients. The data on marijuana and epilepsy remain very mixed and no general statements can be made. The compound CBD, derived from marijuana, may prove most useful, but further research is needed. In addition, marijuana use remains illegal at this time, and its long-term use is associated with other health problems, such as pulmonary and endocrine disorders.

Eastern Herbs

Herbs, as well as other alternative therapies, have historically played a much greater role in Eastern medicine, which often uses mixtures of herbs rather than single agents. As a result, it is difficult to know which of the components may actually be responsible for antiepileptic effects. In addition, published studies on these herbs do not include comparison with a placebo or "blinding" of the experimenters, thus the results may not be scientifically sound.

Qingyangsen is a mixture of Chinese roots that was given to 32 patients with an average of four generalized tonic-clonic seizures per month who were not controlled on AEDs. After 2 to 9 months of treatment, nine patients were reportedly seizure-free without side effects (11). An animal study of this mixture combined with phenytoin showed that it may reduce the production of those proteins in brain cells that may contribute to the occurrence of seizures (12). Another unblinded study treatment using a mixture of 13 Chinese herbs was compared to phenobarbital (1). One hundred patients received the herbal mixture and 40 received phenobarbital. Seizure improvement was similar in the two groups after 8 months of treatment, but fewer side effects were experienced by those using the herbal mixture.

In another study, the herbal preparation *Zhenxianling*, which contains peach flower buds, human placenta, and other ingredients, was given to 239 patients (13). A

>75% reduction in seizures was reported in 66%, and a >50% reduction in another 30% of persons studied.

Two Asian herbal mixtures of the same nine herbs have been reported to have similar antiepileptic efficacy: Japanese *sho-saiko-to* (or *saiko-keishi-to*) and Chinese *chai-hu-keui-chi-tang* (bupleurum-cinnamon combination) (14). These are composed of *Bupleurum falcatum* (thorowax) root, *Paeonia lactiflora* (peony) root, *Pinellia ternata* (ban xia) rhizome, *Cinnamomum cassia* (cassia) bark, *Zingiber officinale* (ginger) rhizome, *Zizyphus jujuba* (jujube) fruit, *Panax ginseng* (Asian ginseng) root, *Scutellaria baicalensis* (scullcap) root, and *Glycyrrhiza uralensis* (licorice, gan cao) rhizome in differing ratios (14). Animal studies show that this herbal mixture may prevent seizures by inhibiting the effects of calcium or by affecting cyclic nucleotides in nerve cells (15). A similar mechanism may explain the antiepileptic affect of *Coleus forskohlii*, an important herb in the Ayurvedic treatment of epilepsy (14). Some human studies on these Oriental herbal mixtures have been reported, but some are unpublished or are in Japanese, and others are not scientifically sound by Western standards. In one study, saiko-keishi-to was given to 24 epileptic patients and reportedly resulted in seizure control in 25% for at least 10 months (16). Approximately 50% showed improvement overall, usually within 1 month. In one unpublished study of the bupleurum-cinnamon mixture, approximately 50% of 35 epilepsy patients were reported cured (17). Sho-saiko-to has rarely been associated with the development of allergic lung inflammation and death, as well as liver injury (14).

TJ-960, another mixture of nine herbs, is the most common and important of the herbal medicines used to treat epilepsy in Japan. Its components include *Paeoniae radix*, *Cinnamomi cortex*, *Bupleuri radix*, *Zingiberis rhizoma*, *Glycyrrhizae radix*, *Ginseng radix*, *Scutellariae radix*, *Pinelliae tuber*, and *Zizyphi fructus* (1). TJ-960 was given to 26 patients with epilepsy and compared with 17 untreated patients (18). After 2 months, 33% of the treated patients showed a 25% reduction in seizures and improvements in cognitive functioning.

Seizures Provoked by Herbs

Although some herbal medicines are considered therapeutic, several herbal medicines may actually worsen seizures. Seizures result from excessive and chaotic activity in the brain, and certain herbs that stimulate brain activity can increase the likelihood of seizures. These herbal medicines may do the opposite of what patients and physicians hope to accomplish.

Ephedra (Ephedra sinica)

Ephedra is also commonly known by its Chinese name, *ma huang*. It is a traditional medicine that has been used for thousands of years in Asia; it was also well known to native Americans in the Midwest. The main active ingredient in ephedra is ephedrine. Ephedrine has stimulating and activating effects, and imitates norepinephrine. It is very similar in chemical structure to amphetamines, which were actually created with ephedrine in mind.

The U.S. Food and Drug Administration (FDA) analyzed cases of adverse events associated with ephedra use between June 1, 1997 and March 31, 1999. A few of these (7 out of 140) cases involved seizures associated with taking ephedra. In many cases, no past history of seizures existed, but seizures were invoked by taking other stimulants in combination with ephedra, such as caffeine or the nonprescription drug phenylpropanolamine. Ephedra stimulates the brain and may worsen seizures, so it is probably best avoided by people who have experienced seizures. It is a main ingredient in the recreational drug herbal ecstasy.

Herbs Containing Caffeine

Caffeine is perhaps the most commonly used stimulant in the world. Several plants produce caffeine and theophylline and theobromine, which are close relatives of caffeine. Most people readily know that coffee (*Coffea arabica* and *C. robusta*) and tea (*Camellia sinensis*) have caffeine in them, but several other herbal medicines also contain caffeine. Cocoa (*Theobroma cacao*) is the main ingredient in chocolate-flavored foods, from candy bars to hot cocoa. There are usually 20 to 60 milligrams of caffeine in an average chocolate bar (200 grams of chocolate). That isn't a lot of caffeine, but eating several pieces of chocolate, particularly dark chocolate, can add up to a significant amount. It also takes the body several hours to process caffeine, so eating several pieces throughout a day can have a cumulative effect. Cocoa also has higher amounts of theobromine in it, which acts in a manner similar to caffeine.

The cola nut (sometimes spelled *kola*) (*Cola acuminata* and *Cola nitida*) comes from Africa and also contains caffeine. As the name suggests, it was part of the original recipe for Coca-Cola®. Two plants from South America, maté (*Ilex paraguariensis*) and guarana (*Paulinia cupana*), also contain caffeine. Maté comes from a holly-like bush and is prepared as a popular tea in Argentina, Paraguay, and Brazil. Guarana is made from the seed of a climbing shrub that grows in the Amazon. It was used as a stimulant by Amazonian natives, but its popularity in developed countries has been growing. People are usually less aware that these plants also contain caffeine.

Caffeine and its relatives stimulate the release of neurotransmitters in the brain, thus increasing brain activity and creating a mentally stimulating effect. Caffeine can prolong seizure activity in several animal studies. Caffeine can also prolong seizures in people who are given electroshock treatments for depression. So, it is probably best for people with seizures to avoid or at least minimize their use of caffeine. It is also important to pay attention to the contents of supplements and foods to avoid the accidental ingestion of caffeine. Many nonprescription weight reduction or energy formulas contain caffeine as a key ingredient.

Ginkgo (Ginkgo biloba)

Ginkgo is a popular herbal medicine for improving memory, and some good research suggests that it may be helpful in this respect. The ginkgo tree has characteristic fan-shaped leaves that are usually processed into an extract and sold in capsule or tablet form. The active ingredients in ginko are *flavinoid glycosides* and *terpene lactones*. It is uncertain how these improve memory, but they may increase brain acetylcholine levels.

The FDA has received seven reports of people experiencing seizures after taking ginkgo. In four of these cases, multiple herbs were taken, but three cases involved ginkgo only. It cannot be determined whether ginkgo actually caused these seizures, or whether the association was due to chance. Many people take ginkgo daily and do not experience seizures; however, ginkgo does activate electrical activity in the brain, which could alter sensitivity to seizures. It may be safer for people diagnosed with epilepsy to avoid taking gingko until more is known about its effects.

Ginseng (Panax ginseng and Panax quinquefolius)

The name *ginseng* typically refers to two plants, Asian ginseng (*Panax ginseng*) and American ginseng (*Panax quinquefolius*). A third plant, Siberian "ginseng" (*Eleutherococcus senticosus*) is unrelated to actual ginseng and little is known about it. American and Asian ginseng have several of the same active ingredients, *ginsenosides*. Both plants have a reputation for treating many different ailments, including memory loss. Although animal research indicates that ginseng may improve memory, very little research has been done to prove or disprove this in humans.

Ginseng can cause several chemical changes in the brain, so it is hard to predict what effect it may have on seizures. Ginseng activates the hypothalamic-pituitary-adrenal stress hormone system. Stress hormones can worsen seizures, and it may best for people with epilepsy to avoid them.

Evening Primrose (Oenothera biennis) and Borage (Borago officinalis)

Evening primrose has become a popular herb for premenstrual syndrome, although whether it really helps is uncertain because the results of research have been inconsistent. Borage has a reputation for treating depression, inflammation, fevers, and coughs, but these effects have never been tested. Both plants are sources of the fatty acid, gamma-linolenic acid, but it is not certain what effect gamma-linolenic acid has on seizures. Some research suggests that these herbs may reduce seizures; some suggests that they may increase them. More research is needed to resolve this issue, so it may be best for patients to avoid evening primrose and borage until more is known about their effects.

Essentials Oils

Essential oils are extracted from a variety of plants and used for aromatherapy, massage, and other purposes. An essential oil may contain hundreds of chemicals in a highly concentrated form. Although it may seem harmless to simply smell something or rub it on the skin, as opposed to swallowing a tablet, chemicals can gain entry into the body and the brain by these routes. The lungs are a very fast way to deliver a drug into the blood-stream; this is what occurs when a person inhales or smokes a drug.

Several essential oils can worsen seizures. In some reported cases, certain oils caused seizures in people who had not experienced seizures previously. Some of these cases involved ingesting the oils by mouth and others through absorption through the skin. The essential oils of greatest concern are: eucalyptus (*Eucalyptus globulus*), fennel (*Foeniculum vulgare*), hyssop (*Hyssopus officinalis*), pennyroyal (*Mentha pulegium* or *Hedeoma pulegioides*), rosemary (*Rosmarinus officinalis*), sage (*Salvia officinalis*), savin (*Juniperus sabina*), tansy (*Tanacetum vulgare*), thuja (*Thuya occidentalis*), turpentine (*Pinus species*), and wormwood (*Artemisia absinthium*). Wormwood is the active ingredient in the alcoholic beverage absinthe, which contains the convulsant chemical thujone. This substance may have caused or worsened Vincent van Gogh's epilepsy and hallucinations (19). Many of these plants are commonly used as cooking spices and may seem harmless at face value; however, unlike normal cooking spices, they are highly concentrated in essential oil form. They should be avoided by people who have seizures.

Other Herbs

Rarely, seizures were reportedly provoked by the herbs bearberry (*Arcostaphylos uva-ursi*), yohimbe (*Pausinystalia yohimbe*), monkshood (*Aconitum* sp.), and water-hemlock (*Cicuta douglasii*) (1). There was one report of a seizure in a person using black cohosh (*Cimifuga racemosa*), but this person was also using evening primrose oil simultaneously. Seizures may also be precipitated by the abrupt discontinuation of herbs with sedative properties, such as valerian and kava.

Herbs That Interact with Prescription Medications

Several herbs may interact with AEDs, for a number of reasons. Some herbs have actions similar to antiepileptic medications, thus excessively magnifying the effects of those medications. For example, the herbs valerian, kava, passionflower, and chamomile may amplify the sedative effects of AEDs. Others may change the way the body breaks down the AEDs, so that the body breaks down the medication too slowly or too quickly.

Herbal Sedatives

The active ingredients in kava are known as *kavalactones*; they have at least two effects that can interact with antiepileptic drugs. Kavalactones magnify the effects of GABA, which slows down (inhibits) activity in the brain. Certain AEDs, such as phenobarbital and benzodiazepines, similarly enhance the action of GABA. Kavalactones also reduce the electrical excitability of brain cells in a manner similar to carbamazepine (Tegretol®) and phenytoin (Dilantin®). Thus, taking kava at the same time as AEDs would likely magnify the effects, causing clouded thinking and excessive sedation.

The active ingredients in valerian are *terpenes* and, similar to kavalactones, these seem to boost the effects of GABA, thereby reducing activity in the brain. Research in humans has shown that valerian has sedative effects. Taking valerian in combination with AEDs could cause oversedation and difficulty in thinking. Specifically, animal studies have shown that valerian has an additive effect when used with barbiturates and benzodiazepines (8).

Passionflower (*Passiflora coerulea* and *Passiflora edulis*) are flowering North American plants that also bear the sweet passionfruit. Native Americans have long used passionflower tea for its sedative and anxiety-reducing effects. The active ingredient in passionflower may be the flavonoid chemical *chrysin*, which acts in a manner similar to the benzodiazepines, such as diazepam and alpraxolam (Xanax®). Both animal and human studies have shown passionflower to have sedative and anxiety-reducing effects. One study showed antiepileptic effects in mice, but this has never been tested in humans. Thus, taking passionflower at the same time as AEDs could magnify their effects.

Two species of chamomile are commonly used, German (*Matricaria recutita*) and Roman (*Chamaemelum nobile*). These are flowering herbs, daisylike in appearance. Chamomile is traditionally used for its relaxing and digestive effects. The active ingredients in chamomile also appear to be flavonoids, as are found in passionflower. Flavonoids work in a manner similar to benzodiazepine medications. The mild sedative effect of chamomile might magnify the side effects of AEDs; however, interactions between chamomile and antiepileptic medications have never been reported. Nevertheless, people taking AEDs and drinking chamomile tea should be aware of a possible additive effect.

St. John's wort (*Hypericum perforatum*) is popular for treating depression, and research supports its efficacy for depression of mild to moderate severity. A few studies show an efficacy similar to that of some prescription antidepressants. St. John's wort may interact with AEDs or increase the liver metabolism of certain drugs, giving them less of an effect than intended. For example, St. John's wort can affect warfarin (used to prevent blood clotting), cyclosporin (used in organ transplants), and indinavir (used to treat HIV). St. John's wort does not appear to affect carbamazepine, but it may lower the levels of other AEDs metabolized in the liver, such as phenytoin and phenobarbital. *Paeoniae radix*, a component of TJ-960 (discussed previously), delays the absorption of phenytoin, and *Shankapushpi*, an Ayurvedic herbal preparation for epilepsy, may lower phenytoin levels (1).

Several herbs can inhibit the liver enzyme cytochrome P450, which is involved in the breakdown of many drugs, including AEDs (e.g., phenytoin, carbamazepine, and phenobarbital). These herbs include garlic, echinacea, licorice, chamomile, wild cherry (*Trifolium pratense*), and dillapiol (1). The resulting elevation in drug levels might cause clinical toxicity.

Using Herbs Wisely

Herbs, although natural, can have significant side effects. In addition, because they are not closely regulated, many side effects may not be reported. There has been concern over kava potentially causing liver damage (8). Twenty-five cases were reported in other countries, and the FDA is investigating cases reported domestically. It is difficult to know whether kava actually caused the liver problems, or whether these cases are chance association. Pacific Islanders have been using kava for hundreds of years, and they do not seem to have an unusual increase in liver disease. Continued monitoring and research will be needed to resolve this issue. Kava may present a greater danger to people with liver disease or those taking additional drugs that can affect the liver, even if it is safe in healthy people.

Most herbs are used to treat minor health problems, as opposed to major diseases, such as epilepsy. Therefore, they should not be considered a substitute for prescribed AEDs. Patients using herbs should notify their physician, due to the risk of interactions with medications. Likewise, herbal practitioners should be advised as to the medical history of those who consult them, including allergies and medications being taken. Notably, 40% of patients using CAMs did not report their use to their physicians (20). Patients should also be aware that it is wise to discontinue herbs at least 2 weeks prior to any surgery, because some herbs may cause bleeding irregularities or may interfere with anaesthesia.

The Regulation of Herbal Medicine

There is a tendency to put great trust in herbs because they are "natural" and, therefore "better" than artificially produced pharmaceutical drugs. Herbs are not considered drugs by the FDA, but rather dietary supplements that are largely unregulated, unlike drugs. As a result, the amount of active ingredient can vary between products manufactured by different companies, and even between batches produced by the same company. A company that produces herbs has to provide a reasonable assurance that their products are not harmful and the company cannot claim that its product cures or prevents a disease. Otherwise, a company can make any other claim about the supposed benefits without supporting evidence. No legal requirement stipulates that herb manufacturers list the contents, side effects, safety, efficacy, or drug interaction information on the label. The FDA can only recall an herb if harmful effects are found. This information highlights the fact that patients should find out as much as possible about an herbal preparation before taking it.

References

1. Tyagi A, Delanty N. Herbal remedies, dietary supplements, and seizures. *Epilepsia* 2003; 44(2):228–235.
2. Nsour WM, Lau CBS, Wong ICK. Review on phytotherapy in epilepsy. *Seizure* 2000;9: 96–107.
3. Spinella M. Herbal medicines and epilepsy: the potential for benefit and adverse effects. *Epilepsy Behav* 2001;2:524–532.
4. Weil A. *Natural Health, Natural Medicine: A Comprehensive Manual for Wellness and Self-Care.* Boston: Houghton Mifflin, 1990.
5. Schulz H, Stolz C, Muller J. The effect of valerian extract on sleep polygraphy in poor sleepers: a pilot study. *Pharmacopsychiatry* 1994;27:147–151.

6. Garges HP. Cardiac complications and delirium associated with Valerian root withdrawal. *JAMA* 1998;280:1566–1567.

7. Fetrow CW, Avila JR. Efficacy of the dietary supplement S-adenosyl-L-methionine. *Ann Pharmacother* 2001;35:1414–1425.

8. *PDA for Herbal Medicine*, 2nd ed. Montvale, NJ: Medical Economics Co., 2000.

9. Gordon E, Devinsky O. Alcohol and marijuana: effects on epilepsy and use by patients with epilepsy. *Epilepsia* 2001;42(10):1266–1272.

10. Ng SK, Brust JC, Hauser WA, et al. Illicit drug use and the risk of new-onset seizures. *Am J Epidemiol* 1990;132:47–57.

11. Ding Y, Xiaoxian H. Traditional Chinese herbs in treatment of neurologic and neurosurgical disorders. *Can J Neurol Sci* 1986;13:210–213.

12. Qing G, Peigen K. Studies of Qingyangshen (II): modulatory effect of co-treatment with Qingyangshen and diphenylhydantoin sodium on rat hippocampal c-fos expression during seizures. *J Tradit Chin Med* 1996;16:48–50.

13. Tiancai W. Effects of Chinese medicine Zhenxianling in 239 cases of epilepsy. *J Tradit Chin Med* 1996;16:94–97.

14. Yarnell E, Abascal K. An herbal formula for treating intractable epilepsy. *Alternative and Complementary Therapies* 2000;203–206.

15. Morello G. Treating epilepsy effectively. *Am J Natural Med* 1996;3(8):14–20.

16. Narita Y, Satowa H, Kokubu T, et al. Treatment of epileptic patients with the Chinese herbal medicine "saiko-keishi-to" (SK). *IRCS Med Sci* 1982;10:88–89.

17. Packer M, Kligler B. Bupleurum for the treatment of epilepsy. *Int J Chin Med* 1984;1(2):55–58.

18. Nagabuko S, Niwa SI, Kumagai N, et al. Effects of TJ-960 on Sternberg's paradigm results in epileptic patients. *Jpn J Psychiatry Neurol* 1993;47:609–620.

19. Arnold WN. Vincent van Gogh and the thujone connection. *JAMA* 1988;260:3042–3044.

20. Eisenberg DM, Davis, RB, Ettner SL, et al. Trends in alternative medicine use in the United States, 1990–1997: results of a follow-up national survey. *JAMA* 1998;280:1569–1575.

CHAPTER 15

Homeopathy

Simon Taffler, DSH, PCH

A new vision of healthcare is emerging in North America and Western Europe: *integrated* healthcare. This vision utilizes conventional, alternative, and spiritual care from a holistic standpoint. Given the primacy of allopathic medicine in the Western world, most healthcare service providers consider the provision of integrated healthcare from within the existing healthcare system. For instance, a general practitioner may use homeopathy to provide a different approach to eliminate symptoms without addressing underlying causes. In my experience, the holistic components of comprehensive medical practices are employed only when conventional approaches fail, but homeopathy is more than a last resort for epilepsy sufferers. Homeopaths should work in conjunction with allopaths as a supportive resource, rather than as practitioners of an adjunct medical practice.

Homeopathic Reality

Professional homeopaths straddle two paradigms, two visions of reality, and two views of health, balance, and harmony. Conventional medical science—with its biochemistry, radiography, and surgery—is a marvelous triumph of technical prowess. Yet, it is representative of a worldview that has fragmented mind, body, and spirit, and the individual, society, and nature. It operates on the assumption that everything consists of matter and that all phenomena are causally determined by mechanistic forces. Therefore, where nonmatter is involved—consciousness for example—such phenomena are regarded as being of secondary importance.

These assumptions, together with the assumed linear relationship between external cause and internal effect, have produced ideas and values that promote a mechanical view of the body, illness, and disease. Materially bound, conventional medicine assumes that anything that cannot be measured, tested in a laboratory, or probed by technical applications simply does not exist. From such a perspective, it is difficult to understand the nature of healing as addressed by homeopathy.

Conversely, homeopathy assumes the body is alive and dynamic, continuously evolving, with growth perceived as the ground of being. It is not a mechanistic, materially based view of reality, but rather an entirely different landscape of connections, of phenomena that cannot be reduced to simple cause and effect.

Homeopathy represents a continuum worldview: the constant flux of dynamic processes between matter-body-mind-soul-spirit. Material things are viewed as embedded in a living universe, which in turn exists within a realm of consciousness that is defined as "the subjective state of being currently aware of something, either within oneself or outside of oneself" (1). In this context, consciousness includes awareness of objects, events, body sensations, memories, daydreams, night dreams, emotional feelings, and inner speech. Ultimately, it is consciousness that experiences moods, stress, disease, and healing. Subjective experiences can only be expressed and articulated by the individual having the experience. Such verbal reports—together with other sensory perceptions from the patient and the practitioner—are the basis of homeopathy.

Thus, in the homeopathic worldview, human beings have the potential to be aware of, identified with, and articulate all states, from matter to spirit. All events are viewed as phenomena in consciousness, with an emphasis on relationship, process, and interconnectedness. Cause and authority are considered internal rather than external. From this perspective, homeopathy addresses our uniqueness—the personal traits and patterns of behavior that constitute each person's absolute individuality.

Many patients with epilepsy suffer from idiopathic epilepsy, where no pathologic basis for seizures has been identified. This is a disorder in which homeopathy can significantly contribute to treatment by addressing all aspects of the disease process. The following description of epilepsy from a patient (in her own words, during a 90-minute consultation) illustrates the level of communication that a homeopath invites from a patient.

I get seizures. They come suddenly and frighten everyone, so I avoid being with people. I like being alone. I hate small rooms; they always feel crowded to me. I've never flown, as the thought of flying in a narrow tube freaks me out. I think that's what may start them off—a feeling of constriction.

Before a seizure starts, I feel a weird sensation, an aura of confusion. Then I heat up. It feels as if hot water is being poured down my neck to my womb. Suddenly, I'm sweating and smell sour. Everything goes yellow. I completely lose my mind—I become literally absentminded. I stop understanding what people are saying. I hear them, but it's all weird sounds. I don't talk, as I know it would be completely unintelligible. Then suddenly, extreme tiredness—pure exhaustion. It's as if I am in a fever dream. All of my senses are mixed up.

After that comes the seizure.

It's a sudden loss of control, total and complete. Everything feels heavy, and then it's like all the lights just turn off. My jaw moves of its own accord and I chew my tongue. I wake up on the floor, often bruised somewhere. My tongue feels heavy; it tastes metallic and is all chewed up. Afterwards, I'm exhausted and need to sleep—but I feel exhausted when I wake up. Sleep generally doesn't regenerate me—being alone does.

The scariest part is knowing it's happening and I can't control it. They started years ago when I was a kid. My parents think it was after I got sunstroke. They are mostly controlled by drugs, but I still get them occasionally.

Commentary

Many allopathic medical practitioners dismiss homeopathy outright. They regard homeopathic medicines, with their diluted strengths, as capable of producing therapeutic benefit only through placebo effect. The author points out, however, that homeopathy is more than the prescribing of medication, and that all healthcare providers can benefit from homeopathy's intensive focus on history-taking and its holistic approach. The case report presented in this chapter illustrates this well. Although no studies evaluate the efficacy of homeopathy for epilepsy, other disorders have been studied in a systematic way. A double-blind crossover study demonstrated the efficacy of a homeopathic preparation for seborrheic dermatitis, when compared with placebo (1). Additionally, homeopathic medications may be beneficial for otitis media in children and to relieve the complications of chemotherapy (2,3). On the other hand, numerous studies were unable to document efficacy of homeopathic medications for numerous illnesses (4).

Based on the available information, we support the holistic approach of homeopathy, especially with regard to risk factor analysis and lifestyle modification for patients with seizures; however, we cannot support the use of homeopathic medicines to treat seizure disorders until well-controlled studies verify their efficacy. Additionally, we caution patients about the serious risks of discontinuing antiepileptic medications to try homeopathic medicines instead.

References

1. Smith SA, Baker AE, Williams JH. Effective treatment of seborrheic dermatitis using a low dose, oral homeopathic medication consisting of potassium bromide, sodium bromide, nickel sulfate, and sodium chloride in a double-blind, placebo-controlled study. *Altern Med Rev* 2002;7(1):59–67.
2. Jacobs J, Springer DA, Crothers D. Homeopathic treatment of acute otitis media in children: a preliminary randomized placebo-controlled trial. *Pediatr Infect Dis J* 2001;20(2):177–183.
3. Oberbaum M, Yaniv I, Ben-Gal Y, et al. A randomized, controlled clinical trial of the homeopathic medication TRAUMEEL S in the treatment of chemotherapy-induced stomatitis in children undergoing stem cell transplantation. *Cancer* 2001; 92(3):684–690.
4. Lewith GT, Watkins AD, Hyland ME, et al. Use of ultramolecular potencies of allergen to treat asthmatic people allergic to house dust mite: double-blind randomized controlled clinical trial. *BMJ* 2002;324(7336):520.

I have always been a tomboy—always loved being out in all weathers. I'm a walker—like the aborigines, I go walkabout. It started when I was a kid; I would just walk off from the playground to be alone.

I'm passionate about plants and gardens. I've won a couple of garden design competitions—hate it when I lose. I want to travel, to fly, and see trees and plants around the world. Otherwise, no particular physical problems, just annual sneezing fits from lily pollen. Some PMS—achy pains in my womb area that go as soon as the blood starts.

The homeopath, employing an holistic approach to this patient, would aim to treat not only the seizures, but the coexisting problems, including claustrophobia, unrefreshing sleep, and premenstrual symptoms.

The Art of Homeopathy

The clinical practice of homeopathy is founded on empirical principles, primarily that substances capable of causing physical and psychologic disorders can be used to remedy similar illnesses. The growth and evolution of homeopathy is based on evidence of verifiable cures using these proven medicines. It is not, as is often thought, the degree of dilution that makes medicines homeopathic, but the similarity (*homeo*) of the disease or suffering (*pathos*) to the pathogenic affects of the medicine. Importantly, their similarity must encompass the basis of the disorder, rather than just immediate symptoms. Details of the patient's physical, emotional, and psychologic characteristics, as well as any factors or circumstances that ameliorate, aggravate, or modify the condition, are matched with the medicine. The concordance between the particular phenomenologically descriptive picture of the given condition and the remedy enable the treatment to be highly personal and constitutionally specific. Therefore, the same disease may require treatment with different medicines for different people, and two different diseases may require the same medicine when the patients are of similar emotional disposition and constitutional makeup.

The underlying assumption in homeopathy is that disease is a process, not a given state. Physical symptoms are seen as an expression of the body in its reaction to an often hidden problem, rather than the disease itself. Homeopathic remedies are viewed as assisting the natural tendency of the vital principal (spirit, soul, mind, and body) to heal itself. All symptoms of ill health are regarded as expressions of disharmony within the whole person and that it is the person who needs treatment, *not* the disease.

The art of the homeopath is, to a large extent, the matching of symptoms with the correct remedy. Mental, emotional, spiritual, and physical symptoms are analyzed and translated into homeopathic prescribing language, or *rubrics*. These translators are organized into repertories and, hence, the translation process is known as *repertorisation*. For the patient described above, who complains of convulsions preceded by absent-mindedness and a sense of confusion, the homeopath would look in a repertory under the rubrics "absent mindedness before epileptic convulsions" and "aura of confusion before epileptic paroxysm" to find the remedies that include these symptoms. To facilitate this repertorisation process and arrive at a remedy, homeopaths refer to reference books known as *Materia Medica* for completeness of the chosen remedy. *Materia Medica* contains collections of symptoms listed according to remedy name. In theory, for any given disease process, there is only one appropriate remedy.

In our example case above, the patient was particularly articulate, which enabled repertorisation with minimal interpretation. The rubrics used were:

- Fear, claustrophobia in narrow places
- Aura from throat to uterus before epileptic paroxysm
- Absentmindedness before epileptic convulsions
- Aura of confusion before epileptic paroxysm
- Perspiration with sour odor
- Metallic taste
- General aggravation or ailments from sunstroke
- Aversion to company, which aggravates, with fondness for solitude
- Pain in the uterus with the menses, ameliorated by the flow of blood

The rubrics indicated—and the *Materia Medica* confirmed—one remedy: Lachesis. This was prescribed over 17 months, during which time the patient slowly reduced her conventional medication as her confidence in homeopathy increased, and a seizure-free state was reached. During the following 3 years she was seizure-free, with no hayfever or premenstrual symptoms; she slept well and overcame her fear of flying after a further 6 months of treatment.

Frequently, a series of remedies must be prescribed before the practitioner and patient arrive at the most relevant prescription. One reason for not prescribing the most appropriate remedy immediately lies in the case-taking and interpretation process. These two processes constitute the art of the homeopath, who uses learned skills and experience to notice similarities in style and form, thus enabling them to see correspondences that patients frequently miss; however, it is not until the patient understands the depth of information required by the homeopath that the correct remedy can be prescribed. In situations in which the patient is unable to fully describe his experiences, such as with children, the practitioner relies on the observations and experiences of family members to fully convey a picture of the epilepsy.

The personal experience of the patient, together with the skills of the homeopath, can lead to a treatment program that assists the facilitation of health goals, such as a life without seizures or a reduction in the toxicity caused by long-term chemically based medication. This is the place where allopathy and homeopathy meet. The combination of symptomatic allopathic treatment with holistic, individualized homeopathic treatment—where no contraindications exist—can lead to an eventual reduction in chemical dependence and epileptic seizures.

The Science of Homeopathy

The complete philosophy and prescribing process of homeopathy was explained and amplified by Samuel Hahnemann (1755–1843) through six editions of his *Organon of the Medical Art*. The principal of the minimum dose was Hahnemann's response to the toxic effect of conventional medicines. He proposed the dilution of medicines in a non-linear, step-by-step, vigorously shaken fashion, whereby the toxic intensity *diminishes* as the energetic effect *increases*. Moreover, he illustrated how this stepwise dilution activates the dynamic effects of substances previously considered medically inert (such as quartz and club moss) or highly poisonous (such as snake venom and arsenic). Homeopaths since Hahnemann have advocated the effectiveness of remedies made from highly attenuated, dematerialized substances and have continued introducing new medicines—approximately 4,000—with 240 specifically for epilepsy.

Despite the efficacy of homeopathy, the prescribing of homeopathic remedies remains controversial. An inability to explain this energetic pharmacology and therapeutic mechanism in conventional scientific terms has inhibited the widespread acceptance of homeopathy as a medical modality for many years. Homeopathy focuses on the individual disease picture and not simply on the physical symptoms revealed by test results or other diagnoses, which means that homeopathy does not lend itself easily to standard clinical trials, because 200 patients may, homeopathically, require 200 different remedies.

Clinical Evidence

Research into homeopathy falls into two categories: (i) research into the mechanism and methodology by which the remedies work, and (ii) research into the clinical effects of homeopathic treatment. There are over 180 trials of homeopathy in the first category, of which 70% are positive. There are, however, no standard clinical trials using homeopathy to treat epilepsy for the reasons previously stated. The majority of published research concerning homeopathy and epilepsy takes the form of case studies, of which over 40 exist. These trial and case studies may be accessed from the Glasgow Homeopathic Hospital Library via their website (2).

Conclusion

Homeopaths advocate for true integration of homeopathy and allopathy in the treatment of epilepsy. Parallel treatment programs, mutually agreed health goals, and ongoing liaisons between practitioners can serve to ensure a smoother path toward the reduction of conventional medicines, as the magnitude and frequency of epilepsy recedes.

Suggested Reading

Kent JT. *Lectures on Homeopathic Philosophy*, 1954.
A classic collection of lectures that clarifies and elaborates on many of the central issues that underpin the principles and practice of homeopathy.

O'Reilly WB, (ed.) *Organon of the Medical Art.* (Sixth edition of Samuel Hahnemann's *Organon der Heilkunst*, 1842.) Redmond, WA: Birdcage Books, 1996.
The latest and best translation of Hahnemann's Organon; the bible of homeopathy.

Sherr J. *The Dynamics and Methodology of Homeopathic Provings*. West Malvern, England: Dynamic Books, 1994.
An outstanding textbook that explains the homeopathic methodology of provings, with a view to ensuring that rigorous procedures are used in all current and future provings.

Vermeulen F. *Concordant Materia Medica.* Haarlem, Netherlands: Merlijn, 1994.
A concordant of the ten best homeopathic *Materia Medica.*

General Homeopathy Books

Koehler G. *The Handbook of Homeopathy.* London: Thorsons, 1983.
An easy-to-read introduction to the principles and practice of homeopathy

Swayne J. *Homeopathic Method. Implications for Clinical Practice and Medical Science.* Churchill
    Livingston, 1998.
An excellent book that explains the principles of homeopathy, emphasizing how homeopaths
    approach their therapeutic task.

Ullman D. *Discovering Homeopathy.* Berkeley, CA: North Atlantic Books, 1991.
A comprehensive introduction to the science and art of homeopathy.

Web Resources

www.homeopathyhome.com
Currently the most comprehensive Internet site regarding homeopathy. Includes a reference
    library of online books, contacts, links, and more.

www.homeopathic.com
Dana Ullman's educationally oriented homeopathic resource site; includes his research articles
    and more.

www.homeopathicresources.com
The Homeopathic Resource Center offers U.S. legal research on the practice of homeopathy,
    together with other useful resources.

Other Resources

National Center for Homeopathy (NCH)
801 N. Fairfax Street, Suite 306, Alexandria, VA 22314
(703) 548-7790
www.homeopathic.org

The North American Society of Homeopaths (NASH)
1122 East Pike Street, #1122, Seattle, WA 98122
(206) 720-7000
www.homeopathy.org

The Society of Homeopaths (SOH)
For more info: SOH, 4a Artizan Road, Northampton, NN1 4HU, England
+44 (0) 1604 621400
www.homeopathy-soh.org

References

1. Farthing GW. *The Psychology of Consciousness.* London: Prentice-Hall, 1992.
2. www.hom-inform.org.

CHAPTER 16

Naturopathic Medicine

NORA JANE POPE, ND

Naturopathic medicine encompasses Western medical diagnosis, combined with treatment and disease prevention using natural therapies. A primary goal of naturopathic medicine is to address the cause of epilepsy, rather than treat symptoms. Naturopathic doctors consider many possible causes or etiologies in dealing with epilepsy. Often these etiologies are multifactorial and can be traced back to microbiology (e.g., parasitic infection), endocrinology (e.g., hormone imbalance), or immunology (e.g., eczema). Other causes can be due to imbalances of a nutritional or energetic nature (e.g., yin and yang or vital force).

Naturopathic doctors (N.D.s) are general practitioners whose medical training covers Western health sciences and diagnosis, as well as a broad spectrum of natural therapies. Since its inception a century ago in the United States, naturopathic medicine has included a diverse list of healing methods, based on the central premise of *vis medicatrix naturae*: through the healing power of nature, the body has intrinsic healing powers as it attempts to achieve balance and homeostasis.

The term *naturopathic* was coined over 100 years ago and means "treating disease by natural means." The first naturopathic medical school was founded in New York City, in 1902, by a husband and wife team, Drs. Louisa and Benedict Lust. They initiated a medical system based on the following six principles:

1. The healing power of nature—*Vis medicatrix naturae*. Nature acts powerfully through healing mechanisms in the body and mind to maintain and restore health. Naturopathic doctors work to support and restore these inherent healing systems when they have broken down, using methods, medicines, and techniques that are in harmony with natural processes.

2. First, do not harm—*Primum non nocere*. Naturopathic doctors use noninvasive treatments that reduce the risks of harmful side effects. They are trained to know which patients they can treat safely and which they need to refer to other health-care practitioners.

3. Find the cause—*Tolle causam*. Every illness has an underlying cause, often due to the lifestyle, diet, or habits of the individual. The naturopathic doctor is trained to find and remove the underlying cause of disease.

4.   Doctor as teacher—*Docere*. Doctor means "teacher" in Latin. A central goal of naturopathic medicine is to inspire responsibility for the individual's success in achieving a healthy lifestyle. Naturopathic doctors appreciate the value of the one-on-one, doctor–patient relationship.

5.   Treat the whole person. Health or disease is the outcome of a combination of physical, emotional, dietary, genetic, and environmental factors. Naturopathic doctors treat the whole person, taking these factors into account.

6.   Preventive medicine. The naturopathic approach to health care can prevent minor illnesses from developing into more serious or chronic degenerative diseases.

Treatment Process

The patient's first visit to an N.D. lasts up to 2 hours. Typically, return visits take an hour. Patients receive a thorough consultation and complete physical examination. Patients are asked to complete a detailed health questionnaire that allows the patient to identify health needs and provides the N.D. with a complete medical history. After the initial consultation, physical examination, and a review of the patient's case, the N.D. will create a treatment program. One or more of six natural therapies may be used in the patient's treatment plan.

Clinical Nutrition

Naturopathic doctors spend a considerable amount of time explaining the benefits of certain foods in the treatment of epilepsy to their patients with seizure disorders. The N.D. takes into account the patient's signs, symptoms, and current prescription medication usage. Blood tests are performed based on this information. Several strategies are used.

Drug-Induced Nutritional Deficiencies

The following drugs deplete important vitamins from the body: phenobarbital, valproic acid, phenytoin, and carbamazepine. The N.D. will recommend either certain foods or nutritional supplements to make up for these losses. Blood tests show that some epilepsy patients have lower levels of a variety of minerals, such as manganese (1), magnesium (2), zinc (3), and vitamin E (4). Supplementation with magnesium or vitamin E may help control seizure activity (4,5).

Uncover Related Physiologic Relationships

Often the N.D. can uncover a physiologic relationship to the patient's seizures when taking the medical history and performing the physical examination. For example, patients with heart disease can benefit from *carnitine*, an amino acid that also shows promise for seizure control. Therefore, if an epilepsy patient has heart disease, a carnitine deficiency should be ruled out as a cause. Another amino acid, *taurine*, has shown promise for seizure control (6) as well as being implicated in cardiovascular disease.

Achieving Balance between Acidity and Alkalinity

As discussed in Chapter 21, the ketogenic diet consists of high fat and low protein, low carbohydrate foods. The goal of the diet is twofold: by forcing the patient to burn fat as fuel instead of carbohydrates, by-products known as *ketone bodies* (such as acetone) are produced. As a result, an acidic environment is created in the patient by metabolic acidosis. This diet can be beneficial, especially if it can be shown that the patient was previously in an alkaline state or had alkalosis (7).

Precautions

Vitamin B3 (niacin) may increase the effect of carbamazepine. An ingredient in black pepper, peperine, increases the effect of phenytoin. Therefore, it is advisable to avoid ingesting these agents when on these medications. Also, phenytoin increases blood levels of copper. Copper is essential in collagen formation, and the author believes this could explain why some patients get overgrown or hyperplastic gums.

Commentary

Surveys have shown that Americans visit alternative care providers, such as naturopaths, chiropractors, massage therapists, herbalists, and acupuncturists, more often than they visit conventional physicians. Other research indicates that nearly 40% of the population has used at least one of these treatment modalities.

Nora Pope provides a clear overview of the field of naturopathic medicine. In her view, the central goal of naturopathic medicine is to address the cause of illness, rather than just treat symptoms. Everyone with epilepsy wants to have the cause treated and eliminated, as do neurologists, but even the most experienced neurologists, using the most sophisticated tests, are unable to find the cause of epilepsy in up to 50% of patients. Seizure medications treat symptoms, rather than the root cause. The other principles of naturopathic medicine are equally attractive: first do no harm, doctor as teacher, treat the whole person, and the healing power of nature. Of course, these values apply to conventional medicine, too, even if all neurologists don't put them into practice.

The naturopathic treatment process, as described in this chapter, includes clinical nutrition, botanical medicine (herbs and dietary supplements), Asian medicine, homeopathic medicine, and lifestyle counseling.

Maintaining good nutrition is indeed important for people with epilepsy. Adequate vitamin D, calcium, and folate intake are particularly key; however, neurologists do not often recommend diets for epilepsy, except the ketogenic diet, which is more effective for children than adults and should be done under the supervision of an experienced physician and nutritionist.

Herbal therapies raise other issues. Studies in patients with epilepsy suggest that nearly 25% have used herbs and that more than two-thirds of this group did not discuss their use of herbs with their neurologists (1). This is of concern, because no herbs have been proven to be beneficial for seizures. In addition, some herbs might lower the amount of seizure medication in the body, thus making seizures more likely. Other herbs might actually cause seizures.

People with epilepsy might take herbs for reasons other than seizure control—for example, as a stimulant, a sleeping aid, a memory booster, or as an antidepressant. While some herbs may have these effects in certain people, there remains the possibility that they will adversely affect seizure control.

Case reports of seizures have been reported in association with the use of ephedra (ma huang), caffeine (coffee, tea, and guarana), gingko, and ginseng (2). St. John's wort might lower the blood levels of certain seizure medications. Herbs with sedating properties, such as kava and valerian, might intensify the sedating side effects of seizure medications.

It is advisable to discuss the pros and cons of taking herbs and dietary supplements with the treating neurologist, in the same way that prescription medicines are discussed. If the reason for seeking out these therapies is to counteract a side effect of seizure medication or to treat a related problem, such as depression, this should be brought to the neurologist's attention, as well, because there may be other ways to help the patient without taking any unnecessary risks. Though some herbs can probably be taken safely by people with epilepsy, none are proved to help seizures. A great deal of further research is needed in this area before any herb can be recommended as safe and effective for seizures.

References

1. Peebles CT, McAuley JW, Roach J, Moore JL, Reeves AL. Alternative medicine use by patients with epilepsy. *Epilepsy Behav* 2000;1:74–77.
2. Spinella M. Herbal medicines and epilepsy: the potential for benefit and adverse effects. *Epilepsy Behav* 2001;2:524–525.

Botanical Medicine

Herbs can be prescribed in their food or herbal tea form, or in a stronger, concentrated botanical form. Naturopathic doctors take into account all possible herb–drug interactions when a patient is on prescription medication. They use several strategies for managing epilepsy with botanical medicine.

Increase Neuronal Inhibition

In experiments in vitro, three herbs show an affinity for gamma aminobutyric acid (GABA) receptors: *Matricaria recutita* (chamomile), *Passiflora incarnata* (passionflower), and valerian. GABA receptors are the same receptors that certain medications target. GABA inhibits the firing of nerve cells. This may be why phenobarbital, clonazepam, and valproic acid help control seizures. The patient may feel a stronger sedative effect if these herbs are taken at the same time as the medications. As a result, the patient may require a lower dosage of drug. The scientific literature has not reported any herb–drug interactions between these three botanicals and the aforementioned antiepileptic drugs. By law, N.D.s cannot change prescription medications, but if patients want to reduce their dosage, N.D.s will work closely with all other medical specialists to do so.

Support Liver Metabolism

Many prescription medications are processed by the liver, which converts drugs into a water-soluble compound that is more easily removed from the body. Liver-friendly (hepatic) herbs can help this process. The N.D. may suggest *Chionanthus virginicus* (fringe tree), gentian, *Leptandra virginica* (Culver's root), and *Cynara scolymus* (artichoke). Silybum (milk thistle) has been reported to prevent liver damage due to phenytoin (Dilantin®) (8).

The following hepatic plants should be avoided by patients taking prescription medication:

*   *Ceanothus americanus* (red root) is an excellent herb for liver support, but it can decrease the absorption of drugs (9).
*   *Rumex crispus* (yellow dock) is a bitter digestive stimulant that is hepatoprotective and treats chronic skin conditions, but it can be hard on the kidneys.
*   *Berberis aquifolium* (Oregon grape) can increase the sedative effects of certain drugs.

Support Kidney Excretion with Diuretic Herbs

If a patient is on an antiepileptic drug that is excreted by the kidneys, herbs that promote urination (diuretics) can be used on a short-term basis to help remove the by-products or metabolites resulting from drug usage more quickly from the body. Two examples are *Equisetum arvense* (horsetail) and *Taraxacum officinale* (dandelion leaf). Dandelion leaf is rich in magnesium, iron, zinc, manganese, potassium, and calcium, which can help balance any potential electrolyte loss. Common foods, such as parsley and blueberries, have a diuretic action and can be consumed on an intermittent basis.

Precautions

As natural products gain more popularity, more interactions are being studied. St. John's wort may interact with phenobarbital, phenytoin, and carbamazepine. If an epilepsy patient feels depressed, other safe products or strategies will be recommended by the N.D.

Asian Medicine

"Same disease. Different causes." This sums up the philosophy of most Asian medical systems.

Balance Yin and Yang

Traditional Chinese medicine (TCM) considers illness to be an imbalance of yin or yang. This imbalance disrupts the *qi* or life force. Acupuncture and Asian herbs address these imbalances. N.D.s consider the patient's history, signs, and symptoms and "symptom picture" to assess whether the treatment should include TCM methods.

Precautions

Asian herbs are gaining more prominence because they can treat multifactorial conditions. For example, patients with eczema or psoriasis have lower blood levels of cyclic AMP. If the patient has eczema and epilepsy, histamine and cyclic AMP levels should be measured. Increasing levels of cyclic AMP not only helps these skin conditions but has also shown antiseizure activity experientially (10). This may be due to its ability to block sodium channels.

Coleus forskolii is an herb from Asia that can increase the body's levels of cyclic AMP (11), and it should be considered if the epilepsy patient has a history of allergic conditions. There are no reported interactions between *Coleus forskolii* and prescription medications, but it is advisable to be cautious if the patient is taking medications that also block sodium channels as well as alter AMP levels.

Homeopathic Medicine

A complete review of homeopathy is presented in Chapter 15. Naturopathic medicine utilizes some homeopathic principles as well.

Support the Patient's Vital Force

Homeopathic medicine views illness as an imbalance in the patient's life or vital force. Samuel Hahnemann, the founder of homeopathic medicine, believed in the healing powers of nature, fresh air, exercise, and a healthy diet to strengthen the patient's immune system. By strengthening the immune system, the N.D. gets a clearer indication of the patient's "symptom picture." This clarity helps the N.D. prescribe more accurately. Many N.D.s use nutritional and herbal strategies as a prelude to homeopathy.

Precautions

Currently, over 500 homeopathic remedies are used to treat epilepsy. All are diluted and therefore nontoxic. None of these remedies interact with any prescription medications, nutritional supplements, botanical medicines, or hormone replacement therapy. Some dramatic results can occur in epileptic patients using homeopathy.

Case Studies

Published cases of epilepsy treated with homeopathy can be found in many American and European scientific journals. An 18-month-old male patient with congenital epilepsy was cured with a homeopathic remedy (12). It took approximately 2 years for his seizures to subside. After 18 months of homeopathic treatment, a 10-year-old female patient with 300 absence seizures a day experienced a fraction of that number after 12 months of treatment (13).

The role of parasitic infections in epilepsy is gaining some attention, and over a dozen homeopathic remedies address this cause. Based on certain physical symptoms, a stool sample should be taken to rule out parasitic infections.

Lifestyle Counseling

An important facet of naturopathic medicine is the encouragement of a healthy lifestyle.

Doctor as Teacher

The N.D. teaches the patient the benefits of a healthy lifestyle so that optimum health is maintained. This appeals to patients who are interested in taking a more active role in their health.

Preventative Medicine: Isolate and Eliminate Seizure Triggers

Epilepsy may have multifactorial triggers. Lack of sleep, stress, caffeine, and dehydration are just a few. Hypoglycemia or low blood sugar is also a common trigger (14). Hormonal imbalances in women have also received more attention in relation to seizures. N.D.s can help patients take greater control of their condition by educating them about these triggers.

Treating Epilepsy and the Menstrual Cycle Naturopathically

Naturopathic doctors have extensive training in the physiology of the menstrual cycle, which can serve to help female patients become more aware of how hormone levels can affect seizures. A healthy menstrual cycle should involve higher estrogen levels in the first half of the cycle and higher progesterone levels in the second half. When some women consistently have more seizures during days 16 to 28 of their cycle, a blood test can determine if a hormonal imbalance exists. Excess estrogen is the culprit in many medical conditions. Hormone replacement therapy is controversial, but N.D.s can help restore hormonal balance naturally by utilizing the following methods.

Nutritional Considerations

Dietary and lifestyle changes can reduce estrogenic effects and increase progesterogenic effects (15). Nutritional and botanical strategies are aimed at balancing the endocrine system by reducing estrogen and increasing progesterone. This strategy can help restore hormonal balance and reduce seizures. Estrogen elimination can be maximized by maintaining liver function and preventing liver toxicity. It is necessary to create healthy intestinal flora and function by increasing motility and function to encourage the growth of the "good" bacteria that decrease estrogen and avoid the growth of the "bad" bacteria that increase estrogen. Finally, lifestyle factors such as stress, exercise, and exposure to environmental toxins, drugs, alcohol, and poor diet compromise liver efficiency and affect the metabolism of hormones (15).

Reduce Estrogen Levels

Phytoestrogens are foods and herbs that contain "plant estrogens" as well as isoflavones or lignans. They have a structure that is similar to estrogen. Isoflavone phytoestrogens can bind to estrogen receptors and lower estrogen levels (16). Also, they increase the blood levels of sex hormone binding globulin (SHBG), also lowering estrogen levels (17).

Phytoestrogens also decrease aromatase, an enzyme involved in estrogen production (18). These foods and herbs encourage the production of "good" estrogen, the estrogen that does not eclipse progesterone production (19).

Sources of isoflavones include soy, legumes, and the herbs *Medicago* (alfalfa), *Melilotus* (clover), and *Glycerrhiza* (licorice root).

Lignans (found in flax seeds) bind to estrogen receptors and suppress estrogen-stimulated responses. Bacteria in the gut convert digested flax to enterodiol and enterolactone (structurally similar to estrogen) in the colon. Enterolactone inhibits aromatase. Therefore, these botanicals and foods should be ingested in the second half of the menstrual cycle to allow the optimum production of progesterone in the patient with elevated estrogen levels.

Increase Progesterone Levels

Progesterone antagonizes many of the metabolic functions of estrogen. Increasing progesterone levels also moderates the estrogen imbalance. Most literature focuses on decreasing estrogen levels, but strategies to increase progesterone levels are also important.

Supplementation with vitamins B6 (20) and E (21), as well as boron and zinc (22) can help with the production of progesterone. Selenium increases plasma progesterone levels in cows (23). Soy foods increase the number of progesterone receptors in normal, noncancerous breast cells (24). Ingesting chaste tree berry (*Vitex agnus castus*) can raise progesterone levels by stimulating the pituitary gland to secrete lutenizing hormone, which, in turn, signals the ovaries to produce progesterone (20).

The highest concentration of beta-carotene in the body is in the corpus luteum, which produces progesterone during the second half of the menstrual cycle. Beta-carotene is required by the corpus luteum for the postovulatory production of progesterone (25). These botanicals and foods should be ingested throughout the menstrual cycle.

Increase Melatonin Levels

Melatonin stimulates progesterone production *and* lowers estrogen levels by binding estrogen receptors (26). Melatonin levels are highest during the second half of the menstrual cycle, and it may be beneficial to increase this hormone to improve the function of the corpus luteum (27). Melatonin is derived from its precursor, serotonin. Banana, tomato, cucumber, beetroot, rice, and corn are high in serotonin (28). Simple lifestyle changes, such as sleeping in a dark room, also increase melatonin levels (29).

Maintain Liver Function

The liver produces bile, which eliminates medications from the body. Vitamin B6 deficiency can cause cholestasis (reduction of bile flow); choline, methionine, and dandelion increase bile flow. Lecithin (choline in concentrated form), L-taurine, and L-methionine (sulphur-containing amino acids) promote bile circulation and increase estrogen excretion from the liver (15). Increasing fiber and using supplements to increase bile flow will increase estrogen excretion into the feces and bile, thereby decreasing estrogen levels (30). Using diet, supplements, and lifestyle changes aids the bowel and liver in hormone metabolism. Liver health is a priority in seizure disorders that are related to hormonal imbalance, because the liver is responsible for the effective excretion of estrogen.

Increasing Motility

If estrogen is not eliminated quickly from the bowel (due to constipation), more estrogen will re-enter the blood stream. Reduced circulating estrogen can be achieved with a vegetarian, high fiber, low saturated fat diet (31). Women who eat a vegetarian, high-fiber diet that is low in saturated fat excrete threefold the amount of estrogen in their feces than their omnivorous, lower-fiber consuming counterparts; they have 15% to 20% lower blood levels of estrogen. A healthy digestive system effectively eliminates estrogen from the body. A diet high in fiber helps move and eliminate waste in the colon. A diet high in fat slows down removal and allows the reabsorption of toxic estrogens. Estrogen becomes water soluble and easily eliminated when combined with glucuronic acid. A high-fat diet increases the activity of beta-glucuronidase, an enzyme responsible for separating (or deconjugating) estrogen from glucuronic acid, thus resulting in estrogen re-entering the bloodstream and remaining in the body. Healthy bacteria prevent the separation of estrogen from glucuronic acid by suppressing intestinal beta-glucuronidase activity (32). The healthy bacteria *Lactobacillus acidophilus* and *Bifidobacterium infantis* can be found in plain yogurt. Supplementation with these bacteria may improve the health of intestinal flora. Fiber also decreases constipation and increases motility.

Environmental Factors

Avoiding environmental chemicals that are known to be estrogenic, such as pesticides, will reduce the estrogen suppression of progesterone production in the body (33). High levels of estrogen from the diet or internal and external environmental sources, create an imbalance in progesterone levels, which can increase seizure activity.

Training and Licensure

Four accredited colleges of Naturopathic Medicine are located in North America: Bastyr University in Seattle (www.bastyr.com) (established in 1978); the Canadian College of Naturopathic Medicine in Toronto (www.ccnm.edu) (established in 1979); National College of Naturopathic Medicine in Portland, Oregon (www.ncnm.edu) (established in 1956); and the Southwest College of Naturopathic Medicine in Tempe, Arizona (www.scnm.edu). All four institutions are graduate schools that require either a bachelor's degree or a minimum of 3 years of undergraduate studies. A naturopathic medical program includes four and a half years of studies in the medical sciences, diagnosis, natural therapies, and over 1,500 hours treating patients. Graduates of this program earn the title *Naturopathic Doctor* (N.D.). The curriculum covers clinical nutrition, Western and Eastern botanical medicine, homeopathy, counseling, acupuncture, traditional Chinese medicine, minor surgery, obstetrics, and several different physical therapies, such as hydrotherapy, physiotherapy, massage, and manipulation. All four schools listed above engage in ongoing research into natural therapies.

To become licensed, naturopathic doctors must pass two sets of North American Board Exams administered by the National Board of Naturopathic Examiners: first, the five basic medical science exams, including anatomy, physiology, biochemistry, microbiology, and pathology; and second, the 10 clinical science exams, which include physical and clinical diagnosis (PCD), laboratory diagnosis, clinical nutrition, botanical medicine and pharmacology, emergency medicine, minor surgery, Chinese medicine and acupuncture, homeopathy, physical medicine, and counseling psychology. In addition to these Board Exams, N.D.s must pass state or provincial licensing exams.

Financial Considerations and Length of Treatment

Fees for naturopathic treatments vary. An initial visit can range from $120 to $250. Laboratory tests cost extra (e.g., a complete red blood cell count test costs approximately $15 to $25, depending on your geographical area).

The first two visits are scheduled closely together; the third visit may occur a month later, depending on the recommended treatment.

Follow-up appointments can range from $75/hr to $125/hr.

Length of treatment is difficult to assess. Some cases resolve completely in 2 years. Some require longer management.

Conclusion

Epilepsy has been treated with natural medicine for centuries. The goal of the naturopathic doctor is to treat the whole person using safe therapies that address the root cause illness. As the layperson becomes more aware of the options in treating epilepsy, it is crucial that complementary and alternative therapies are used with respect and with curative goals.

References

1. Hurley LS, et al. Influence of manganese on susceptibility of rats to convulsions. *Am J Physiol* 1963;204:493–496.
2. Jooste PL, et al. Epileptic-type convulsions and magnesium deficiency. *Aviation Space Envir Med* 1979;50:734–735.
3. Barbeau A, et al. Zinc, taurine and epilepsy. *Arch Neurol* 1974;30:52–58.
4. Ogunmekan AO. Vitamin E deficiency and seizures in animals and man. *Can J Neurol Sci* 1979;6:43–45.
5. Pfeiffer C. *Mental and Elemental Nutrients.* New Canaan, CT: Keats; 278, 402–408.
6. Van Gelder NM. A central mechanism of action for taurine osmoregulation, bivalent cations, and excitation threshold. *Neurochem Res* 1983;8:687–699.
7. Barborha CJ. Ketogenic diet treatment of epilepsy in adults. *JAMA* 1928;91:73–78.
8. Fintellman V. Toxic-metabolic liver damage and its treatment. *Zeitsch Phytother* 1986;(3):65–73.
9. Brinker F. *Drug Interactions and Contraindications.* Eclectic Medical Publications, 1998.
10. Ferrendelli JA. Roles of biogenic amines and cyclic nucleotides in seizure mechanism. *Ann Neurol* 1984;16s:89–103.
11. Seamon KB, Forskolin. A unique diterpene activator of c-AMP generating systems. *J Cyclic Nucleotide Res* 1981;7:201–224.
12. Dimitriadis G. A case of congenital severe hypotonia with epilepsy. *Homoeopath* 1996;June(1):572–575.
13. Leckridge B. I love my work. *Homeopath* 2001;June(1):34–35.

14. Tyson F, et al. A study of blood sugar in epileptics. *Am J Med Sci* 1935;190:164–169.

15. Hoffman RL. The holistic M.D.: estrogen dominancy syndrome. *Conscious Choice: J Ecology and Natural Living* 1999;12(9):33,35,37.

16. Kuiper GG. Interaction of estrogenic chemicals and phytoestrogens with estrogen receptor beta. *Endrocrinology* 1998;139(10):4252–4263

17. Pino AM. Dietary isoflavones affect sex hormone-binding hormone in post-menopausal women. *J Clin Endrocrinol Metab* 2000;85(8):2797–2800.

18. Wang C, et al. Lignans and flavonoids inhibit aomatase enzyme in human preadipocytes. *J Steroid Biochem Mol Biol* 1994;50(3-4):205–212.

19. Xu J, et al. Isoflavonoids and chronic disease: mechanism of action. *Biofactors* 2000;12(1-4):209–215.

20. Reichert R. Comparing vitex and vitamin B6 for PMS. *Quarterly Review of Natural Medicine* 1998;19–20.

21. London RS, et al. Endrocrine parameters and alpha-tocopherol therapy in patients with mammary dysplasia. *Cancer Res* 1981;41:3811–3813.

22. Carr C. Keep your (hormonal) balance. *Conscious Choice: J Ecology and Natural Living* 1998;11(2):55.

23. Kamada, et al. Effect of dietary selenium supplementation on the plasma progesterone concentration in cows. *J Vet Med and Sci* 1998;60(1):133–135.

24. McMichael-Philips DF, et al. Effects of soy supplementation on epithelial proliferation in the histologically normal human breast. *Am J Clin Nut* 1998;68(suppl 6):1431S–1435S.

25. Hudson T. Wild yam, natural progesterone, unraveling the confusion. *Townsend Letter for Doctors and Patients* 1996 July 31;3:228–233.

26. Tamarkin L, Baird CJ, Almeida O. Melatonin: A coordinating signal for mammalian reproduction? *Science* 1985;227:714–720.

27. Brun J, Claustrat B, David M. Urinary melatonin, LH, oestradiol, progesterone excretion during the menstrual cycle or in women taking oral contraception. *Acta Endocrinol* (Copenh) 1987;116(1):145–149.

28. Dubbels R, et al. Melatonin in edible plants identified by radioimmunoassay and by high performance liquid chromatography-mass spectrometry. *J Pineal Res* 1995;18:28–31.

29. Kaur SD. Understanding the hormone puzzle. In: Kaur SD: *A Call to Women.* Kingston: Quarry Press Inc., 2000:57–90.

30. Biskind MS. Diminution in ability of liver to inactivate estrone in vitamin B complex deficiency. *Science* 1941;94:462.

31. Sherwood L, Gorbach SL, Goldin BR. Diet and the excretion and enterohepatic cycling of estrogens. *Prev Med* 1987;16:525–531.

32. Proctor C. Women's Health (lecture). Canadian College of Naturopathic Medicine. March 2001.

33. Foster WG, et al. Hexachlorobenzene (HCB) suppresses circulating progesterone concentrations during the luteal phase in the cynomolgus monkey. *J Appl Toxicol* 1992;321:293–297.

CHAPTER 17

Traditional Chinese Medicine

Shaobai Wang, MD, NYS, LAc and Yanmei Li, MD

Traditional Chinese medicine (TCM) is the study of human physiology and pathology, and the prevention, diagnosis, and treatment of human diseases. It is a system that consists of the clinical and theoretical investigation of the physiology and pathology of organs and functions. Current TCM practice is based on the cosmologic principles of Chinese philosophy, including holism, differentiation, yin/yang, and the five elements. Herbal medicine, acupuncture, and moxibustion are the treatment methods employed in TCM, in order of frequency. TCM has a more than 2,500-year history consisting of the development of major theories and clinical investigations that have been carried out by generations of practitioners and investigators. The theoretical basis for TCM is beyond the scope of this chapter. A detailed discussion may be found in the work of Bensky, et al. (1–3).

Traditional Chinese medicine deserves serious consideration as a treatment option for patients with epilepsy. The TCM approach to the classification and treatment of epilepsy may appear very different from the concepts and findings of conventional Western medicine. Nevertheless, based on modern clinical and experimental research, TCM treatments for epilepsy are as effective as current standard pharmacotherapies and with far fewer adverse effects. In many cases where conventional medications have had little or no effect, TCM herbal treatment provides significant benefits. Moreover, increasing scientific evidence demonstrates the pathophysiologic mechanisms of TCM treatment for epilepsy. TCM is not a "magic pill," but rather a system of scientifically and clinically proven treatments whose proper administration requires an experienced TCM practitioner.

Before reviewing selected research studies demonstrating the effectiveness of TCM herbal treatments for epilepsy, it is important to clarify two key principles unique to TCM: holism and differentiation.

The TCM concept of *holism* considers the individual person as being comprised of and subject to the elements and forces of nature as a whole. At the same time, each individual is considered as a unified, interconnected "whole" comprised of mind, body, and spirit. In practice, this approach leads the TCM practitioner to consider the physical, mental, and emotional state of the patient on the one hand and, in addition, the patient's relation to his environment, including climate, diet, and daily activities. Diagnostically, holism leads the practitioner to assess the health of the patient in all areas, in addition to the specific presenting seizure disorder. With herbal treatments, holism in the TCM treatment approach addresses not only the seizure disorder, but tonifies or balances all the physiologic functions, so that the individual patient's whole functioning is supported. Finally, the TCM practitioner also addresses the prevention of illness, with guidance on diet, exercise, and daily activities, to help prevent the further development or reoccurrence of illness.

The *principle of differentiation* allows a properly trained TCM practitioner to find the differentiating patterns of signs and symptoms of illness—which have been identified in TCM practice over the centuries—that are manifest in each case. Such factors extend beyond the circumscribed pattern of clinical signs of a seizure disorder typically focused on and treated in Western medicine. Such differentiating clinical factors include, for example, particular disorders of digestion, respiration, elimination, and neuromuscular tone, to name a few. According to the principle of differentiation, various pathologic factors and their mechanisms are responsible for or contribute to disease formation; these factors may be different in different patients, albeit their common diagnosis of epilepsy. Thus, using the clinical process of differentiation, the appropriate treatment (herbs and acupuncture) specific to each case is then administered. As a result, TCM herbal treatment regimens for epilepsy are much more individualized than those of Western medicine.

Modern Research on TCM Herbal Treatment in Epilepsy

As practiced in China today, TCM relies on herbal formulas as the principal treatment method for all diseases, including epilepsy. Acupuncture is used as a supplemental treatment (4). During the past few decades, many studies in China have examined the clinical effectiveness and pathophysiologic effects of the TCM herbal formulas used in treating epilepsy. One focus of modern research has been to compare the effectiveness of TCM herbal treatment to conventional Western pharmacotherapies. Although conventional medications can provide a more rapid initial clinical response, TCM can provide a long-term clinical benefit equivalent to conventional medications, but with significantly fewer side effects (5). In China, it is common to use Western medications initially and then replace or supplement these by TCM herbal formulas.

Li et al. (6) randomly divided 306 patients into two groups. One hundred fifty-three patients received the TCM herbal formula *Wuhuzhuifeng San*; the control group was treated with phenytoin sodium, sodium valproate, carbamazepine, and clonazepam, either singly or in combination. A clinical cure—defined by more than 2 years without seizures—was achieved in 67 TCM treatment cases and in 60 patients taking conventional medications. Seventeen cases in the TCM treatment group and 23 controls showed significant clinical improvement; 19 cases in the treatment and 36 cases in the control showed no therapeutic effects. Overall, marked clinical improvement and/or cure was achieved in the TCM treatment group more often than in the medication group (p<0.01). Xiao et al. (7) used the herbal formula *Fuxian San* to treat 148 cases; the control group was treated with phenytoin sodium. Clinical improvement was seen in 97.3% of the TCM treatment group, but only in 70% of the controls (p<0.01). When the comparison was restricted to those patients with a duration of illness equal to or longer than 10 years, the rate of clinical improvement was 96% in the treatment group and 63.9% in the phenytoin group, with a statistically significant difference (p<0.001). Similar findings were reported by other investigators who compared TCM herbal formulas to phenytoin sodium and clonazepam (8,9). Recently, Du et al. (10) and Wang et al. (11) reported no significant difference between *Huabaodingjian San*, a TCM herbal formula, and sodium valproate for seizure control and EEG improvement.

Studies also show good clinical outcomes with TCM herbal treatments for several types of epilepsy. A prospective study on the effectiveness of the TCM formula

Commentary

More than $1 billion is spent on herbal remedies each year in the United States alone. As with Ayurvedic medicine, it would be unwise to dismiss a system of medicine that has existed for thousands of years. Evidence continues to accumulate demonstrating the antiepileptic effects of many herbal medicines, both experimentally and in small clinical trials; however, many remedies are compounds containing several substances, thus making it difficult to determine which agents are active, or equally important, toxic.

One TCM herbal formula, *Chai-Hu-Long-Ku-Mu-Li-Tan* (1), with clear antiepileptic potential, was studied in a well-accepted animal model and found to exert an antiepileptic effect through the stabilization of brain cell membranes and by its ability to inhibit the release of glutamate (an excitatory neurotransmitter responsible for brain excitability and seizures). Although there is no doubt about the potential usefulness of a medication with these properties, no data exist on dosing, toxicity, or interactions of this compound with other medications. Therefore, without proper safety data available, it is impossible for physicians to encourage the use of these herbal preparations. Additionally, although many of these agents are sold as dietary supplements or herbal remedies, they carry the same risks and benefits as the medications approved by the FDA.

For a comprehensive overview of herbal medicines for epilepsy, see the review by Tyagi and Delanty (2).

References

1. Wu HM, Huang CC, Li LH, et al. The Chinese herbal medicine Chai-Hu-Long-Ku-Mu-Li-Tan (TW-001) exerts anticonvulsant effects against different experiemental models of seizure in rats. *Jpn J Pharmacol* 2000;82(3):247–260.
2. Tyagi A, Delanty N. Herbal remedies, dietary supplements, and seizures. *Epilepsia* 2003;44(2):228–235.

Zhenxianling (plus umbilicus plaster) was used for both tonic-clonic and other forms of epilepsy. Wang (12) reported that in 239 patients treated for 6 months to 2 years, 95.4% of the patients showed therapeutic benefit ranging from mild improvement to complete cure during 6 months to 3 years of follow-up. Zhang (13) reports similar results with the formula *Jiaojichujian Wan*, in 476 patients with different types of epilepsy. After 1 year, 304 patients achieved a clinical cure; 167 cases obtained significant clinical improvement; and only 5 cases were unchanged. The overall effectiveness of this herbal formula was 98.9%. In a series of 42 patients with petit mal epilepsy treated with the modified formula *Longdanxiegan Tang*, Li (14) reported clinical improvement in 88.9%. Deng (15) reported that 91.7% of 36 petit mal patients obtained clinical benefit from the original formula, *Longdanxiegan Tang*, with improvements in EEG and a decrease in seizure frequency.

TCM herbal treatments may also benefit patients in whom prior treatment either has failed or has been of limited benefit. After administering the formula *Bushen Tang* to 12 such unresponsive cases, Yang (16) reported that four improved significantly; three achieved moderate improvement; and improvement was mild in only three. Furthermore, in seven cases, EEGs nearly normalized. *Xianfukang*, another TCM formula used for chronic and unusually difficult cases, was found by Liu et al. (17) to provide significant improvement in 25 of 60 patients studied, with most of the remaining cases showing moderate to slight improvement. In addition, post-traumatic epilepsy (PTE) has also been alleviated by TCM herbal treatments. Zeng (18) reported clinical cures in 32 out of 40 PTE cases (80%). More recently, Liu (19) reported clinical cures in 14 of 37 patients with PTE, and significant improvement in 17.

A growing body of research explores the mechanism of action of TCM herbal formulas. Much of this work has been with animal models. For example, He et al. (20) used rat and mouse models to study the effect of the herbal formula *Caoguozhimu Tang* in epilepsy. This formula raised the seizure threshold in four standard epilepsy models. Similarly, Hu et al. (21), used a strychnine hydrochloride-induced and electrical convulsion mouse model and reported that TCM herbal formulas may inhibit cerebral cortex epileptic electrical discharges. Future studies hope to identify the precise physiologic and pharmacologic mechanisms of TCM herbal formula treatments for epilepsy.

History of Epilepsy Treatment Using TCM

In China, 2,000 years ago, prenatal (congenital) factors were recognized as important in the development of epilepsy. Epilepsy subtypes were differentiated and herbal formulas were first used 400 years ago. The symptoms of epilepsy were described then just as they are today. At present, the diagnosis is made by interpreting clinical symptoms, supplemented with EEG and other modern tests, as needed.

TCM has its own schema for the differentiation of epilepsy, the most widely used of which includes four differentiation types. Other approaches to the differentiation of epilepsy identify more types, but these different schemas for the differentiation of epilepsy are not necessarily incompatible. They differ in how broadly a particular clinical form is defined and whether particular clinical variations should be considered as separate major forms or subtypes. Even after thousands of years, such diagnostic considerations still persist in modern Western medicine.

Because conditions and situations vary within the same patient, so do the clinical presentations. In all cases, the treatment formula is modified according to the patient's overall situation. The TCM treatment approach for epilepsy is threefold. First, treat the seizure disorder with herbs and acupuncture, as determined by the clinical diagnosis and differentiation. Second, following improvement and/or remission of seizures, regulate the overall functions of the organs and channels with the use of herbs, acupuncture, and moxibustion. Third, encourage the patient to adopt daily life guidelines to prevent relapse.

Prevention of illness is highly emphasized in TCM. Preventive measures are incorporated into TCM herbal treatment, in which specific herbal combinations are administered to support the overall strength of the body, while at the same time others herbs are selected to treat the particular disorder. In addition, lifestyle preventive measures are also recommended for the overall prevention of illness. These include good personal hygiene, a well-balanced selection of food, good eating habits, the importance of restorative sleep, and proper regulation of mood and physical activity—all prescribed and guided by the practitioner. Regular exercise for both the prevention and treatment of illness is most important and exemplified by such traditional Chinese practices as Tai Chi and Qi Gong, which are enjoying increasing popularity in recent years.

Conclusion

TCM is a comprehensive system of medical theory and practice that, in many respects, is very different from modern Western medicine. TCM should be given serious consideration as a safe and effective treatment alternative for epilepsy, whether conventional medical interventions have been successful or not. Just as with Western medicine, TCM practice and treatment requires specialized training and clinical expertise, and only properly credentialed practitioners should be consulted. When used improperly, either by self-administration or by unqualified persons, herbal medicine and acupuncture may have no effect, or may even cause unexpected side effects.

Acknowledgments

The author wishes to thank the following people for their assistance in the preparation of this chapter:

Mark Ast, Ph.D., Long Island Jewish-North Shore Health Systems, New York

Peter Holt, M.D., Columbia University, New York

Donald Kotler, M.D., Columbia University, New York

Jianqi Liu, M.D., Ph.D., Helsinki University Central Hospital, Helsinki, Finland

Steven F. Moss, M.D., Brown University, Providence, RI

Marc Rubins, D.C., Glen Cove, New York

References

1. Bensky D, et al. *Chinese Herbal Medicine Formulas and Strategies.* Seattle: Eastland Press, 1990.
2. Bensky D, et al. *Chinese Herbal Medicine Materia Medica.* Seattle: Eastland Press, 1993(a).
3. Bensky D, et al. *The Foundation of Traditional Chinese Medicine.* Seattle: Eastland Press, 1993(b).
4. Lin H, et al. The latest development in treatment of epilepsy by acupuncture. *Tianjin TCM* 2001;3:55.
5. Li Z, et al. The development of the epilepsy treatment by herbal medicine. *Hunan Guiding J TCM* 7:205.
6. Li Y. A report on 153 cases of epilepsy treated by modified Wuhuzhuifeng San. *TCM Forum* 1997;4:26.
7. Xiao Y, et al. A report on 148 cases of epilepsy treated by Fuxian San. *New TCM* 1992;10:42.
8. Gao Z, et al. Dianxianmin capsule treated 50 epilepsy cases. *Hebei TCM* 1993;5:17.
9. Tang Z, et al. Xinjia Baohe Wan is effective for epilspsy. *Sichuan TCM* 1993;12:26.
10. Du W, et al. An observation on the treatment of children's epilepsy by Huanbaodingjian Wan. *Practical Integrate J Western Medicine and TCM* 1997;9:841.
11. Wang W, et al. A double-blinded control research on the treatment of epilepsy by Wuchong San and sodium valproate. *Practical Integrate J Western Medicine and TCM* 1997;9:841.
12. Wang T. Zhanxianling treated 239 cases of epilepsy patients. *The J TCM* 1993;4:32.
13. Zhang A. A report on TCM herbal formula treatment of 476 cases of epilepsy. *Shandong TCM Journal* 1992;6:14.
14. Li X, et al. The herbal treatment of petit mal epilepsy based on TCM liver and spleen theories. *Liaoning TCM Journal* 1998;77:310.
15. Deng S. Clinical observation on 36 petit pal cases treated by tonifying method. *The J TCM* 1997;7:418.
16. Yang W. Difficult epilepsy cases treated by TCM herbal formula. *Liaoning TCM Journal* 1989;7:18.
17. Liu Z, et al. Clinical observation on difficult epilepsy cases treated by Xianfukang. *Hubei TCM Journal* 1998;2:32.
18. Zeng J. Regulating blood stasis method treating traumatic epilepsy. *New TCM Journal* 1987;6:35.
19. Liu Y. 37 traumatic epilepsy case treatment based on differentiation. *Hunan TCM Guide* 1997;3:6.
20. He J, et al. A study on pharmacodynamics of Caoguozhimu Tang with anti-epilepsy rat and mouse model. *Beijing TCM University Journal* 1997;2:37.
21. Hu J, et al. (1985). Clinical and experimental study on modified TCM herbal formula for epilepsy. *Tianjin TCM* 1985;6:14.

CHAPTER 18

Acupuncture

KARL O. NAKKEN, MD, PhD

At the National Center for Epilepsy in Norway, our patients express an interest in non-traditional therapies, either as an alternative or as a supplement to antiepileptic drugs, epilepsy surgery, and vagus nerve stimulation. This interest applies especially to those who still have seizures and/or disabling side effects from medication, despite optimal treatment. In their desperation, they turn to nontraditional treatments, such as acupuncture—the Chinese practice of puncturing the body at certain points to cure disease or relieve pain.

In traditional Chinese medicine, acupuncture practitioners treat many diseases, including epilepsy (1,2). Several publications have described the suppression of seizures, both in experimental animal models (2–5) and in humans (6–8), as a result of acupuncture. In humans, the efficacy of electroacupuncture (6), scalp needling (7), and catgut embedding in acupuncture points (9) has been reported in treating epilepsy.

The mechanisms by which acupuncture may influence seizure control are not clear, although enhanced neurotransmitters, such as endorphins, serotonin, and gamma aminobutyric acid (GABA), have been proposed (4,10–12).

To determine the efficacy of acupuncture in patients with difficult-to-treat epilepsy, we initiated a controlled clinical trial, the first to our knowledge within this field (13).

Patients

Thirty-nine adult patients recruited from the outpatient population at the National Center for Epilepsy, a tertiary referral center, entered the study. All had difficult-to-treat partial or generalized epilepsy. Mean age was 39 years; mean age at onset of epilepsy was 11.5 years; mean duration of epilepsy was 27.5 years; and mean number of seizures per week in the baseline period was 2.5. During the 12-week baseline period, but before randomization, five patients withdrew from the study because they found participation inconvenient. Thus, 34 patients were randomized into two treatment groups. At baseline, these groups were comparable with regard to age, gender, duration of epilepsy, age at onset of epilepsy, seizure frequency, and proportion of patients who had previously received acupuncture.

Study Design

The study included a baseline period of 10 weeks, a treatment period of 8 weeks, and a follow-up of 12 weeks. The patients were divided into two groups by four-block randomization: one acupuncture group with 18 patients and one control group with 16 patients. (In block randomization, the unit of randomization is not the individual, but a large group.) Two Chinese acupuncturists, both senior staff members of the Shanghai University of Traditional Chinese Medicine, gave the treatment. All the patients were also diagnosed according to the principles of traditional Chinese medicine. One of five diagnoses was given to each patient. As outpatients, all received 20 treatments (three treatments per week for 3.5 weeks, 1 week pause, and another series of treatments over 3.5 weeks). Each treatment lasted about 30 minutes. The patients' antiepileptic medication was held stable throughout the study, and both patients and epileptologists were blinded.

Acupuncture Technique

The acupuncture group was given bilateral needling of the acupoints LR3, LI4, and GV20, in addition to one or two points based on individual diagnoses. The needles were traditional Chinese acupuncture needles, diameter 0.3 millimeters and length 25 to 55 millimeters, placed at variable depths. The needles were rotated or stimulated manually to obtain the needling sensation (*Te chi*). As part of the individualized treatment, the patients also could have scalp needling or electroacupuncture using a standard transcutaneous nerve stimulation apparatus with acupuncture needles as electrodes. For electroacupuncture, we used an Elpha 2000 instrument (3 hertz, 3–20 milliamperes).

The patients in the control group received sham (imitation) acupuncture. They were given bilateral needling of three sham acupoints chosen by a group of Chinese and Norwegian acupuncturists: S1–2.5 cun to the side of the umbilicus, S2–3 cun above the midpoint of the patella, and S3–1 cun below the midpoint between LI15 and TE14. (*Cun* is an individual system of measurement used in traditional Chinese medicine; it is familiar to acupuncturists around the world.) We chose these points on the basis of minimum expected effect. In the sham group, we used thinner needles (0.25 millimeters in diameter, 13 millimeters in length, less than 5 mm depth) that were not stimulated, either manually or electrically.

Effect Parameters

For effect parameters, we used seizure frequency, duration of seizure-free periods, electroencephalography (EEG) with automatic spike detection, and health-related quality of life—QOLIE-89. (QOLIE-89 is the Quality of Life in Epilepsy Inventory. The inventory measures five factors: psychosocial, satisfaction, epilepsy-related effects, role, physical performance, and cognition.) We assessed these parameters in the three periods noted, registered any deviation from the results in the baseline period, and analyzed them statistically.

Commentary

In addition to the anecdotal reports of the efficacy of acupuncture for epilepsy, several laboratory studies have shown intriguing effects of acupuncture on the brain, compelling us to investigate this treatment modality for our patients with seizure disorders. Using a rat epilepsy model, Yang and colleagues demonstrated a reduction in the activity of the enzyme nitric oxide synthase, which produces the potential neurotoxin nitric oxide, after acupuncture treatment [1]. Using acupuncture, other investigators inhibited seizures in an experimental model of temporal lobe epilepsy [2]. In contrast, acupuncture increased seizure activity in one animal epilepsy model [3]. Whether acupuncture technique alone explains the contradictions in these studies is unclear.

It is unwise to dismiss the potential attributes of any therapy, such as traditional Chinese herbal medicine or Ayurvedic medicine, that has been used for thousands of years. As with all standard and complementary therapies, however, studies such as the one presented here by Dr. Nakken are critical in determining the truth about the efficacy of these treatments. The study failed to show a beneficial effect of acupuncture for patients with uncontrolled seizures when compared with a well-matched control group that received sham treatments. The increase in the number of seizure-free weeks during and after the treatment period in the sham group suggests a possible placebo effect.

Dr. Nakken points out that his study was limited by the small subject number, treatment variation between patients, and heterogeneous patient groups (the study included patients with all different epilepsy types). The study was also conducted in patients with difficult-to-control seizures. It is possible that a mild therapeutic benefit of acupuncture could go unnoticed in such a group. We applaud Dr. Nakken and his colleagues, however, for conducting one of the few controlled clinical studies of any complementary therapy. It is now up to acupuncture advocates to conduct a larger, well-controlled study to assess the benefits of acupuncture for the treatment of epilepsy.

References

1. Yang R, Huang ZN, Cheng JS. Anticonvulsion effect of acupuncture might be related to the decrease of neuronal and inducible nitric oxide synthases. *Acupun Electrother Res* 2000;25(3-4):137–143.
2. Gusel' VA, Vol'f NL, Ferdman LA. Effect of acupuncture on the activity of experimental epileptogenic foci in the hippocampus of rabbits. *Biull Eksp Biol Med* 1985;99(1):27–29.
3. Chen RC, Huang YH, How SW. Systemic penicillin as an experimental model of epilepsy. *Exp Neurol* 1986;92(3):533–540.

Results

At baseline, no significant difference was observed between the sham group and the acupuncture group for any of the effect parameters. Compared to the baseline condition, we saw a slight reduction in seizure frequency in both groups during the treatment and in the follow-up period; however, we saw no statistically significant differences between the groups regarding reduction in seizure frequency. There was a slight trend toward a greater seizure reduction during the treatment and follow-up period among those with a low seizure frequency in the baseline period. The number of seizure-free weeks increased slightly during the treatment and follow-up period in both groups, but compared to the baseline condition, this change reached statistical significance in the sham group only, and not in the acupuncture group.

We were not able to detect any treatment-induced differences in the EEG changes within each group or between the two groups. Compared to the baseline condition, the two intervention groups had no significant differences in score changes on any of the QOLIE-89 scales. Separate analysis of the two groups showed no significant changes from baseline to postintervention and to follow-up in any QOLIE-89 dimension, either in the sham or acupuncture group (14).

Limitations of Study

The choice of placebo or intervention for the control group in trials of acupuncture is controversial. In 28 controlled trials, 28 different acupuncture placebos were used (15), making comparisons between studies difficult. In this study, we chose needling as treatment of the control group using a minimalist approach: piercing the skin outside the usual acupuncture points, using fine needles without any stimulation, and not obtaining the needling sensation. Nevertheless, we can still not exclude the physiologic effects of sham acupuncture.

The small sample size in our study enabled us to detect differences between the groups of 1 SD, normally a very large difference. (SD, standard deviation, is a common descriptive measure of the spread or dispersion of data results from a scientific study.) With a larger sample size, we might have detected smaller differences at the chosen power level. There were variations in the treatments given and acupoints used within the groups; however, these differences are a part of traditional Chinese acupuncture. The patients studied had chronic and drug-refractory epilepsies; they varied with regard to seizure type and frequency, and clearly were not representative of the total population of patients with epilepsy. The follow-up time in our study may have been too brief to detect longitudinal changes in seizure severity and frequency or quality-of-life aspects.

Conclusion

In a randomized controlled clinical trial with two parallel treatment arms, we assessed the effect of acupuncture and sham acupuncture as adjunctive treatment on seizure frequency, EEG results, and health-related quality of life in patients with intractable epilepsy. A slight reduction in seizure frequency occurred in both groups, which did not reach a level of statistical significance. A slight increase in number of seizure-free weeks also occurred in both groups, which reached statistical significance only in the sham group. Neither of the two groups had statistically significant changes in EEG or in health-related quality-of-life aspects.

Thus, in our study, we were not able to demonstrate a beneficial effect of acupuncture in patients with difficult-to-treat epilepsy.

References

1. Lai CW, Lai YH. History of epilepsy in Chinese traditional medicine. *Epilepsia* 1991;32:299–302.
2. Wu D. Suppression of epileptic seizures with acupuncture: efficacy, mechanism and perspective. *Am J Acupunct* 1988;16:113–117.
3. Cantera B, Mendoza C, Hernandez I, et al. EEG study on acupuncture treatment preceding induced epileptic seizures. *Am J Acupunct* 1992;20:43–46.
4. Wu D. Mechanism of acupuncture in suppressing epileptic seizures. *J Trad Chin Med* 1992;12:187–192.
5. Klide AM, Farnbach GC, Gallagher SM. Acupuncture therapy for the treatment of intractable, idiopathic epilepsy in five dogs. *Acupunct Electrother Res* 1987;12:71–74.
6. Shi Z, Gong B, Jia Y, et al. The efficacy of electroacupuncture on 98 cases of epilepsy. *J Trad Chin Med* 1987;7:21–22.
7. Chen K, Chen G, Feng X. Observation of immediate effect of acupuncture on electroencephalograms in epileptic patients. *J Trad Chin Med* 1983;3:121–124.
8. Yang J. Treatment of status epilepticus with acupuncture. *J Trad Chin Med* 1990;10:101–102.
9. Weimin Z. Clinical observation on 865 cases of epilepsy treated by catgut embedding in acupoints. *Chin J Acupunct Moxibustion* 1990;3:159–164.
10. Sjölund B, Terenius L, Eriksson M. Increased cerebrospinal fluid levels of endorphins after electro-acupuncture. *Acta Physiol Scand* 1977;100:382–384.
11. Han J. Central neurotransmitters and acupuncture analgesia. In: Pomeranz B, Stux G, (eds.) *Scientific Bases of Acupuncture.* New York: Springer Verlag, 1989.
12. Pomeranz B. Acupuncture research related to pain, drug addiction and nerve regeneration. In: Pomeranz B, Stux G, (eds.) *Scientific Bases of Acupuncture.* New York: Springer Verlag, 1989.
13. Kloster R, Larsson PG, Lossius R, et al. The effect of acupuncture in chronic intractable epilepsy. *Seizure* 1999;8:170–174.
14. Stavem K, Kloster R, Røssberg E, et al. Acupuncture in intractable epilepsy: lack of effect on health-related quality of life. *Seizure* 2000;9:422–426.
15. Kubiena G. Überlegungen zum Placeboproblem in der Akupunktur. *Wien Klin Wochenschr* 1989;101:362–367.

PART IV

Nutritional Approaches

CHAPTER 19

Nutrition and Epilepsy

MARK RUDDERHAM, ND, RACHEL LAFF, BA, AND ORRIN DEVINSKY, MD

Nutrition plays a central role in health and disease processes. The body draws all of its resources except oxygen from the diet. What we consume and how much we consume determines these resources and can influence health and disease. The traditional balanced diet recommended by the American Dietetic Association (ADA) consists of a mixture high in carbohydrates, moderate in protein, and low in fats. Some researchers are criticizing this once accepted food pyramid model that was the framework for a healthy diet for nearly 30 years. Studies on the Atkins diet, a high protein, low carbohydrate diet, support its utility as an effective means for weight loss, but no evidence relates its effects on seizures or long-term safety (1). The ketogenic diet, which is high fat and extremely low in carbohydrates, can help control seizures in some patients (see Chapter 21). Fasting rarely provokes seizures, and actually may reduce seizure frequency by putting the body in a state of ketosis (2,3). Hypoglycemia could possibly provoke seizure activity, although it is not common (4,5).

Scientific data on the relationship between diet and epilepsy are very limited. Specific metabolic deficiencies rarely cause epilepsy, as in the case of pyridoxine (vitamin B6) deficiency. Such seizures usually occur very early in life and are exquisitely responsive to pyridoxine therapy. Mitochondrial disorders result from abnormalities in the energy producing organelle. Tissues such as the heart and brain, which have high energy demands, are sensitive to mitochondrial dysfunction. Certain diets (e.g., more frequent meals and snacks with some glucose and electrolytes) and supplements (e.g., antioxidants) may help some patients with mitochondrial disorders and secondarily improve seizure control (6,7). Even in this special and uncommon case, however, little evidence links dietary changes and improved seizure control.

For the vast majority of epilepsy patients, no evidence links dietary changes and either improvement or exacerbation of seizure activity. Many anecdotal reports arise from individual patients or families that certain foods (e.g., those with high sugar content) or additives (e.g., aspartame) can trigger seizures. Little evidence supports these associations when scientifically studied (8,9). Similarly, some patients with epilepsy take antioxidants and free radical scavengers, such as omega-3 fatty acids and vitamin E (10,11). Although some evidence suggests that this class of compounds may reduce cancer risk and slow the progression of neurodegenerative disorders such as Alzheimer's and Parkinson's disease (12,13), no evidence shows that antioxidants reduce seizure activity or the negative long-term effects of epilepsy, such as impaired short-term memory. In many physical data and laypeople's assessment, however, the benefits of nutritional and vitamin supplements outweigh the risks.

The more we understand the biochemical pathways behind disease, the more we understand the biochemical pathways behind healthy functioning. Further, as research and technology improve our ability to design effective medications, we gain important insights into what diet and nutrition provide for maintaining good health. Our knowledge of the neurochemical basis behind epilepsy is growing, but we must translate and supplement this with information about how epilepsy impacts the body's use of specific nutrients. Amino acids, vitamins, and minerals are essential components of daily metabolism, and may be affected to varying degrees by epilepsy. Studies are beginning to look at both the preventative and therapeutic roles nutrition can play in the treatment of epilepsy. Because of the broad spectrum of causes for epilepsy, treatments must be chosen carefully, and the findings of one particular study may not apply to all people with epilepsy.

Amino Acids

Amino acids are the building blocks for proteins. The body relies upon approximately 22 different amino acids, nine of which are essential, meaning the body cannot produce them on its own. Amino acids occur naturally in most foods, with high concentrations in animal-based foods, such as meat, fish, and eggs. Once eaten, digested, and absorbed by the body, amino acids play many diverse roles—from directing cell division to composing muscle fiber and influencing brain chemistry. Simplistically, epilepsy can be viewed as the result of an imbalance of excitatory and inhibitory processes in a nervous system that produces too much excitation or too little inhibition. Concentrations of glutamate and aspartate, the primary excitatory amino acid neurotransmitters, increase in the brain during and shortly after a seizure (14). Inhibitory amino acid neurotransmitters, such as gamma aminobutyric acid (GABA), glycine, and taurine, "damp down" electrical activity. In theory, with these inhibitory neurotransmitters, dietary supplementation (in forms that readily cross the blood–brain barrier) could reduce seizure activity.

Gamma Aminobutyric Acid

The inhibitory amino acid neurotransmitter, GABA, is produced in the brain via the following reaction:

Alpha-ketoglutarate $\longrightarrow$ Glutamate $\longrightarrow$ GABA
Glutamate Dehydrogenase   Glutamate Decarboxylase

Alpha-ketogrutarate and other substrates are converted to glutamate by the enzyme glutamate dehydrogenase; then the resulting glutamate is converted to GABA via the enzyme glutamate decarboxylase. Glutamate is an excitatory amino acid neurotransmitter and GABA is inhibitory. One possible neurochemical basis for the development of epilepsy is that the glutamate dehydrogenase enzyme is overactive and the glutamate decarboxylase enzyme is underactive, thus resulting in an excess of glutamate compared to GABA. Too much excitation and not enough inhibition can result in a seizure.

GABA metabolism has been a primary area of drug research for epilepsy. Several relatively new antiepileptic drugs (AEDs) have been licensed that utilize different approaches towards elevating levels of GABA in the brain (15). Vigabatrin is a drug that blocks the action of the enzyme GABA transaminase, which is responsible for breaking down GABA. Inhibiting GABA degradation results in an increase of GABA levels in the brain. Tiagabine is a drug that increases GABA levels by blocking the reuptake of GABA by neurons and glia cells. This increases the amounts of GABA present to act on other

Commentary

This chapter provides an overview on how foods and dietary supplements may influence epileptic activity. We are what we eat. Nutrition is important for health. Brain cells require certain amino acids, vitamins, essential minerals, and fats for their normal function. A strong intuitive sense tells us that nutritional supplements or certain diets can influence epilepsy activity. Chapter 20 on the Use of Fatty Acids in the Diet, by Drs. David Mostofsky and Schlomo Yehuda and Chapter 21 on the Ketogenic Diet, by Dr. John Freeman, provide evidence for the role of fats. Very good scientific evidence suggests that the ketogenic diet does improve seizure control for some patients with epilepsy. In the case of the fatty acid supplements, the animal data strongly suggest a therapeutic trial in humans, and we await the results.

Overall, the data are scant on nutrition and epilepsy, but often a strong desire exists on the part of people with epilepsy or their family to improve seizure control by some nutritional change. This chapter provides a brief overview on what we know about the role of amino acids, essential minerals, fatty acids, and other dietary substances in modulating seizure activity. The authors correctly point out that, for the majority of nutritional supplements that are advocated to improve seizure control (e.g., taurine, vitamin E, omega-3 fatty acids), there are simply insufficient data. We don't know if they help. If they do, is there a certain group (partial vs. generalized epilepsies) that responds? The success of the ketogenic diet highlights the potential benefits of nutrition. Antioxidants could theoretically help prevent some of the long-term neuronal damage that occurs in some patients with years or decades of recurrent seizures. Such studies will be difficult to do because it may take many years to see a benefit. The research is needed, however, because well-designed prospective and controlled studies can help answer these and other important questions about the role of nutrition and dietary supplements for people with epilepsy.

neurons. Gabapentin was designed as a GABA molecule attached to a ring that would allow the molecule to pass through the blood–brain barrier and influence brain activity. Gabapentin appears to influence the GABA system in the brain, but the precise mechanism is not nearly as simple as its original design, which was to stimulate GABA receptors. The differences in the mechanisms of action that these drugs take explain why different drugs cause different side effects (16).

The use of GABA is a logical choice to treat epilepsy; however, it is not well absorbed across the blood–brain barrier, a protective layer of tightly sealed cells that excludes most molecules from entering the brain based on size, charge, and composition. Increased dietary levels of GABA will not penetrate the brain in a substantial enough amount to impact seizure activity (17). Researchers are experimenting with agents that increase the permeability of the blood–brain barrier, such as nitric oxide or other free radicals, to see if this could cause a rise in GABA levels inside the brain (17,18). Some recommend that GABA be dosed in the range of several grams per day to treat epilepsy, although no evidence shows that this therapy has any effect on seizure activity.

Carnosine

Carnosine is an amino acid involved with GABA activity in the brain. It is most easily found and measured as homocarnosine, a dipeptide metabolite of GABA and histidine, another amino acid (19). It is unclear exactly how carnosine is directly involved with seizure activity in the brain. Carnosine appears to directly bind to GABA, forming homocarnosine. Zinc and copper levels inside neurons may also be modulated by carnosine activity (20).

Contradictory findings exist regarding the role of homocarnosine in patients with epilepsy. One study reported higher homocarnosine levels in children with uncontrolled epilepsy and febrile seizures compared with children with medically controlled epilepsy (21). Other studies found that homocarnosine levels were higher in patients who responded to AED therapy (22–24). In these cases, homocarnosine levels appeared to increase as GABA levels increased following drug therapy. These studies show that homocarnosine levels vary according to GABA levels, but do not necessarily correlate with seizure control (19,24). A study examined homocarnosine levels and seizure control in 14 patients with juvenile myoclonic epilepsy and 12 patients with complex partial seizures. Higher homocarnosine, but not GABA, levels were associated with better seizure control (25). One unblinded study reported positive findings in patients taking dietary supplemental carnosine as an adjunctive therapy. After 10 weeks of carnosine supplements, five of seven subjects had improved EEG patterns with decreased spike-wave discharges (20). Although formal testing was not done, blinded therapists reported improved cognition, behavior, and language function in all seven patients. More rigorous studies are needed to confirm or refute these findings in small pilot studies. The role of homocarnosine as a therapeutic agent for epilepsy remains unproven but warrants further study.

Taurine

Taurine is classified as a conditionally essential amino acid because it is an amino acid that the body needs and is unable to synthesize on its own, yet it is not used for proteins. Taurine functions as a free amino acid or simple peptide and plays an important role in mammalian development. Taurine is involved in several different metabolic processes including detoxification, cell membrane stabilization, and the regulation of cellular calcium levels (26). These are all important metabolic processes involved in the maintenance and function of neuronal activity. How critical a role taurine plays in these processes remains uncertain. In the brain, taurine is an inhibitory neurotransmitter. It appears that a genetic variation in taurine metabolism is present in some cases of epilepsy (27). It has not proven to be very effective as a preventive antiepileptic agent because only a small fraction of taurine in the blood system will cross the blood–brain barrier. Increased levels of taurine are associated with reduced seizure susceptibility; decreased levels of taurine are associated with more spontaneous seizure activity (28). These trends do not indicate, however, that taurine can be used as an effective antiepileptic therapy (28).

Several studies suggest that taurine has a mild anticonvulsant effect in humans. An unblinded study done on 25 children with intractable epilepsy reported complete seizure control in only one case. A greater than 50% decrease of seizure frequency occurred in one case, a less than 50% decrease in frequency in four cases, but no effect in 18 cases (29). Another unblinded study on nine patients with intractable seizures who were treated with taurine showed only transient effects. Seizures disappeared for about 2 weeks in five patients; seizure frequency was temporarily reduced by 25% in one patient. No effect on seizure activity occurred in the remaining three cases (30). Thus, there is little theoretical basis for the use of taurine to treat epilepsy.

In one study, magnesium-deficient mice with audiogenic seizures (magnesium deficiency in mice both causes and increases audiogenic seizures) were treated with three different types of magnesium supplementation: magnesium acetyltaurinate (a combination of magnesium with the inhibitory neurotransmitter taurine), magnesium pyrrolidone-2-carboxylate (PCMH), and magnesium chloride (31). Only treatment with magnesium acetyltaurinate showed lasting effects for seizure control. Audiogenic seizures recurred 6 hours after treatment in the mice given PCMH and magnesium chloride. The mice supplemented with magnesium acetyltaurinate showed seizure control for up to 72 hours after treatment. This study indicates that taurine, in the magnesium acetyltaurinate form, may be effective in treating some types of seizure disorders. In human studies, the dosage for adults is around 2000 mg/day of taurine. No significant side effects due to taurine treatment have been reported.

Carnitine

Carnitine is a transport molecule that helps make energy available to cells and removes waste products. We obtain approximately 75% of the carnitine we need from meat and dairy products; the body produces the rest. Patients who are treated with valproic acid can develop carnitine deficiency (32,33). Clinically significant carnitine deficiency is uncommon, however. The most serious problems occur rarely in children (and extremely rarely in adults) with inborn errors of carnitine metabolism that make them especially susceptible to the effects of valproate (34). Possible symptoms of carnitine deficiency include fatigue, muscle weakness, enlarged heart, irregular heartbeat, frequent infection, seizures, poor muscle tone, slow growth, chronic vomiting, chronic fever, hyperammonemia, and hypoglycemia. Carnitine does pass through the blood–brain barrier. Van Wouwe, in his 1995 article, recommends that carnitine deficiency during valproic acid therapy can be reversed within a week by supplementation at 15 mg/kg body weight (33).

Carnitine can play a protective role in the brains of mice. When supplemented with carnitine prior to being exposed to a seizure-provoking agent, brain energy metabolites were preserved and seizures were reduced (35). Similar results are not reported in human studies. A double-blind placebo-controlled crossover study on 47 children taking valproic acid or carbamazepine found no difference in parental reports of improved seizure control or reduced side effects with carnitine supplementation (36). Due to the costliness of carnitine supplements and the lack of systematic evidence supporting its efficacy, these researchers do not recommend administering carnitine prophylactically to alleviate common side effects (36). In 1998, a panel of pediatric neurologists concluded that carnitine supplementation is recommended for patients with specific carnitine deficiency syndromes, especially infants and children on long-term valproate treatment (37). Carnitine's role in maintaining metabolic stability remains imprecisely defined, and these findings have yet to be reproduced in human subjects. Further studies are warranted to better define the stabilizing effect carnitine might have in the brain.

Glycine

Glycine is the simplest of the amino acids and acts as an inhibitory neurotransmitter in the central nervous system. Different forms of glycine have been tested for their anticonvulsant properties. One study found that trimethylglycine, dimethylglycine, and methylglycine reduced the number of seizures induced by strychnine in animal models (38). In humans, one study found no difference between dimethylglycine and placebo treatment for a group of 19 patients (39). The majority of the literature reports that dimethylglycine has no significant therapeutic effect in reducing seizure activity in humans (40,41). Some researchers suggest, however, that in selected individuals, dimethylglycine supplementation at 100 mg twice a day may have some benefit (42).

Vitamins

Antioxidants

Antioxidants include vitamins C, E, and A, and selenium and the carotenoids. These are made up of molecules that help prevent damage to the integrity of the cell and its components. Free radicals are the molecular by-products of metabolic processes that disrupt cellular functioning in numerous ways, including injury to the cell membrane and mitochondria. Hypothetically, free radicals can contribute to seizure activity by many different pathways; we highlight two here. In one pathway, free radicals inactivate glutamine synthase, an enzyme responsible for breaking down glutamate. This causes a build-up of glutamate, an excitatory neurotransmitter. An excess of excitatory neurotransmitter can induce seizure activity. Another pathway free radical agents can take is to inactivate glutamate decarboxylase, an enzyme responsible for converting glutamate to GABA. This results in a lack of GABA, the primary inhibitory neurotransmitter. A decrease in inhibitory neurotransmitters can also result in seizure activity (43). Due to its cell damaging effects, free radical activity may be involved in neurodegenerative diseases such as Alzheimer's and Parkinson's disease (13).

One study found that epilepsy patients have increased oxidative stress when compared with nonepileptic controls (43). In this study, 29 patients with epilepsy were compared with 50 normal controls. In addition, 10 patients who were seizure-free for 1 year, but who were still being treated with phenobarbital, were evaluated. Erythrocyte glutathione reductase (an antioxidant) and plasma vitamin C and A levels were significantly lower in the group of patients with epilepsy compared with normal controls. In the 10 seizure-free patients, erythrocyte glutathione reductase was significantly higher than pretreatment levels, and plasma vitamin A, E, and C levels were normal. This suggests that seizure activity may directly impact oxidative blood levels, and that antioxidants should be supplemented to compensate for the increase in free radicals.

Antioxidants are easily supplemented and levels can be restored with a beneficial effect on seizure activity. Fruits, vegetables, and whole grains (in particular), and sweet potatoes, carrots, and spinach are major sources of antioxidants. A double-blind placebo-controlled study on 24 patients with medically refractory epilepsy found that patients treated with 400 IU/day of vitamin E in addition to their regular medication experienced a significant reduction in seizures. The placebo group experienced no change in their seizure activity (10). One study demonstrated in patients with refractory epilepsy that an antioxidant supplement did not eliminate seizures, but reduced seizure frequency (44). Another study on aged rats with induced epileptogenic foci found that antioxidant supplements reduced the amount of reactive oxidant species (free radicals) in the brain (45). Antioxidant vitamins may work as a group. Thus, some nutritionists suggest dosing with a complete antioxidant formula to achieve maximal benefit.

Vitamin B6

Vitamin B6 plays an essential role in the metabolism and regulation of amino acids. It is a necessary component of many enzymes that process amino acids, assembling them into proteins and hormones, and taking them apart. It is found in foods such as potatoes, bananas, bran cereals, lentils, turkey, and tuna. The enzyme glutamate decarboxylase that converts glutamate to GABA depends upon vitamin B6. If there is too little vitamin B6 in the body, the enzyme cannot function properly, thereby increasing seizure activity due to decreased GABA levels. A vitamin B6 deficiency that causes seizures is well documented but extremely rare. The role of routine vitamin B6 supplementation in children or adults with epilepsy is not established, and no controlled studies support it. Typical adult doses of 50 mg to 150 mg of vitamin B6 are used therapeutically. Excessive amounts can damage sensory nerves, resulting in numbness in hands and feet (46,47). More research is needed to determine the extent of the therapeutic efficacy vitamin B6 can provide in controlling seizures.

A rare genetic vitamin B6 dependency disorder causing severe neonatal seizures and associated mental disability requires lifelong supplementation of B6 (48). Seizures return immediately when vitamin B6 therapy is discontinued. Some researchers postulate that the developmental outcome of the child depends on the dosage of vitamin B6. More research is needed to determine what the optimal dose is, if any, to control seizures and assure positive future development.

Minerals

Minerals are inorganic elements needed for various functions in the body. The body relies on 16 essential minerals, such as calcium for bone growth and maintenance, and iron for oxygenating the blood. Trace elements, such as zinc, copper, and manganese, have important functional roles in the nervous system. One study evaluating trace elements in hair found differences in mineral levels in patients with epilepsy versus controls. The average copper, magnesium, and zinc levels in the hair were significantly lower in epilepsy patients (49). Serum analysis showed no differences in the average magnesium and zinc levels in patients treated with anticonvulsants and those not receiving drug therapy. These findings suggest that AED therapy does not impact trace mineral levels, but rather it is the condition of epilepsy, underlying causes, or other factors that cause these differences. Low levels of zinc, magnesium, and copper in the hair of patients with epilepsy indicate the need for supplementation (49).

Manganese toxicity can cause tremor and seizures. Withdrawal from manganese supplementation quickly resolves seizure activity (50). In contrast, an old Anglo-Saxon prescription for "devil sickness" (epilepsy) was lupine, a plant exceptionally high in manganese. The suspected anticonvulsant properties of manganese made lupine a recommended treatment for epilepsy during that period (51). These two examples demonstrate that, as with many minerals, a certain range of concentration is needed for proper functioning. Both manganese intoxication and manganese deficiency result in seizure activity.

Manganese deficiency is more commonly reported in the literature than toxicity. Manganese is found in grain products, nuts, legumes, and leafy greens. Manganese supplementation should be given at 50 to 100 mg/d (42). Average daily intake in the United States from food sources is 3 mg. Doses greater than 100 mg may cause nausea. Manganese may interfere with the absorption of copper, iron, and zinc. The high levels of copper, zinc, calcium, and magnesium that have been found in patients with epilepsy may inhibit the absorption of manganese.

Magnesium deficiency is common in people with epilepsy. Magnesium is needed for calcium absorption, and an adequate ratio of calcium and magnesium is needed for normal nerve functioning. Magnesium is also important for the body to be able to utilize vitamin B6. Two unblinded studies found that magnesium supplements improved seizure control (52). In one study, 450 mg of daily magnesium supplements controlled seizures in all 30 patients. In another study, 450 mg of daily magnesium supplementation improved seizures in 29 of 30 children with tonic-clonic or absence seizures. Magnesium is generally used for seizures associated with toxemia of pregnancy, acute nephritis in children, and migraine (53,54). Magnesium is best found in green vegetables, nuts, seeds, and some whole grains. Although magnesium supplementation has demonstrated some positive results, controlled blinded studies are needed to confirm the accuracy of these findings.

Zinc deficiency and copper excess during pregnancy may pose a risk to the early development of the brain. This may be a cause for the development of epilepsy. Zinc and copper have an antagonistic relationship. Zinc levels are lower in patients with epilepsy, and the use of AEDs may also contribute to zinc deficiency. Copper deficiency may cause seizures; however, copper levels are higher in patients treated for epilepsy, possibly due to copper complexes formed by the activation of AEDs. The zinc–copper ratio is not fully understood. Some researchers theorize that seizures occur when the zinc–copper ratio falls suddenly in the absence of taurine (42). A 10 to 1 through 30 to 1 ratio of zinc to copper is recommended (55). Zinc at 15 to 50 mg/d is an appropriate adult dose. Copper can be administered at 1 to 3 mg/d. The best dietary sources of zinc are oysters, lean meats, poultry, fish, and organ meats. It can also be found in dairy products, eggs, whole grains, nuts, and seeds. Good sources of dietary copper are seafood, organ meats, whole grains, nuts, raisins, legumes, and chocolate.

Melatonin

Melatonin is a hormone, produced by the pineal gland, that affects the sleep/wake cycle. It also helps protect the body from free radicals. Melatonin's action on free radicals may help boost overall immunity, including the body's own cancer prevention system. In addition, melatonin helps maintain the brain's balance of excitatory and inhibitory neurotransmitters, stabilizing its electrical activity. One study demonstrated that melatonin helps reduce seizure activity in mice. When melatonin was injected 0 to 30 minutes before the seizure-inducing medium, the mice experienced no seizures (56). Although we can't extrapolate these findings to humans, this study does support further study in epilepsy patients.

Melatonin levels in the body vary during the course of the day in a circadian cycle. In a study of patients with intractable temporal lobe epilepsy, melatonin levels were lower than normal subjects prior to having a seizure and were three times higher than normal after a seizure (57). Based on the animal and human data, melatonin supplements could potentially improve seizure control. The melatonin surge after a seizure could be a compensatory action by the brain to prevent further seizure activity and could also contribute to postictal lethargy. Another study found that melatonin had effects as an AED and sleep stabilizer. Dosing of 5 to 10 mg a night can normalize sleep patterns and positively influence seizure activity in children with sleep disturbance and epilepsy (58). One clinical study reports high doses of melatonin as an additional AED necessary for seizure control in a child resistant to other AEDs. Reduction of melatonin was associated with an increase in seizures. Restabilization occurred only after restoring the melatonin dosage (59). Another preliminary clinical study showed that melatonin improved seizure control in 5 out of 6 children with severe intractable epilepsy. In this study, both nocturnal and daytime seizures improved (60). In contrast, another study reported melatonin to have a proconvulsive effect on nocturnal seizures. Melatonin levels in the body surge at night, in most individuals at around 2 A.M. (56). Increased melatonin secretion at night or premenstrually may play a role in nocturnal epilepsy. AEDs such as the benzodiazepines that block melatonin secretion, may help treat these seizure types (61).

Melatonin supplements are readily available where nutritional supplements are sold; however, some researchers question the safety of melatonin use. Although promising studies show the beneficial effects of melatonin on electrical activity in the brain, a lack of controlled clinical data exists. More research is needed to distinguish the effects of melatonin therapy versus a placebo effect, and more clinical trials are needed to confirm its efficacy. Also, possible improvements in seizure activity may reflect improvement in sleep efficiency or duration. More research is needed to understand the fluctuating nature of this hormone and its potential proconvulsive or anticonvulsive effects at different points in the sleep/wake cycle. Melatonin could be an effective adjunct to other AEDs in lowering the dosage and side effect burden of these drugs, because it is not known to cause significant side effects or interfere with other AEDs (59,62).

Conclusion

Nutritional therapies remain an attractive naturalistic approach to controlling epilepsy. Apart from the ketogenic diet—and treatment of very rare disorders such as pyridoxine-deficient seizures with vitamin B6—no dietary therapies have been established in relieving seizure activity. Similarly, no clear evidence suggests that any foods or supplements increase seizure activity. Nutritional therapies depend on the type of epilepsy a person has. Their effects in the body may vary from prevention of seizures to protection of the areas of the brain where the seizure takes place. A full diagnostic workup before the administration of any treatment is critical in enhancing outcome. Therapies should be administered one at a time to monitor and evaluate their efficacy. When administering nutritional supplements concurrent with medications, it is important to understand how the two treatments will interact. Hopefully, future research will increase our understanding of the biochemistry and physiology of the nutrients involved in epilepsy and the pharmacology of the drugs used in the management of the disease. Future research directed towards understanding these mechanisms will hopefully translate into therapeutic nutritional approaches to treat patients with epilepsy.

References

1. Westman EC, Yancy WS, Edman JS, et al. Effect of 6-month adherence to a very low carbohydrate diet program. *Am J Med* 2002;113(1):30–36.
2. Freeman JM, Vining EP. Seizures decrease rapidly after fasting: preliminary studies of the ketogenic diet. *Arch Pediatr Adolesc Med* 1999;153(9):946–949.
3. Mahoney AW, Hendricks DG, Bernhard N, et al. Fasting and ketogenic diet effects on audiogenic seizures susceptibility of magnesium deficient rats. *Pharmacol Biochem Behav* 1983;18(5):683–687.
4. Malouf R, Brust JC. Hypoglycemia: causes, neurologic manifestations, and outcome. *Ann Neurol* 1985;17(5):421–430.
5. Naritoku DK. Hypoglycemia and seizures. http://www.siumed.edu/neuro/epilepsy/QNA/QNAframes/hypoglycemiajs.html. Accessed April 4, 2003.
6. Gropman AL. Diagnosis and treatment of childhood mitochondrial diseases. *Curr Neurol Neurosci Rep* 2001;1(2):185–194.
7. Gold DR, Cohn BH. Treatment of mitochondrial cytopathies. *Semin Neurol* 2001;21(3):309–325.
8. Butchko HH, Stargel WW, Comer CP, et al. Aspartame: review of safety. *Regul Toxicol Pharmacol* 2002;35(2 Pt 2):S1–93.
9. Rowan AJ, Shaywitz BA, Tuchman L, et al. Aspartame and seizure susceptibility: results of a clinical study in reportedly sensitive individuals. *Epilepsia* 1995;36(3):270–275.
10. Ogunmekan AO. Vitamin E deficiency and seizures in animals and man. *Canadian J Neurologic Science* 1979;6:43–45.
11. Schlanger S, Shinitzky M, Yam D. Diet enriched with omega-3 fatty acids alleviates convulsion symptoms in epilepsy patients. *Epilepsia* 2002;43(1):103–104.
12. Maynard M, Gunnell D, Emmett P, et al. Fruit, vegetables, and antioxidants in childhood and risk of adult cancer: the Boyd Orr cohort. *J Epidemiol Community Health* 2003;57(3):218–225.
13. Weisburger JH. Lifestyle, health and disease prevention: the underlying mechanisms. *Eur J Cancer Prev* 2002;11(suppl) 2:S1–7.
14. Raevskii KS, Avakian GN, Kudrin VS, et al. Features of neurotransmitter pool in cerebrospinal fluid of patients with epilepsy. *Zh Nevrol Psikhiatr Im S S Korsakova* 2001;101(6):39–41.
15. Czuczwar SJ, Patsalos PN. The new generation of GABA enhancers. Potential in the treatment of epilepsy. *CNS Drugs* 2001;15(5):339–350.
16. Treiman DM. GABAergic mechanisms in epilepsy. *Epilepsia* 2001;42(suppl 3):8–12.
17. Shyamaladevi N, Jayakumar AR, Sujatha R, et al. Evidence that nitric oxide production increases γ-amino butyric acid permeability of blood-brain barrier. *Brain Research Bulletin* 2002;57(2):231–236.
18. Oztas B, Kilic S, Dural E, et al. Influence of antioxidants on the blood-brain barrier permeability during epileptic seizures. *J Neurosci Res* 2001;66(4):674–678.
19. Henry TR, Theodore WH. Homocarnosine elevations: A cause or a sign of seizure control? *Neurology* 2001;56:698–699.
20. Chez MG, Buchanan CP, Komen JL. L-carnosine therapy for intractable epilepsy in childhood: effect on EEG. *Epilepsia* 2002;43(7):65.
21. Takahashi H. Studies on homocarnosine in cerebrospinal fluid in infancy and childhood. Part II. Homocarnosine levels in cerebrospinal fluid from children with epilepsy, febrile convulsions or meningitis. *Brain Dev* 1981;3(3):263–270.
22. Petroff OA, Hyder F, Collins T, et al. Acute effects of vigabatrin on brain GABA and homocarnosine in patients with complex partial seizures. *Epilepsia* 1999;40(7):958–964.

23. Petroff OA, Hyder F, Rothman DL, et al. Effects of gabapentin on brain GABA, homocarnosine, and pyrrolidinone in epilepsy patients. *Epilepsia* 2000;41(6):675–680.

24. Pitkanen A, Matilainen R, Ruutiainen T, et al. Levels of total gamma-aminobutyric acid (GABA), free GABA and homocarnosine in cerebrospinal fluid of epileptic patients before and during gamma-vinyl-GABA (vigabatrin) treatment. *J Neurol Sci* 1988;88(1-3):83–93.

25. Petroff OA, Hyder F, Rothman DL, et al. Homocarnosine and seizure control in juvenile myoclonic epilepsy and complex partial seizures. *Neurology* 2001;56(6)709–715.

26. Birdsall TC. Therapeutic applications of taurine. *Altern-Med-Rev* 1998;3(2);128–136.

27. Collins BW, Goodman HO, Swanton CH, et al. Plasma and urinary taurine in epilepsy. *Clin Chem* 1988;34(4):671–675.

28. Durelli L, Mutani R. The current status of taurine in epilepsy. *Clin Neuropharmacol* 1983;6(1):37–48.

29. Fukuyama Y, Ochiai Y. Therapeutic trial by taurine for intractable childhood epilepsies. *Brain Dev* 1982;4(1):63–69.

30. Konig P, Kriechbaum G, Presslich O, et al. Orally-administered taurine in therapy-resistant epilepsy. *Wien Klin Wochenschr* 1977;89(4):111–113.

31. Bac P, Herrenknecht C, Binet P, et al. Audiogenic seizures in magnesium-deficient mice: effects of magnesium pyrrolidone-2-carboxylate, magnesium acetyltaurinate, magnesium chloride and vitamin B-6. *Magnes Res* 1983;6(1):11–19.

32. Thom H, Carter PE, Cole GF, et al. Ammonia and carnitine concentrations in children treated with sodium valproate compared with other anticonvulsant drugs. *Dev Med Child Neurol* 1991;33(9):795–802.

33. Van Wouwe JP. Carnitine deficiency during valproic acid treatment. *Int J Vitam Nutr Res* 1995;65(3):211–214.

34. Coulter DL. Carnitine, valproate, and toxicity. *J Child Neurol* 1991;6(1):7–14.

35. Igisu H, Matsuoka M, Iryo Y. Protection of the brain by carnitine. *Sangyo Eiseigaku Zasshi* 1995;37(2):75–82.

36. Freeman JM, Vining EP, Cost S, et al. Does carnitine administration improve the symptoms attributed to anticonvulsant medications?: a double-blinded crossover study. *Pediatrics* 1994;3(6 Pt 1):893–895.

37. De Vivo DC, Bohan TP, Coulter DL, et al. L-carnitine supplementation in childhood epilepsy: current perspectives. *Epilepsia* 1998;39(11):1216–1225.

38. Freed WJ. Prevention of strychnine-induced seizures and death by the N-methylated glycine derivatives betaine, dimethylglycine and sarcosine. *Pharmacol Biochem Behav* 1985;22(4): 641–643.

39. Gascon G, Patterson B, Yearwood K, et al. N,N dimethylglycine and epilepsy. *Epilepsia* 1989;30(1):90–93.

40. Haidukewych D, Rodin EA. N,N-dimethylglycine shows no anticonvulsant potential. *Ann Neurol* 1984;15(4):405.

41. Roach ES, Gibson P. Failure of N,N-dimethylglycine in epilepsy. *Ann Neurol* 1983;14(3):347.

42. Department of Neurology, Massachusetts General Hospital. *Epilepsy and Nutritional Supplementation.*

43. http://neuro-www.mgh.harvard.edu/forum/EpilepsyF/11.22.973.29AMEpilepsyNutritio. Accessed April 4, 2003.

44. Sudha K, Rao AV, Rao A. Oxidative stress and antioxidants in epilepsy. *Clinica Chimica Acta* 2001;303:19–24.

45. Hung-Ming W, Liu CS, Tsai JJ, et al. Antioxidant and anticonvulsant effect of a modified formula of chaihu-longu-muli-tang. *Am J Chin Med* 2002;30(2-3):339–346.

46. Komatsu M, Hiramatsu M. The efficacy of an antioxidant cocktail on lipid peroxide level

and superoxide dismutase activity in aged rat brain and DNA damage in iron-induced epileptogenic foci. *Toxicology* 2000;148(2-3):143–148.

47. Dordain G, Deffond D. Pyridoxine neuropathies. Review of the literature. *Therapie* 1994;49(4):333–337.

48. Morra M, Philipszoon HD, D'Andrea G, et al. Sensory and motor neuropathy caused by excessive ingestion of vitamin B6: a case report. *Funct Neurol* 1993;8(6):429–432.

49. Gupta VK, Mishra D, Mathur I, et al. Pyridoxine-dependent seizures: a case report and a critical review of the literature. *J Paediatr Child Health* 2001;37:592–596.

50. Ilhan A, Uz E, Kali S, et al. Serum and hair trace element levels in patients with epilepsy and healthy subjects: does the antiepileptic therapy affect the element concentrations of hair? *European J Neurology* 1999;6:705–709.

51. Komaki H, Maisawa S, Sugai K, et al. Tremor and seizures associated with chronic manganese intoxication. *Brain & Development* 1999;21:122–124.

52. Dendle P. Lupines, manganese, and devil-sickness: an Anglo-Saxon medical response to epilepsy. *Bull Hist Med* 2001;75(1):91–101.

53. Murphy P. Magnesium and manganese: raising the seizure threshold. *Epilepsy Wellness Newsletter* Spring, 1999.

54. Ahsan SK, al-Swoyan S, Hanif M, et al. Hypomagnesemia and clinical implications in children and neonates. *Indian J Med Sci* 1998;52(12):541–547.

55. Johnson S. The multifaceted and widespread pathology of magnesium deficiency. *Med Hypotheses* 2001;6(2):163–170.

56. Haas EM. Zinc. Available at: http://www.healthy.net/asp/templates/article.asp?PageType=article&ID=2071. Accessed April 4, 2003.

57. Mohanan PV, Yamamoto HA. Preventive effect of melatonin against brain mitochondrial DNA damage, lipid peroxidation and seizures induced by kainic acid. *Toxicol Lett* 2002;129(1-2):99–105.

58. Bazil CW, Short D, Crispin D, et al. Patients with intractable epilepsy have low melatonin, which increases following seizures. *Neurology* 2000;55:1746–1748.

59. Fauteck J, Schmidt H, Lerchl A, et al. Melatonin in epilepsy: first results of replacement therapy and first clinical results. *Biol Signals Recept* 1999;8(1-2):105–110.

60. Molina-Carballo A, Munoz-Hoyos A, Reiter RJ, et al. Utility of high doses of melatonin as adjunctive anticonvulsant therapy in a child with severe myoclonic epilepsy: two years experience. *J Pineal Res* 1997;23(2):97–105.

61. Peled N, Shorer Z, Peled E, et al. Melatonin effect on seizures in children with severe neurologic deficit disorders. *Epilepsia* 2001;42(9):1208–1210.

62. Sandyk R, Tsagas N, Anninos PA. Melatonin as a proconvulsive hormone in humans. *Int J Neurosci* 1992;63(1-2):125–135.

63. Asif Ali Siddiqui M, Nazmi AS, Karim S, et al. Effect of melatonin and valproate in epilepsy and depression. *Indian J Pharmacology* 2001;33:378–381.

CHAPTER 20

The Use of Fatty Acids in the Diet for Seizure Management

DAVID I. MOSTOFSKY AND SHLOMO YEHUDA

All antiepileptic drugs (AEDs) share a common feature: they supply specially designed chemicals to the brain that are able to change the neurophysiology of the brain, thereby controlling the bioelectrical discharges that cause seizures. The need to control seizures is self-evident. In addition to the clinical and observable behavior changes that define an epileptic seizure, animal studies have shown that a seizure can impair important functions of the hippocampus (a brain structure that is involved with memory, execution of logical tasks, and emotion, among other functions) causing, for example, disturbances in learning to avoid and escape from an unpleasant environment (1–4). At the cellular and biochemical level, functional changes in the hippocampus following a seizure include a decrease in both the short and the persisting electrical activity of the cells' activity (1,5–7), as well as structural changes, such as loss of neurons in critical areas of the hippocampus (3). AEDs are imperfect and their effects are not uniform for every patient. Often, no single AED can control seizures. The more one has to add to the cocktail of AEDs to better control seizures, the more likely the patient will suffer from side effects. The less serious side effects may take the form of drowsiness, clouded learning and cognitive ability, stomach upset, and hyperactivity. Sometimes seizures turn out to be especially resistant to conventional treatment, leading frustrated patients and their caregivers to consider unconventional therapies, many of which have little or no sound scientific basis or credibility. Not everything that is unconventional is necessarily useless or fraudulent, however. Among the more popular proposed alternative treatments for epilepsy—for which some degree of support exists—are the use of behavior modification, hypnosis, exercise, and EEG biofeedback (8). These activities have been shown to help numerous patients, but true randomized clinical trials—the only ones that serious critics of any experiment are prepared to accept and be convinced by—remain to be conducted. Currently, the existing data are largely based on small sample studies and anecdotal reports.

An exception to the widespread criticism of alternative treatment is the use of the ketogenic diet (see Chapter 21), although it is outside of this discussion of the therapeutic potential for fatty acids (FAs) in epilepsy. For all the other techniques, however, rigorous clinical trial methodologies to convincingly demonstrate the benefits of such alternative or complementary techniques are not yet available. In contrast to the pharmacologic attempts at seizure control, the theoretical rationale for alternative or complementary techniques is limited, although many of the significant advances in medicine have resulted from accidental discoveries of things that work with an understanding of why they work, coming much later, if at all.

This chapter proposes a treatment alternative for epilepsy that is based on dietary intake, although considerable research with human subjects must be done before a conclusion can be reached or the treatment can become part of mainstream neurologic practice. Special dietary supplementation is advocated—not necessarily as the primary or sole treatment of choice—but as an adjunct or add-on therapy. Even in the absence of large-scale human studies, a scientific rationale exists for this alternative treatment. Laboratory experiments have been conducted over a number of years, using animal subjects, that back up this approach. Furthermore, the risk of side effects for most patients is practically nonexistent, and the cost of following such a program is economically acceptable. This approach includes a type of chemical supplementation not usually associated with AEDs. Fatty acids are available in some of the foods commonly eaten. Indeed, these specific chemical formulations are known as *essential fatty acids* (EFAs). They are essential because, as opposed to many animals who can manufacture these chemicals, the only way humans receive them is via diet. (Additional notes on fatty acid biochemistry are provided at the end of this chapter. Only an elementary introduction is included, but interested readers can find simple descriptions of fatty acid biochemistry in a number of well written books targeted for the nonspecialist audience: see *Smart Fats* by Michael Schmidt and *Fats That Heal; Fats That Kill* by Udo Erasmus.)

The promising relationships between epilepsy and seizure on the one hand and fatty acids on the other hand are complex and not obvious. This is especially true for a class of fatty acids known as *polyunsaturated fatty acids* (PUFAs), which serve as neuroprotectors and neural stabilizers. The PUFAs directly affect the passage of brain chemicals through the neuronal cell membrane. The property of allowing flow through the membrane can be quantified and expressed as the *membrane fluidity index*. Because of this pivotal role in regulating neuronal functions, PUFAs affect many complex activities in the brain and, not surprisingly, they can influence epileptic seizure activity. The aim of this chapter is: (i) to present the evidence that essential fatty acids play major roles in epilepsy and seizures; (ii) to demonstrate that essential fatty acid treatment may help prevent or limit the number and severity of the seizures; and (iii) to offer an hypothesis to understand this property of the essential fatty acids.

Essential Fatty Acids

Few topics in nutrition cause as much controversy and concern—and are as frequently misunderstood—as fats. The repeated cautionary warnings from the medical profession have dramatically reduced the amount of fat we eat to minimize the risks associated with cardiovascular diseases, diabetes, and other chronic disorders. Deficiencies in fat intake, however, can also contribute to health hazards, including an increased risk of infection, dysregulation of cyclic and rhythmic activity, and impaired cognitive and sensory functions (especially in infants). Symptoms of essential fatty acid deficiency may include fatigue, skin problems, immune weakness, gastrointestinal disorders, heart and circulatory problems, growth retardation, and sterility. In addition to these symptoms, a lack of dietary essential fatty acids has been implicated in the development or aggravation of breast cancer, prostate cancer, rheumatoid arthritis, asthma, depression, schizophrenia, and attention deficit/hyperactivity disorder (ADHD). This list of possible health complications resulting from PUFA deficiency in the diet is by no means exhaustive.

A consensus has emerged from research suggesting that the *balance* of the different fat types is more important than the *amount* of fat consumed. The type of dietary fat affects the behavior of each cell and determines how well it can perform its vital functions and its ability to resist disease. Within the class of essential fatty acids, two PUFAs—linoleic and α-linolenic acids—are necessary for good health. These EFAs must be provided by nutritional intake, and they have beneficial effects when available in moderation. Excesses of these otherwise beneficial fatty acids should, however, be avoided. In contrast to PUFAs, a high intake of *saturated* and hydrogenated fats are linked to an increase in a number of health risks, including degenerative diseases, cardiovascular disease, cancer, and diabetes.

Commentary

This chapter discusses a dietary approach to the treatment of epilepsy, proposed as an add-on to seizure medications. The authors are quick to point out, rightly so, that considerable research with human subjects lies ahead before it will be clear if this diet works and what its side effects are, if any.

The diet involves the ingestion of essential fatty acids (EFAs), and a detailed overview is given for readers unfamiliar with these supplements. The scientific rationale for the possible role of EFAs in the treatment of epilepsy is then explained, followed by a summary of an animal experiment that evaluated the effect of fatty acids on seizures.

As the authors conclude, sufficient justification exists at this time for undertaking additional research on the effects of dietary EFAs on people with epilepsy. This research would hopefully clarify the benefits and risks of this treatment and whether patients with certain types of seizures are more likely to benefit than others.

The authors end by recommending that people with seizures supplement their diet with polyunsaturated fatty acids (PUFAs). Readers should note that this recommendation is not based on controlled clinical studies and that this is not a recommendation generally made by neurologists or epilepsy specialists for the treatment of seizures. Therefore, it is prudent for any interested patients to first discuss this approach with their neurologist.

Omega-6 and Omega-3 Fatty Acids

Linoleic acid (LA) is a member of the family of omega-6 (T-6 or n-6) fatty acids; α-linolenic acid is an omega-3 (T-3 or n-3) fatty acid. These terms refer to characteristics in the chemical structure of the fatty acids. Other omega-6 fatty acids can be manufactured in the body using linoleic acids as a starting point. These include gamma-linoleic acid (GLA), dihomo-gamma-linoleic acid (DHGLA), and arachidonic acid (AA). Similarly, other omega-3 fatty acids that are manufactured in the body using α-linolenic acid as a starting point include eicosapentaenoic acid (EPA) and docosa-hexaenoic acid (DHA). Many fatty acids are sold as supplements in natural food and health stores, and these ingredients are commonly featured on the label.

The brain has two sources for all n-3 and n-6 acids. These PUFAs are comprised of more than 18 carbons in their chain. One source is the elongation process of linoleic acid and α-linolenic acid that takes place in the blood–brain barrier (BBB) and in most cells in the brain. The other source of PUFA is from the diet itself. The fatty acids that come from the diet must cross the BBB, although we do not know how most PUFAs cross the BBB. A better understanding of this issue is very important to understand the pathologic processes that occur in aging and other pathologic states. A more detailed review and discussion of this problem and its ramifications can be found elsewhere (9). (See Figure 20.1.)

EFAs are necessary for energy production, the transfer of oxygen from the air to the bloodstream, and the manufacture of hemoglobin. They are also involved in growth, cell division, and nerve function. EFAs are found in high concentrations in the brain and are essential for normal nerve impulse transmission and brain function.

Among the significant components of cell membranes are the phospholipids, which contain fatty acids. The type of fatty acids in the diet determines the type of fatty acids available to the composition of cell membranes. A phospholipid made from a saturated fat has a different structure, and is less fluid, than one that incorporates an unsaturated and essential fatty acid. In addition, linoleic and α-linolenic acids *by themselves* have an effect on the neuronal membrane fluidity index. They decrease the cholesterol level in the membrane, thus increasing membrane fluidity. Poor membrane fluidity makes it difficult for brain cells to function normally and increases the susceptibility of cells to injury and death. These consequences for cell function are not restricted to absolute levels of FAs, but depend on the *relative* amounts of omega-3 fatty acids and omega-6 fatty acids in cell membranes.

We have hypothesized five categories of PUFA functions that are common to different brain functions, including modifications of: (i) membrane fluidity; (ii) activity of enzymes bound to the membrane that break down FA into other forms of FA; (iii) number and properties of receptors that are able to make use of the incoming chemicals; (iv) function of ion channels that allow molecules of a chemical to flow through the cell; and (v) production and activity of neurotransmitters (responsible for the passage of nerve progress and stimulation) that block or activate other chemicals and interfere with electrical activity (10,11). Numerous studies of the neurobiologic properties of EFAs confirm

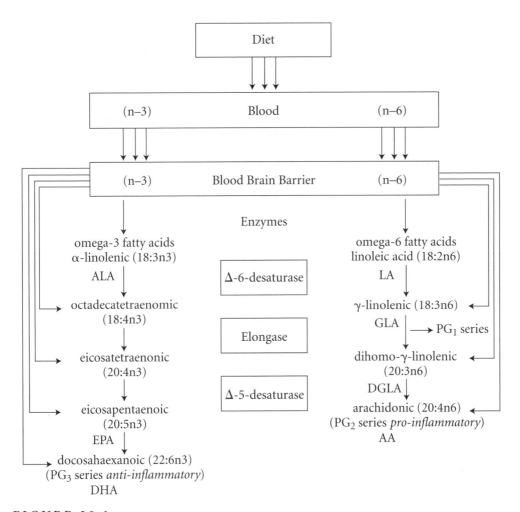

FIGURE 20.1

Some of the major essential fatty acids and their metabolites. Note that following dietary intake, the derivative fatty acids from both LA and ALA may be supplied to the body directly from the blood, or they may first have to cross the blood–brain barrier.

their important role in a variety of normal and pathologic brain functions (12). These FAs are important to retinal function, learning and memory mechanisms, thermoregulation, pain, stress, and sleep. We demonstrated that a specific mixture of α-linolenic acid (n-3) and linoleic acid (n-6) in a ratio of 1:4 had significant effects on humans and animals. The compound improved the quality of life of Alzheimer's patients and exerted beneficial effects in intact aged rats, as well as in rats that were experimentally rendered learning deficient. It improved the memory, thermoregulation, and sleep in humans and in rats, and ameliorated the symptoms of induced multiple sclerosis in rats (10). Furthermore, we demonstrated that this compound protected rats who were injected with a convulsant agent (13). In the case of epilepsy, seizures are understood to occur when a sudden change occurs in brain function and storms of uncontrolled neuronal firing occur. Such changes in neuronal firing result from temporary changes in the neuronal membrane, which in turn are responsive to the activity of FAs.

The relationship between lipids and FA metabolism on the one hand and epilepsy on the other has previously been described (14). The global category of the PUFAs and n-3 FAs, in particular, are regarded as neuroprotectors because they protect the brain from ischemia and other insults. They are also membrane stabilizers, since they are beneficial for cardiac tissue and in raising the seizure threshold (15). The biochemical relationships between lipids (fats) and acid levels (FA metabolism) during and after experimentally induced epilepsy were reported (16). Seizures cause a gross disturbance in FA metabolism and inhibit the biochemical pathway (17–22). One of the effects of a seizure is the brief disruption of the BBB mechanism (22–24), which is critical for the production of other PUFAs. Treatment with n-3 fatty acid alleviates symptoms of convulsions in epilepsy patients (25), thereby preserving the status of the biochemicals necessary for normal brain function.

A well-known application of FAs for treating epilepsy is the ketogenic diet, used for children with refractory seizures (26–28). The powerful and dramatic therapeutic results from the ketogenic diet continue to be reaffirmed by many clinical investigations (6,29–31). Although this diet was developed independent of considerations regarding PUFAs, in 2001, Stafstrom (32) described a "PUFA diet" with effects similar to a ketogenic diet.

Possible modes of action for the involvements of brain lipids include (14):

- Lipids are important constituents of the neuronal membrane, and changes in lipid composition may alter membrane activities.
- Lipids may offset the dangerous effects of substances that induce epilepsy (such as iron, which increases other lipid decomposition).
- Lipids may offer a stability in the membrane fluidity that helps control epilepsy.
- Lipids may control the change in neuronal membrane phospholipid metabolism that may result from the high level of excitatory amino acid receptors in the epileptic focus and that leads to frequent and uncontrolled electrical firing.
- Although a genetic link may exist between epilepsy and PUFA deficit (33), the addition of PUFA to the diet may provide some measure of correction.
- Some of the EFAs may be neuroprotective, similar to the protective cardiac effects of EFAs. This was shown in a study in which α-linolenic acid, but not palmatic acid or GLA (a form of LA), protected against ischemic-induced neuronal death and prevented seizures induced by a powerful convulsant agent (kainic acid) and its associated neuronal death (5,34).

A potentially significant advantage to adopting the FA treatment program for seizure control—if the animal data are substantiated in human clinical trials—would be that it could offset other undesired properties of standard AEDs that cause side effects, such as tremors, gastrointestinal distress, effects on the bone (35), auditory hallucinations (36), and demyelination (37). In addition, a striking consequence of the AEDs is the frequently reported impairment of cognitive performance. Both recurrent seizures and AEDs may cause cognitive deficits. Many AEDs can cause cognitive problems (29,31,38–40) in patients with epilepsy as well as healthy volunteers (41). In humans, AEDs can adversely affect declarative memory (31) and long-term memory (42), suggesting an insult to the hippocampus and perhaps other brain structures.

The hippocampus undergoes changes following a seizure, including decreased levels of serotonin (43), acetylcholine (44), brain-derived factors (45), amino acid and energy metabolism (46), as well as enzymatic changes (47). These may contribute to mood changes (including depression), sexual functioning, and maintaining a balance for many normal activities of the body's systems. Furthermore, induced seizures increased the arachidonic acid (AA) and platelet-derived factors (17)—the latter being a potent, biologically active phospholipid in the adaptive properties of the synapses, which are critical for the transmission of nervous system signals.

Recently, we compared the antiseizure and cognitive effects of carbamazepine (CBZ) and the FA compound we developed (9). Although both drugs blocked the induced seizure activity, only the FA ameliorated PTZ-induced learning deficits. The administration of CBZ also increased cortisol levels. The beneficial effects of the FA preparation correlated with its reduction of cortisol levels (48). We theorized that interacting effects and multiple pathways affect seizures, cognitive performance, and cortisol following either CBZ or FA. Both compounds reduce seizure frequency or severity; however, CBZ decreased learning performance and increased cortisol. The FA may improve learning and decrease cortisol levels (Figure 20.2).

The possible explanation of our results is complicated. Several variables play a role in this situation, including the BBB during and after seizures. In 1986, Cornford and Oldendorf (23) demonstrated that seizures disturb BBB functions, especially in the glucose transport required for cellular function. Studies confirmed these findings and also found changes in the rates of penetration of glucose and oxygen, as well as structural changes in the BBB (49). Oztas and colleagues found that, during a seizure, vast amounts of AA (20:4n6) are released. The importance of the increased AA level is twofold:

- AA is a powerful generator of free radicals (chemicals that are destructive in brain chemistry). Thus, AA opens a vicious cycle in which a seizure induces an increase in AA level, leading to an increase in the free radical level that causes damage to the frontal cortex and hippocampus, eventually intensifying the next seizure. Recently, Farooqui, et al. (50) described the role of AA in kainic acid-induced neurotoxicity. Stimulation of kainic acid receptors causes a rapid release of AA. This increased level of AA modifies the membrane fluidity index and membrane permeability.
- AA prolongs the period required for complete recovery from a seizure (51). Pretreatment and treatment with n-3 fatty acids may protect the brain from the damaging effects of excessive AA level. The effects of n-3 fatty acids are opposite to n-6 fatty acids activity, and n-3 fatty acids may actually inhibit n-6 fatty acids activity (52).

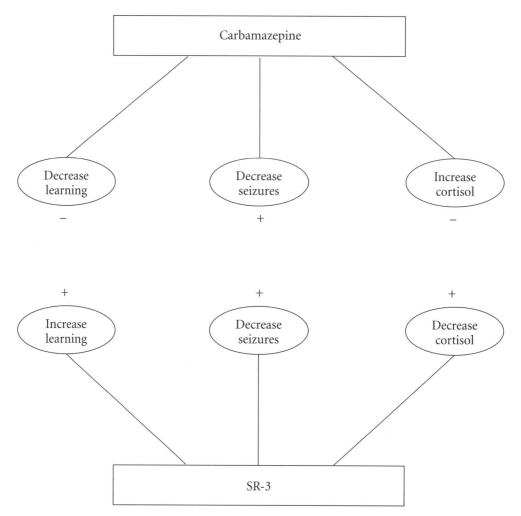

FIGURE 20.2

The separate effects of carbamazepine and SR-3 on learning, seizures, and cortisol level. A favorable effect is noted by a + sign; an adverse effect is noted by a − sign.

The role of cortisol in seizures needs further clarification. A seizure is a stressful situation and immunologic markers of stress increase immediately after seizures; (53) cortisol levels increase in response to stress (54–56). Ionic channels (and cortisol) are involved in the neurophysiology of seizures; however, a detailed discussion about the role of particular ionic channels (K+, Na+, or Ca++) in epilepsy is beyond the scope of this review.

Conclusion

The possible protective effects against seizures provided by PUFAs, especially fatty acids of the n-3 group (EPA and DHA), are documented. Some additional support can be found in a review on the beneficial effects of a ketogenic diet (57). Similarly, the role of FAs in increasing the threshold for electrically induced seizures is well established (58). In mice, n-3 fatty acids can block PTZ-induced unhealthy brain excitation and stimulation that produces convulsions in various hippocampal neurons (34). Similar results show that DHA (an n-3 fatty acid type) can inhibit epileptic activity in the hippocampus of rats (12). Of equal interest is that n-3 fatty acids (i.e., linolenic acid) are neuroprotective (15).

The relative potency of each individual FA as a neuroprotective agent is unknown. Some investigators have proposed that even with adequate LA and ALA levels, seizure patients may lack the sufficient enzymatic activity necessary to metabolize these FAs, and that supplementation with EPA and/or DHA may be the more attractive design for clinical experimentation. Our data suggest that the optimal effective combination of FA in a ratio of 1:4 of α-linolenic to linoleic acid might comprise the first order study in a program of dietary supplementation.

A sufficiently reliable and scientific basis exists for undertaking randomized clinical trials to more precisely evaluate the practical value of FA supplementation as a therapy for epilepsy. The practical reality for the success of such a program would require 2 to 4 months of daily intake of FA substances (2 to 4 g per day). Assuming there are no problems with blood thinning, diabetes, or other related medical contraindications, the only side effect is stomach discomfort that may occur during the first few days. A variety of choices and suppliers for FA supplements is available in most pharmacies, supermarkets, and natural food stores at a reasonable cost. Look for these keywords on the label: *omega-3*, *DHA*, and *EPA*. Usually, the cost of these nonprescription nutritional products will not be reimbursed by insurance plans. Finally, the patient, along with caregivers, primary care physician, and neurologist should all be updated on the program of diet supplementation. The outcomes of the program, with respect to general behavioral status, sleep improvement, and any other reactions or impressions, should be recorded at regular intervals. If the PUFA diet reduces seizure frequency or severity, an authorized reduction in AEDs may be considered by the neurologist. Without waiting for the results of formally designed randomized clinical trials, however, the safety of dietary PUFA supplementation—when taken in the recommended dosages—is sufficient to warrant implementation at this time.

Notes on the Chemistry of Essential Fatty Acids

Fats (lipids) and fatty acids, in a manner similar to many organic chemicals, are represented by combinations of various carbon, oxygen, and hydrogen elements that are linked together by one or two bonds. Each carbon has four binding sites. In the carbon chain, two sites will be taken up by other carbons (i.e., the two adjacent carbons on the chain). In a saturated fat, the other two sites are taken up by hydrogen atoms. Saturated fats are typically solid at room temperature, such as lard and butter, and are generally of animal origin. Saturated fats are generally burned as fuel by our bodies.

Unsaturated fats have two adjacent carbons held together by a biochemical "double bond." These fats are generally liquid at room temperature and are of plant origin (olive oil, corn oil, etc.). Unsaturated fats can be classified as "omega three" fatty acids (or T-3 or n-3) or "omega six" fatty acids (or T-6 or n-6), depending on the location of the double bond relative to the end of the chain. These types of fatty acids are essential, meaning that our bodies cannot make them, and they must be included in the diet. These fats are not burned for fuel. Instead, they are used as structural components. The omega-6 fatty acids are used as the main structural components of cells. Omega-3s are used in the structure of the retina and central nervous system.

The connections among the different elements may take different shapes. In the case of PUFAs, they form a chain composed of a long-chain fatty acid containing two or more double bonds. They occur throughout the animal, plant, algae, fungi, and bacteria kingdoms and have potential promise for therapeutic and nutritional applications. They may also be produced commercially from selected seed plants and some marine sources.

PUFAs are grouped into two series on the basis of the position of the terminal double bond, either three positions or six positions from the terminal carbon atom of the fatty acid chain. Some examples are: n-3-series PUFA, (e.g., ALA and DHA); and n-6-series PUFA, (e.g., GLA and AA). They are involved in the structure and composition of membranes (in the form of phospholipids) and other biophysical activities, including the regulation of the architecture, dynamics, phase transitions, permeability of membranes, and the control of membrane-associated processes.

The importance of PUFA metabolism and eicosanoid function for humans was recognized when it was discovered that AA is the precursor for prostaglandins, which are associated with pain phenomena. Eicosanoids are a diverse group of hormones that are fundamental to the proper maintenance of many functions, including blood pressure, inflammatory reactions, and immune response. They are produced mainly through the metabolism of AA and EPA.

Present-day eicosanoid-related ailments can be traced to changes in human nutrition. Research indicates that 10,000 years ago, the intake of PUFAs was evenly balanced between 3-series and 6-series PUFAs. Since then, reductions in 3-series PUFAs have created an imbalance in most modern societies. This can be attributed to the move away from a hunter-gatherer culture, and the increased consumption of certain plants and animal products, resulting in a large rise in 6-series PUFA with a correspondingly reduced level of 3-series PUFA.

The importance of balanced PUFA intake has been recognized by health organizations throughout the world over the past decade. A consensus now exists that PUFAs should constitute a minimum of 3%, and preferably 10% to 20%, of the total lipid intake, and that the n-6 to n-3 ratio should ideally be around 4:1 or 5:1. Although the biologic effects of eicosanoids are undisputed, the same cannot be said for their PUFA precursors, and most of the proposed pharmacologic effects for PUFAs are unconfirmed. In addition, the importance of PUFA intake in the genesis and progression of diseases, relative to other factors such as nutrition, genetic determinants, and environmental influences, remains unclear.

Evidence for the possible medical effects of PUFA deficiencies—coupled with the growing acceptance of pharmafoods or "neutriceuticals" by consumers—has brought these compounds to the attention of food and pharmaceutical companies, which have been quick to exploit markets in the biomedical and pharmafood areas. A variety of specialty PUFA lipids are being studied for a multitude of medical applications, ranging from antiaging, antithrombotic, antiinflammatory, anticholesterolemic, and anticancer drugs to immunostimulant and immunosuppressant therapeutics. Their efficacy has not yet been conclusively proven. An increase has also occurred in the unregulated applications for esters, glycerides, and phospholipids, such as health food additives for foods, nutritional formulas, and cosmetics ingredients. The most obvious commercial impact of PUFAs has been in health supplements, with a host of plant- and fish-derived GLA, EPA, and DHA products now available in the marketplace for uncontrolled dietary use. These nonprescription preparations may be effective for some health problems, such as depression.

This raises the question as to whether PUFAs should be treated as special nutritional products or as pharmaceuticals. There is a basis for considering them as food components because they occur in foodstuffs; yet they are biologically active, and because serious disease states may result from eicosanoid imbalances, there is justification to regard them as biomedical additives.

Acknowledgments

We would like to thank the William Farber Center for Alzheimer Research and Rose K. Ginsburg Chair for Research into Alzheimer's Disease for their support. We are also grateful to Dr. Debra Morley for her assistance in the preparation of this chapter.

References

1. Ruthrich H, Grecksch G, Krug M. Effects of piracetam on pentylenetetrazol-kindling development, hippocampal potentiation phenomena and kindling-induced learning deficit. *Naunyn Schmiedeberg's Arch Pharmacol* 1999;360:413–420.
2. Rossler AS, Schroder H, Dodd RH, et al. Benzodiazepine receptor inverse agonist-induced kindling of rats alters learning and glutamate binding. *Pharmacol Biochem Behav* 2000;67:169–175.
3. Becker A, Braun H, Schroder H, et al. Effects of enadoline on the development of pentylenetetrazol kindling, learning performances, and hippocampal morphology. *Brain Res* 1999;823:191–197.
4. de Feo MR, Mecarelli O, Palladini G, et al. Long-term effects of early status epilepticus on the acquisition of conditioned avoidance behavior in rats. *Epilepsia* 1986;27:476–482.
5. Lauritzen I, Blondeau N, Heurteaux C, et al. Polyunsaturated fatty acids are potent neuroprotectors. *EMBO J* 2000;19:1784–1793.
6. Sankar R, Sotero de Menezes M. Metabolic and endocrine aspects of the ketogenic diet. *Epilepsy Res* 1999;37:191–201.
7. Ruthrich H, Grecksch G, Krug M. Development of long-lasting potentiation effects in the dentate gyrus during pentylenetetrazol kindling. *Int J Neurosci* 2001;19:247–254.
8. Mostofsky DI, Loyning Y, (eds.) *The Neurobehavioral Treatment of Epilepsy.* Hillsdale, NJ: Erlbaum Press, 1993.
9. Yehuda S, Rabinovitz S., Carasso RL, et al. The role of polyunsaturated fatty acids in restoring the aging neuronal membrane. *Neurobiology of Aging* 2002;23:843–853.

10. Yehuda S, Rabinovitz, S, Mostofsky, DI. Essential fatty acids are mediators of brain biochemistry and cognitive functions. *J Neurosci Res* 1999;56:565–570.

11. Yehuda S, Mostofsky DI, (eds.) *Chronic Fatigue Syndrome.* New York: Plenum Press, 1997.

12. Mostofsky DI, Yehuda S, Salem N, (eds.) *Fatty Acids: Physiologic and Behavioral Functions.* New York: Humana Press, 2001.

13. Yehuda S, Carasso RL, Mostofsky DI. Essential fatty acid preparation (SR-3) raises the seizure threshold in rats. *European J Pharm* 1994;254:193–198.

14. Yehuda S, Rabinovitz S, Mostofsky DI, et al. Essential fatty acids preparation rehabilitates biochemical and cognitive functions in EAE rats. *European J Pharm* 1997;328:23–29.

15. Blondeau N, Widmann C, Lazdunski M, et al. Polyunsaturated fatty acids induce ischemic and epileptic intolerance. *Neurosci* 2002;109:231–241.

16. Lauritzen L, Hansen HS, Jorgensen MH, et al. The essentiality of long chain n-3 fatty acids in relation to development and function of the brain and retina. *Prog Lipid Res* 2001;40:1–94.

17. Bazan NG. The neuromessenger platelet-activating factor in plasticity neurodegeneration. *Prog Brain Res* 1998;118:281–291.

18. Pediconi MF, Rodriguez de Turco EB, Bazan NG. Reduced labeling of brain phosphatidylinositol, triacylglycerols, and diacylglycerols by [1-14C] arachidonic acid after electroconvulsive shock: potentiation of the effect by adrenergic drugs and comparison with palmitic acid labeling. *Neurochem Res* 1986;11:217–230.

19. Van Rooijen LA, Vadnal R, Dobard P, et al. Enhanced inositide turnover in brain during bicuculline-induced status epilepticus. *Biochem Biophys Res Commun* 1986;136:827–834.

20. Flynn, CJ, Wecker L. Concomitant increases in the levels of choline and free fatty acids in rat brain: evidence supporting the seizure-induced hydrolysis of phosphatidylcholine. *J Neurochem* 1987;48:1178–1184.

21. Visioli F, Rodriguez de Turco EB, Kreisman NR, et al. Membrane lipid degradation is related to interictal cortical activity in a series of seizures. *Metab Brain Dis* 1994;9:161–170.

22. Birkle DL. Regional and temporal variations in the accumulation of unesterified fatty acids and diacylglycerols in the rat brain during kainic acid-induced limbic seizures. *Brain Res* 1993;613:115–122.

23. Cornford EM, Oldendorf WH. Epilepsy and the blood-brain barrier. *Adv Neurol* 1986;44:787–812.

24. Cervos-Navarro J, Kannuki S, Nakagawa Y. Blood–brain barrier (BBB). Review from morphological aspect. *Histol Histopathol* 1988;3:203–213.

25. Schlanger S, Shinitzky M, Yam D. Diet enriched with omega-3 fatty acids alleviates convulsion symptoms in epilepsy patients. *Epilepsia* 2002;43:103.

26. Freeman JM, Vining EPG, Pillas DJ, et al. The efficacy of the ketogenic diet—1998: a prospective evaluation of intervention in 150 children. *Pediatrics* 1998;102:1358–1363.

27. Stafstrom CE. Animal models of the ketogenic diet: what have we learned, what can we learn? *Epilepsy Res* 1999;37:241–259.

28. Vining EPG. Clinical efficacy of the ketogenic diet. *Epilepsy Res* 1999;37:181–190.

29. Ben-Menachem E. New antiepileptic drugs and non-pharmacological treatments. *Curr Opin Neurol* 2000;13:165–170.

30. Likhodii SS, Musa K, Mendonca A, et al. Dietary fat, ketosis, and seizure resistance in rats on the ketogenic diet. *Epilepsia* 2000;41:1400–1410.

31. Helmstaedter C, Kurthen M. Memory and epilepsy: characteristics, course and influence of drugs and surgery. *Curr Opinion Neurology* 2001;14:211–216.

32. Stafstrom CE. Effects of fatty acids and ketones on neural excitability: Implications for epilepsy and its treatment. In: Mostofsky DI, Yehuda S, Salem N, (eds.) *Fatty Acids: Physiologic and Behavioral Functions.* New York: Humana Press, 2001:273–290.

33. Søvik O, Mansson JE, Bjorke Monson AL, et al. Generalized peroxisomal disorder in male twins: fatty acid composition of serum lipids and response to n-3 fatty acids. *J Inherit Metab Dis* 1998;21:662–670.

34. Xiao Y, Li X. Polyunsaturated fatty acids modify mouse hippocampal neuronal excitability during excitotoxic or convulsant stimulation. *Brain Res* 1999;846:112–121.

35. Valmadrid C, Voorhees C, Litt B, et al. Practice patterns of neurologists regarding bone and mineral effects of antiepileptic drug therapy. *Arch Neurol* 2001;58:1352–1353.

36. Matthews SC, Miller BP. Auditory hallucinations associated with topiramate. *J Clin Psychiatry* 2001;62:653.

37. Behrens S, Pohlmann-Eden B. Reversible phenytoin-induced extrapontine myelinolysis. *Nervenartz* 2001;72:453–455.

38. Goldberg JF, Burdick KE. Cognitive side effects of anticonvulsants. *J Clin Psychiatry* 2001;62:27–33.

39. Huppertz HJ, Quiske A, Schulze-Bonhage A. Cognitive impairments due to add-on therapy with topiramate. *Nervenartz* 2001;72:275–280.

40. Katoh-Semba R, Takeuchi IK, Inaguma Y, et al. Induction of brain-derived neurotrophic factor by convulsant drugs in the rat brain: involvement of region-specific voltage-dependent calcium channels. *J Neurochem* 2001;77:71–83.

41. Martin R, Meador K, Turrentine L, et al. Comparative cognitive effects of carbamazepine and gabapentin in healthy senior adults. *Epilepsia* 2001;42:764–771.

42. Borowicz KK, Kleinrok Z, Czuczwar SJ. Influence of D(-)CPP and (+/-)CPP upon the protective action of conventional antiepileptic drugs against electroconvulsions in mice. *Pol J Pharmacol* 2000;52:431–439.

43. Dailey JW, Reith ME, Yan QS, et al. Anticonvulsant doses of carbamazepine increases hippocampal extracellular serotonin in genetically epilepsy-prone rats: dose response relationships. *Neurosci Lett* 1997;227:13–16.

44. Serra M, Dazzi L, Cagetti E. Effects of pentylenetetrazol-induced kindling on acetylcholine release in the hippocampus of freely moving rats. *J Neurochem* 1997;68:313–318.

45. Becker A, Grecksch G, Brosz M. Antiepileptic drugs B their effects on kindled seizures and kindling-induced learning impairments. *Pharmacol Biochem Behav* 1995;52:453–459.

46. Erakovic V, Zupan G, Varljen J, et al. Altered activities of rat brain metabolic enzymes caused by pentylenetetrazol kindling and pentylenetetrazol-induced seizures. *Epilepsy Res* 2001;43:165–173.

47. Davies B, Kearns IR, Ure J, et al. Loss of hippocampal serine protease BSP1/neuropsin predisposes to global seizure activity. *J Neurosci* 2001;21:6993–7000.

48. Yehuda S, Mostofsky DI, Rabinovitz S. Anticonvulsant efficiency, behavioral performance, and cortisol levels: A comparison of carbamazapine and a fatty acid compound. *Psychoneuroendocrinology* 2004;29:113–124.

49. Oztas B, Kili, Ô, Esen D, et al. Influence of antioxidants on the blood-brain barrier permeability during epileptic seizures. *J Neurosci Res* 2001;66:674–678.

50. Farooqui AA, Ong WY, Lu XR, et al. Neurochemical consequences of kainite-induced toxicity in brain: involvement of arachidonic acid release and prevention of toxicity by phospholiopase A_2 inhibitors. *Brain Res Rev* 2001;38:61–78.

51. Keros S, McBain CJ. Arachidonic acid inhibits transient potassium currents and broadens action potentials during electrographic seizures in hippocampal pyramidal and inhibitory interneurons. *J Neurosci* 1997;17:3476–3487.

52. Yehuda S, Rabinovitz S, Mostofsky DI. PUFA: mediators of the nervous, endocrine, and immune systems. In: Mostofsky DI, Yehuda S, Salem N, (eds.), *Fatty Acids: Physiologic and Behavioral Functions*. New York: Humana Press, 2001;403–420.

53. Penkowa M, Molinero A, Carrasco J, et al. Interleukin-6 deficiency reduces the brain inflam-

matory response and increases oxidative stress and neurodegeneration after kainic acid-induced seizures. *Neurosci* 2001;102:805–818.

54. Dirik E, Sen A, Anal O, et al. Serum cortisol and prolactin levels in childhood paroxysmal disorders. *Acta Paediatr Jpn* 1996;38:118–120.

55. Motta E. Epilepsy and hormones. *Neurol Neurochir Pol* 2000;33:31–36.

56. Tunca Z, Ergene U, Fidaner H, et al. Re-evaluation of serum cortisol in conversion disorders with seizure (pseudoseizure). *Psychosomatics* 2000;41:152–153.

57. Bough KJ, Eagles DA. Comparison of the anticonvulsant efficacies and neurotoxic effects of valproic acid, phenytoin, and the ketogenic diet. *Epilepsia* 2001;42:1345–1353.

58. Voskuyl RA, Vreugdenhil M, Kang JX, et al. Anticonvulsant effect of polyunsaturated fatty acids in rats, using the cortical stimulation model. *Eur J Pharmacol* 1998;341:145–152.

CHAPTER 21

The Ketogenic Diet

John M. Freeman, MD

Despite the many new antiepileptic drugs (AEDs), approximately 20% to 30% of children and adults continue to have seizures that are difficult to control. Some are candidates for epilepsy surgery to remove a seizure focus. Many must continue trying different medications. The ketogenic diet represents a promising, alternative therapeutic approach to improved seizure control for some children, and it is a potential but untested therapy for adults. A schematic diagram of the course of seizures and epilepsy—and the role of the ketogenic diet—is shown in Table 21.1 (1).

The classic ketogenic diet: high in fat, adequate in protein, and low in carbohydrates, was developed in the 1920s. The diet was initially designed to mimic the effects of starvation, which had been shown to have dramatic and long-lasting effects on the control of seizures. After the discovery of *phenytoin*, the classic ketogenic diet was used less frequently. The results of the study listed in Table 21.1 document the continued efficacy of the diet in children with uncontrolled seizures. Additionally, an article in *Pediatrics* in 2000, by LeFevre and Aronson stated, "This improvement is in the range of, or greater than, that reported with the addition of newer antiepileptic drugs" (1).

A healthcare practitioner working with a knowledgeable dietician must carefully calculate the contents of the diet to achieve and maintain the *individual* ideal body weight for the child. The diet *must* be supplemented with multivitamins, calcium, and trace minerals, and it must *only* be used under medical supervision.

The ketogenic diet achieves more than a 50% decrease in seizure frequency in more than 50% of the children initiated (Table 21.1). It seems equally effective at various ages, in different seizure types, and appears to have a dramatic effect in many children with the atonic/myoclonic seizures of Lennox-Gastaut syndrome, a serious, rare epilepsy beginning between the ages of 1 and 6 years (2,3). The diet is tolerated in adolescents when sufficiently effective. Its effectiveness in adults remains to be determined.

The ketogenic diet mimics starvation by restricting carbohydrate ingestion and replacing 90% of the calories with fat. In the absence of sufficient carbohydrates, the fatty acids are incompletely oxidized, resulting in increased levels of beta-hydroxybutyrate (B-OHB). Elevated blood B-OHB is thought to be critical for achieving seizure control, but the precise correlation (if any) of blood level of B-OHB with seizure control remains to be determined. The mechanisms by which the ketogenic diet exerts its anticonvulsant effects are still unknown.

TABLE 21.1

Outcomes of the Ketogenic Diet—Johns Hopkins 1998

Number Initiating	Seizure Control and Diet Status	3 months	6 months	12 months
Total	Seizure-free	4 (3%)	5 (3%)	11 (7%)
N = 150	>90%	46 (31%)	43 (29%)	30 (20%)
	50%-90%	39 (26%)	29 (19%)	34 (23%)
	<50%	36 (24%)	29 (19%)	8 (5%)
	Continue diet	125 (83%)	106 (71%)	83 (55%)

The ketogenic diet, if supplemented with vitamins, calcium, and trace minerals, appears to be nutritionally adequate and permits normal linear growth, even while restricting weight gain. Kidney stones occur in 5% to 8% of children and often can be prevented by increased fluids and alkalinization of the urine with citrates. A mild dyslipidemia is common, with mean cholesterol of 220 mg/dL, and high-density lipoproteins (HDLs) of 50 mg/dL.

Commentary

The high fat, low carbohydrate ketogenic diet is widely used by most comprehensive epilepsy centers as an adjunct to standard medical therapy for children with medically refractory seizures. There is little doubt that the diet provides complete or partial seizure control for a subgroup of patients, particularly children with myoclonic seizures. Just how the diet works is still poorly understood. Some basic researchers believe that ketones (biochemicals produced from the breakdown of fats when carbohydrates are absent) are antiepileptic (1). Other researchers attribute the antiepileptic effect of the ketogenic diet to the reduction of calories and dispute the need for ketone production (2). Unfortunately, no clinical studies in children compare the ketogenic diet to a low-calorie, high-carbohydrate diet for seizure control.

The success rate at Johns Hopkins—greater than 50% reduction in seizures in more than 50% of patients—is higher than many other centers report. An Italian multicenter study found that a 50% or greater reduction of seizures was found in 27% at 6 months and 9% at 1 year after initiation of the diet (3). At Connecticut Children's Medical Center, 23% had a >50% reduction of seizures at 1-year followup (4). At the Cleveland Clinic, 24% of patients with focal seizures and 42% of patients with generalized seizures enjoyed this benchmark of seizure control at 1-year followup (5). Many did not reach the 1 year mark on the diet.

Those who have tried the diet know that it requires enormous commitment from the family and patient. As Dr. Freeman points out, even a small amount of carbohydrate can reverse the ketotic state and possibly reduce the effectiveness of the diet. This requires constant vigilance by patients and care-givers to ensure that children do not stray from the diet; even medicines and dietary supplements must be free of carbohydrate additives. The initiation of the diet may be especially difficult for young children and infants, because the diet may result in very low blood glucose levels, dehydration, and metabolic derangements. Most physicians elect to initiate the diet in the hospital, where careful monitoring of vital signs and blood studies can take place.

The long-term safety of the diet has always been of concern to physicians. Issues such as growth retardation and atherosclerosis have not been studied in great detail, but are less of a concern when the diet is employed for a limited duration (usually less than 2 years). Studying the group thought to be at greatest risk for complications—infants—Nordli and his colleagues found normal growth parameters for nearly all 32 infants placed on the diet (6). Well-controlled, long-term longitudinal studies of other health risks of the diet have not been completed. Serious adverse events can occur, including cardiac disorders and death from acute pancreatitis (7,8).

In summary, the ketogenic diet is a reasonable adjunct and, in some cases, an alternative to antiepileptic medications and surgery for childhood seizures. Its usefulness in adults is less clear, although preliminary results suggest that in medically refractory cases, it can reduce the burden of seizures and antiepileptic drugs in some patients (9). Its main limitations are the rigorous dietary requirements, the need for constant surveillance of ketosis and possible complications, and quality of life alteration, especially for older children.

References

1. Likhodii SS, Burnham WM. Ketogenic diet: does acetone stop seizures? *Med Sci Monit* 2002;8(8):HY19–24.
2. Eagles DA, Boyd SJ, Kotak A, et al. Calorie restriction of a high-carbohydrate diet elevates the threshold of PTZ-induced seizures to values equal to those seen with a ketogenic diet. *Epilepsy Res* 2003;54(1):41–52.
3. DiMario FJ Jr, Holland J. The ketogenic diet: a review of the experience at Connecticut Children's Medical Center. *Pediatr Neurol* 2002;26:288–292.
4. Coppola G, Veggiotti P, Cusmai R, et al. The ketogenic diet in children, adolescents and young adults with refractory epilepsy: an Italian multicentric experience. *Epilepsy* Res 2002;48:221–227.
5. Maydell BV, Wyllie E, Akhtar N, et al. Efficacy of the ketogenic diet in focal versus generalized seizures. *Pediatr Neurol* 2001;25:208–212.
6. Nordli DR Jr, Kuroda MM, Carroll J, et al. Experience with the ketogenic diet in infants. *Pediatrics* 2001;108(1):129–133.
7. Best TH, Franz DN, Gilbert DL, Nelson DP, Epstein MR. Cardiac complications in pediatric patients on the ketogenic diet. *Neurology* 2000;54:2328–2330.
8. Stewart WA, Gordon K, Camfield P. Acute pancreatitis causing death in a child on the ketogenic diet. *J Child Neurol* 2001;16:682.
9. Sirven J, Whedon B, Caplan D, et al. The ketogenic diet for intractable epilepsy in adults: preliminary results. *Epilepsia* 1999;40:1721–1726.

The following are the other important aspects of the diet (4):

- Eating even small amounts of carbohydrates makes the diet ineffectual. For example, sugar—even in toothpaste—is prohibited.
- The diet may work for all kinds of seizures, but it has had the most desired results in atonic, tonic, and myoclonic seizures.
- The diet is usually begun in a hospital, so that the blood sugar level and fluid status can be monitored.
- High-fat foods (i.e., mayonnaise, butter, and cream) make up 80% to 90% of the diet; protein is at least 1 gram per kilogram of body weight; carbohydrates make up the remaining calories and are kept to a minimum (about 2 to 10 grams per day).
- There is no evidence that children develop atherosclerosis from the diet.
- The diet, if effective, is usually continued for about 1 to 3 years, and then is discontinued gradually.

As we begin to learn how the ketogenic diet works for difficult-to-control seizures in childhood, we will, perhaps, develop new understanding of the mechanisms underlying epilepsy and be able to develop less burdensome forms of AEDs.

Suggested Reading

Freeman JM, Kelly M, Freeman JB. *The Ketogenic Diet: A Treatment for Epilepsy.* New York: Demos Medical Publishing, 2000.

Freeman JM, Vining EPG. Seizures rapidly decrease after fasting: preliminary studies of the ketogenic diet. *Arch Pediatr Adolesc Med* 1999;153:946–949.

Freeman JM, Vining EPG, Casey JC, et al. The ketogenic diet revisited. In: Schmidt D, Schachter SC, (eds.) *Epilepsy: Problem Solving in Clinical Practice.* London: Martin Dunitz, 2000; Chap. 24.

Swink TD, Vining EPG, Freeman JM. The ketogenic diet. 1996. *Adv Pediatr* 1997;44:297–329.

References

1. LeFevre F, Aronson N. Ketogenic diet for the treatment of refractory epilepsy in children: a systematic review of efficacy. *Pediatrics* 2000;105(4):E46. URL: http://www.pediatrics.org/cgi/content/full/105 /4/e46.
2. Freeman JM, Vining EPG, Pillas DJ, et al. The efficacy of the ketogenic diet–1998: a prospective evaluation of intervention in 150 children. *Pediatrics* 1998;102:1358–1363.
3. Hemingway C, Freeman JM, Pillas DJ, et al. The ketogenic diet: a 3- to 6-year follow-up of 150 children prospectively enrolled. *Pediatrics* 2001;108:898–905.
4. Devinsky O. *Epilepsy: Patient and Family Guide*, 2nd edition. Philadelphia: F. A. Davis, 2001.

PART V

Alternative Medical Therapies

CHAPTER 22

Hormonal Therapy

Alan R. Jacobs, MD

The mainstay of hormonal therapy for epilepsy in women is natural progesterone. Important issues for women are related to estrogen, birth control pills, and menopausal hormone replacement therapy, and issues related to reproductive hormone disorders.

The clinical observations that led to the idea of using progesterone to treat epilepsy were reports by over one-third of women with seizure disorders that their seizures were more frequent and/or more severe at certain times in their menstrual cycles on a recurrent basis. This is known as *catamenial* epilepsy. Herzog et al. have documented three specific patterns of catamenial epilepsy with seizures exacerbating around the time of menses, around midcycle when ovulation occurs, and a third pattern involving the whole second half of the menstrual cycle between ovulation and menstruation (the luteal phase) (1).

These patterns are thought to occur because of the effects that estradiol and progesterone have on neurons, and because of the cyclic variations of the blood levels of these hormones during the menstrual cycle. Estradiol has an excitatory effect on neurons by increasing their metabolism and firing rates and by effecting chemical influences on them (2). In animal and human experiments, estradiol promotes seizure occurrence (3).

Progesterone has the opposite effects on neurons, reducing their metabolism and firing rates and suppressing experimental and clinical seizures (4). The most common pattern of catamenial epilepsy occurs premenstrually, at a time when estrogen levels are high relative to progesterone and when progesterone is withdrawing, which itself can provoke seizures (5). The midcycle pattern of exacerbation around ovulation occurs when a surge of estrogen occurs prior to the rise in progesterone. In some women, a third luteal phase pattern occurs when the second 2 weeks of the cycle are characterized by normal estrogen levels, but low or inadequate progesterone levels. Thus, estrogen-to-progesterone ratios are higher than normal, and seizures are more frequent throughout the whole 2 weeks preceding menstruation.

Catamenial epilepsy is treated with natural progesterone, not synthetic progestins, such as those found in birth control pills or medroxyprogesterone acetate (Provera®). One theory as to why natural progesterone works whereas synthetics do not has to do with its main metabolite, allopregnanalone, which is even more potent as a barbiturate-like, antiseizure chemical in the brain (6). The synthetic progestins do not break down to such a chemical. Prometrium® is now available as an FDA-approved form of micronized natural progesterone. It comes in 100 mg and 200 mg pills. Oral micronized progesterone has a 6- to 8-hour half-life in the bloodstream. Therefore, it is typically given three times daily. The important issue is when in the menstrual cycle to take progesterone. In general, progesterone is begun at the time of ovulation, typically on day 14 of a 28-day cycle, to offset the surge in estrogen that naturally occurs at this time. It is continued, for example, as 200 mg every 8 hours, all the way through the luteal phase of the cycle until the 28th day. To keep the estrogen-to-progesterone ratio favorable and to avoid causing progesterone-withdrawal effects, the hormone is tapered by one pill per day until off, usually tailing 2 days into the next cycle. With the onset of menses, the new cycle starts as day 1 and the progesterone begins again on the next day 14. This 2-weeks on and 2-weeks off pattern is usually easy to adapt to and does not interfere with a woman's natural cycle or prevent ovulation, as do birth control pills. This therapy has been used successfully to treat certain anxious, irritable forms of premenstrual syndrome. This makes sense, because the temporal lobe limbic areas that are most responsive to estrogen and progesterone are highly prone to seizures and are also involved in emotional processing.

Several open-label studies treating seizures with progesterone were done by Herzog et al. The first was in 1986, in which six out of eight women with catamenial intractable partial complex seizures and inadequate luteal phase progesterone cycles (the type 3 pattern) experienced a 68% decline in their average monthly seizure frequency over 3 months (7). A larger study in 1993, with similar subjects, showed 19 of 25 women experienced a 54% average monthly decline for complex partial seizures and a 58% decline for secondary generalized seizures over 3 months (8). In October 2000, the National Institutes of Health (NIH) began funding a multicenter, double-blind, placebo-controlled clinical trial known as Progesterone Therapy for Women with Epilepsy, with Dr. Herzog as the principal investigator.

Progesterone has dose-dependent side effects, most commonly sedation and occasional sadness. It is rare, however, for women to not tolerate doses of progesterone that provide efficacy for their seizures. Progesterone and the liver-inducing antiepileptic drugs (AEDs; e.g., carbamazepine, phenytoin, and phenobarbital) compete for the same metabolic sites in the liver. Thus, taking such an AED will lower the serum levels of progesterone due to more rapid metabolism. Yet, we have also seen women who have seizure exacerbations early in their menstrual cycle (e.g., days 2, 3, and 4) due to the rapid decline in estrogen and progesterone levels that naturally occurs at that time, which allows the liver to metabolize the AEDs rapidly. Thus, serum drug levels drop. This is easy to document by obtaining trough blood AED levels premenstrually (e.g., on day 26) and during menses (day 2 or 3). If a drop is found, doses can be increased during week 1 of each cycle.

Many neurologists and other doctors lack an awareness of the hormonal influences on epilepsy. Hopefully, the successful completion and publication of the NIH study will greatly increase this awareness. Currently, the most powerful argument a woman can

Commentary

For centuries, some women with epilepsy have noted a connection between the occurrence of their seizures and a specific period of time in their menstrual cycle. Until relatively recently, these observations were generally dismissed by physicians. A good deal of scientific research has now shown a connection between the female hormones estrogen and progesterone, which fluctuate during the menstrual cycle, and the tendency for seizures to occur. Furthermore, some women with epilepsy do not have normal menstrual cycles, and these women are perhaps most likely to have a hormonal connection to their seizures.

What are the clues that a woman may have seizures related to the sex hormones? As discussed by Dr. Jacobs, seizures may tend to occur either mid-cycle, premenstrually, or during the last half of the cycle. Seizures can occur at other times as well, for example, during periods of stress or sleep deprivation. They can occur, at times, randomly within the menstrual cycle in women with catamenial epilepsy. The diagnosis of catamenial epilepsy is made by the consistently increased seizure frequency during certain periods of the cycle. Another clue is that seizures may have begun in association with puberty or that periods are irregular.

Women should discuss these issues with their neurologist and carefully track their seizures and menstrual cycles on a calendar. If a consistent relationship exists between seizures and the menstrual cycle, then further testing or a referral to a specialist in this area might be recommended to confirm the problem. Testing might take a few months to complete.

The treatment options for women with catamenial epilepsy that are available by prescription are discussed by Dr. Jacobs. Work to date, especially with progesterone, has been promising. The long-term benefits and adverse effects of such hormonal therapies are not well documented. More definitive studies are underway to determine the effectiveness and tolerability of progesterone for catamenial epilepsy. Also, although the comment that synthetic progestins do not have antiseizure properties is supported by some data, insufficient data exist to make any definitive statements about their relative efficacy or safety in women with epilepsy. It is possible that their efficacy is similar or varies by the type of catamenial epilepsy present. Women who plan to take herbs or dietary supplements with estrogenic actions (such as soy estrogen) should discuss these plans with their neurologist because of the possible exacerbation of seizures.

make that she has catamenial epilepsy is to use a calendar to record her menses and track whether and when seizures occur in relation to the day of her cycle. The patterns are easy to document when they exist. Seizure counts from three consecutive cycles are usually sufficient to diagnose catamenial epilepsy.

The decision to consider a woman with epilepsy as a candidate for hormonal therapy begins first and foremost by establishing a history of one of the three catamenial patterns of seizure occurrence:

- Seizures tending to occur ± 3 days surrounding the onset of menses (premenstrual, or type 1)
- ± 3 days surrounding ovulation at mid-cycle (periovulatory, or type 2)
- For the 3 weeks beginning around ovulation and continuing into menses, with the second week of the cycle being the only seizure-free time (inadequate luteal phase cycles, or type 3)

A 2:1 ratio of seizures occurring at one of these times compared to other random times is sufficient to diagnose catamenial epilepsy (1). The next step in the evaluation is to explore the reproductive history for any symptoms of dysfunction, such as irregular menstrual cycle lengths, skipping menses, infertility, or changes in libido or sexual function. If a review of these symptoms is positive, serum levels of reproductive hormones can be measured to look for conditions such as polycystic ovarian syndrome, hypothalamic amenorrhea, low or high androgens, or even perimenopause. Referral to a gynecologist or reproductive endocrinologist may be appropriate at this point. Establishing seizure types is also of great interest here, because temporal lobe partial seizures, with or without secondary generalization, are most likely to occur in a catamenial pattern, but other seizure types occasionally occur in these patterns. Finally, treatment with natural progesterone (e.g., Prometrium®) is begun as described above, usually without changing other anticonvulsant medications while evaluating the response to therapy. Seizure calendars are continued for one to three cycles to allow doctor and patient to judge efficacy and side effects.

Hormonal influences on seizures are high at other times and settings in the reproductive lives of women with epilepsy. The first is around menarche, the onset of menstruation in young women in their early teens. During this time, when the hormonal cycles are establishing themselves, ovulation can be sporadic for the first 6 months or so. Thus, many early cycles are anovulatory; without normal ovulation, no progesterone is produced. This leads to a persistent state of unopposed estrogen effect on the brain, exacerbating seizures. A second setting for seizure increase is when women take oral contraceptive pills (OCPs), because the estrogens in the OCPs are seizure-provoking, but the progestins are synthetic and do not have the antiseizure properties of natural progesterone. Currently, no OCPs contain natural progesterone. Finally, perimenopause and postmenopausal hormone replacement are both associated with seizure exacerbation (9). In the later years of perimenopause, as actual menopause draws nearer, ovulation becomes more sporadic and, thus, progesterone becomes scarcer and scarcer. This again leads to relative estrogen excess, and seizures intensify. The standard hormone replacement therapy (HRT) given at this time utilizes various estrogens, all containing seizure-provoking properties, but synthetic progestins that lack antiseizure properties. Thus, the classic Premarin® and Provera® combination is similar to taking unopposed estrogen as far as seizures are concerned. All these settings can be remedied by using natural progesterone (e.g., Prometrium®) to offset the unopposed estrogen influence.

In women, hormones affect seizures and seizures also affect hormones. Menstrual dysfunction, infertility, and reproductive disorders, such as polycystic ovarian syndrome, are all more common in women with temporal lobe seizures than in women without epilepsy. Altered temporal lobe function due to epilepsy probably disrupts the normal controls that the temporal lobe usually has over hormonal secretion from the pituitary gland (10). These hormonal changes are often associated with a lack of ovulation and, thus, diminished progesterone secretion, leading to higher ratios of estrogen to progesterone, which promotes seizures. Again, progesterone treatment can help normalize progesterone levels and reduce seizures. With less frequent seizures, temporal lobe controls over hormones can be more normal and menstrual disorders can resolve.

Reproductive hormone disorders also occur in men with temporal lobe epilepsy, who can also benefit from hormonal treatments of their seizures (11). These disorders include lowered sex drive, reduced potency, and even infertility. Several mechanisms may be responsible. Temporal lobe seizure discharges can disrupt the regulation of pituitary hormone secretion. Second, the resulting disruption can elevate estrogen levels and decrease testosterone levels, exacerbating seizures and reducing sex drive, potency, and feelings of well-being in men. Finally, AEDs can reduce testosterone levels and raise estrogen levels. Treating epileptic men with testosterone and testolactone, which prevents the conversion of testosterone into estrogen, improves sexual function (12). A trend toward improving seizure control using this hormonal treatment is also noted.

To conclude, a significant subset of women with seizure disorders suffer from catamenial epilepsy. Moreover, the hormonal fluxes accompanying menarche, OCP use, and menopause may adversely affect an even larger group of women with epilepsy. The biological underpinnings of these phenomena are being actively studied. For example, Reddy et al. at the Epilepsy Research Branch of NIH are using a rat model of catamenial epilepsy to test the efficacy of newer specific treatments with neuroactive steroids (13). One such compound being evaluated is known as *ganaxalone*, a synthetic analog of allopregnanalone, the main metabolite of progesterone in the brain, which has potent antiseizure effects. Pharmaceutical companies are avidly investigating neurosteroids as promising treatments for seizures, anxiety disorders, mood disorders, and other related disorders. All of this, along with a general shift of interest and funding by government and private institutions toward women's issues in healthcare, should lead to more awareness of hormonal influences on seizures and effective treatments for catamenial epilepsy.

References

1. Herzog AG, Klein P, Ransil BJ. Three patterns of catamenial epilepsy. *Epilepsia* 1997; 38(10):1082–1088.
2. Smith SS. Estradiol administration increases neuronal responses to excitatory amino acids as a long-term effect. *Brain Res* 1989;503:354–357.

3. Hardy RW. Unit activity in Premarin-induced cortical epileptogenic foci. *Epilepsia* 1970;11:179–186.

4. Blackstrom T, Zetterlund B, Blom S, et al. Effects of intravenous progesterone infusions on the epileptic discharge frequency in women with partial epilepsy. *Acta Neurol Scand* 1984;69:240–248.

5. Moran MH, Smith SS. Progesterone withdrawal I. *Brain Res* 1998;807(1-2):84–90.

6. Smith SS, Gong QH, Hsu FC, et al. GABA(A) receptor alpha 4 subunit suppression prevents withdrawal properties of an endogenous steroid. *Nature* 1998;392(6679):926–930.

7. Herzog AG. Intermittent progesterone therapy and frequency of complex partial seizures in women with menstrual disorders. *Neurology* 1986;1607–1610.

8. Herzog AG. Progesterone therapy in women with complex partial and secondary generalized seizures. *Neurology* 1995;45(9):1660–1662.

9. Harden CL, Pulver M, Ravdin LD, et al. Effect of menopause and perimenopause on the course of epilepsy. *Epilepsia* 1999;40(10):1402–1407.

10. Herzog AG. Reproductive endocrine considerations and hormonal therapy for women with epilepsy. *Epilepsia* 1991;32(suppl 6):S27–S33.

11. Herzog AG, Seibel MM, Schomer DL, et al. Reproductive endocrine disorders in men with partial seizures of temporal lobe origin. *Arch Neurol* 1986;43:347–350.

12. Klein P, Jacobs AR, Herzog AG. A comparison of testosterone versus testosterone and testolactone in the treatment of reproductive/sexual dysfunction in men with epilepsy and hypogonadism. *Neurology* 1998;50:782–784.

13. Reddy DS, Rogawski MA. Enhanced anticonvulsant activity of ganaxolone after neurosteroid withdrawal in a rat model of catamenial epilepsy. *J Pharmacol Exp Ther* 2000;294(3):909–915.

CHAPTER 23

Transcranial Magnetic Stimulation

Michael Orth, MD and Michael R. Trimble, MD

Normal brain function relies on a carefully balanced network of excitatory and inhibitory nerve cells. An imbalance in this system can lead to hyperexcitability of the brain—in particular, the cortex—and consequent seizures. Seizures result from excessive firing and synchronization of neurons within the seizure focus. This firing cannot be contained by the surrounding inhibitory neurons and eventually leads to the impairment of the normal functioning of this part of the brain. If the epileptic focus lies within the motor cortex, the seizure will cause abnormal motor activity, for example, of an arm or a leg. Subsequently, the electrical activity may spread to other parts of the brain, resulting in more symptoms and, eventually, loss of consciousness.

Treatment of epilepsy with antiepileptic drugs (AEDs) aims to stabilize the balance of synaptic excitation and inhibition of neurons. With medical treatment alone, 70% to 80% of patients with epilepsy enter 5-year remission, while 20% to 30% develop chronic intractable epilepsy (1). In some of these patients, particularly those whose seizures arise from well-defined lesions, such as hippocampal sclerosis, surgery is an alternative treatment option. Surgery, however, carries the risk of complications, and the rate of success varies (2). It is therefore desirable to develop alternative forms of treatment for intractable epilepsy.

History of Electrical and Magnetic Stimulation of the Brain

About two decades ago, researchers discovered that electrical stimulation of the motor areas of the brain through the intact scalp (transcranial electrical stimulation [TES]) (3) could activate motor neurons. A brief electrical shock over the motor cortex elicited a relatively synchronous response of the corresponding muscle that could be recorded with electrodes; however, TES also activated pain fibers in the scalp and was therefore quite painful. A few years later, using magnetic instead of electrical stimuli (transcranial magnetic stimulation [TMS]) (4), researchers showed it was also possible to stimulate the brain in a way similar to that of TES, but with little or no pain.

Since then, TMS, as a noninvasive technique, has been used as a diagnostic tool in various neurologic disorders. In principle, the technique uses a magnetic field generated by an electrical current flow in an insulated wire coil applied to the outside of the scalp (5). The stimulation is usually experienced as a slight, nonpainful prick on the scalp, similar to a poke with a fingernail. The magnetic pulses, in turn, induce a small electrical current in the brain up to 2 to 3 centimeters beneath the scalp, depending on the stimulus intensity (6) (Figure 23.1). When applied over the motor cortex, TMS pulses can activate the large, fast-conducting descending motor neurons connecting the motor cortex with the spinal cord and, eventually, the corresponding muscle. This results in a twitch of the corresponding muscle that can be recorded as a motor evoked potential (MEP) by electromyography (EMG)—for example, a small hand muscle.

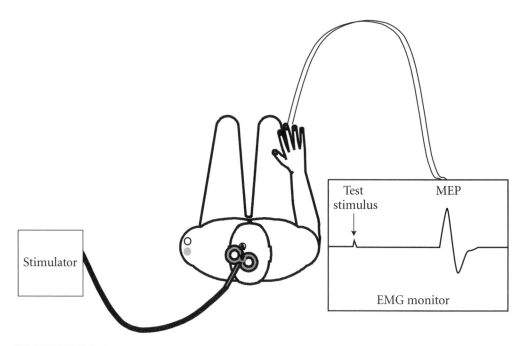

FIGURE 23.1

Schematic illustration of experimental setup in transcranial magnetic stimulation. MEP, motor evoked potential; EMG, electromyography.

Transcranial Magnetic Stimulation as an Investigative Tool in Epilepsy

TMS can measure a number of parameters that help assess the state of excitability of the motor cortex. The motor threshold—the smallest intensity needed to produce an EMG response (contracting muscle fibers)—reflects the neuronal excitability of motor neurons (7). In patients with untreated primary generalized epilepsy, the motor threshold is lower than that in healthy subjects (8), suggesting that this is a reflection of cortical hyperexcitability in the patients with the illness. In contrast, treatment with AEDs has been associated with increasing motor thresholds.

Commentary

Although TMS has a proven role as a research tool in epilepsy, its role as a treatment for epilepsy is unproven. Experimental evidence shows promising effects of low frequency TMS on epileptogenic brain regions (1). In 1999, Tergau and colleagues reported the first clinical application of the technique in nine patients with partial epilepsy, demonstrating a short-term reduction in seizure frequency of 70% for one patient with very frequent seizures (2).

A well-controlled study of TMS at the National Institutes of Health (NIH), however, failed to demonstrate a significant reduction in seizure frequency (3). The study examined the effects of twice daily stimulation in 24 patients for 1 week. Although the effect on seizure frequency did not reach statistical significance, the authors believed a mild and short-lived response did occur. Additionally, the effects may have been more significant for patients with seizure foci in brain regions more accessible to the field of the magnet. Clearly, more study is necessary to determine which patients may benefit from TMS, how long and how often to perform treatments, and whether the amount of seizure reduction is worth the time involved. Low-frequency TMS may be slightly uncomfortable, but it is usually well tolerated and appears not to produce any long-term adverse effects.

References

1. Akamatsu N, Fueta Y, Endo Y, et al. Decreased susceptibility to pentylenetetrazol-induced seizures after low-frequency transcranial magnetic stimulation in rats. *Neurosci Lett*. 2001;310(2-3):153–156.
2. Tergau F, Naumann U, Paulus W, Steinhoff BJ. Low-frequency repetitive transcranial magnetic stimulation improves intractable epilepsy. *Lancet* 1999;353:2209.
3. Theodore WH, Hunter K, Chen R, et al. Transcranial magnetic stimulation for the treatment of seizures: a controlled study. *Neurology* 2002;59:560–562.

Investigators have shown that TMS activates predominantly horizontally oriented intracortical inhibitory or facilitatory interneurons (9). A measurement of the effectiveness of intracortical inhibitory mechanisms (the same mechanisms presumed to reduce seizure spread), at least in the motor cortex, is possible using a paired-pulse technique (9). In this model, a conditioning stimulus precedes the test stimulus. The interval between the conditioning and the test stimulus determines whether the amplitude of the test stimulus increases (facilitation) or decreases (inhibition). A differential increase in motor cortex excitability or decreased inhibition of the affected hemisphere has been shown in patients with focal epilepsy (10). Thus, TMS is a valuable noninvasive tool to assess cortical excitability.

Transcranial Magnetic Stimulation as a Treatment for Epilepsy

TMS has also actively modified cortical and corticospinal excitability with trains of stimuli, known as *repetitive TMS* (rTMS). rTMS produces effects that outlast the stimulation train. Slow rTMS (1 Hertz) decreases cortical excitability in humans (11), similar to the long-term depression of synaptic transmission observed in animals after single-Hertz-range electrical stimulation (12). This raises the possibility that low-frequency rTMS may influence the hyperexcitability observed in patients with epilepsy. Bolstering the "inhibitory defenses" using low-frequency rTMS may help correct the imbalance between excitation and inhibition thought to contribute to the generation of seizures. In experimental animals with a low seizure threshold, low-frequency electrical stimulation elevated the seizure threshold (13). In addition, a pilot study demonstrated that low-frequency rTMS, applied over the vertex (the crown of the head), can decrease seizure frequency in unselected patients with intractable seizures (14), possibly by reducing cortical hyperexcitability.

Thus, evidence exists that low-frequency rTMS has an anticonvulsant effect, and trials are ongoing in both the United Kingdom and the United States to assess its feasibility as a treatment for epilepsy.

Precautions

TMS and rTMS have been used safely in thousands of individuals around the world. These therapies can be harmful, however, in people who have a pacemaker, an implanted medication pump, a metal plate in the skull, or metal objects inside the eye or skull—for example, after brain surgery or from a shrapnel wound. The effects of magnetic stimulation on the fetus are unknown, and so we advise against its use in pregnancy. Theoretically, rTMS can cause seizures, but this has been rare in practice and difficult to produce on purpose, even in epilepsy patients. Since the introduction of agreed on safety guidelines (6), there have been no reports of seizures. In addition to seizures, the only known risk of rTMS is headache, which always goes away promptly using nonprescription medication.

Conclusion

TMS is an exciting tool for research into the pathophysiology of epilepsy and the mechanisms of action of anticonvulsant drugs. It can help improve our understanding of the basic mechanisms in epilepsy and, thus, aid the development of AEDs. In addition, evidence indicates that low-frequency rTMS may have an anticonvulsant effect, and further study is needed. We are now studying the treatment response of patients with epilepsy to various low-frequency rTMS protocols. Depending on the validity of the results of this and similar studies, rTMS may develop into an alternative noninvasive treatment for epilepsy.

References

1. Juul-Jensen P, Foldspang A. Natural history of epileptic seizures. *Epilepsia* 1983;24:297–312.
2. Engel J Jr. Clinical neurophysiology, neuroimaging, and the surgical treatment of epilepsy. Review. *Curr Opin Neurol Neurosurg* 1993;6:240–249.

3. Merton PA, Morton HB. Stimulation of the cerebral cortex in the intact human subject. *Nature* 1980;285:227.

4. Barker AT, Jalinous R, Freeston IL. Noninvasive magnetic stimulation of human motor cortex. *Lancet* 1985;1(8437):1106–1107.

5. Rothwell JC, Thompson PD, Day BL, et al. Stimulation of the human motor cortex through the scalp. *Exp Physiol* 1991;6:159–200.

6. Wassermann EM. Risk and safety of repetitive transcranial magnetic stimulation: report and suggested guidelines from the International Workshop on the Safety of Repetitive Transcranial Magnetic Stimulation, June 5-7, 1996. *Electroencephalogr Clin Neurophysiol* 1998;108:1–16.

7. Ziemann U, Lonnecker S, Steinhoff BJ, et al. Effects of antiepileptic drugs on motor cortex excitability in humans: a transcranial magnetic stimulation study. *Ann Neurol* 1996;40:367–378.

8. Reutens DC, Berkovic SF, Macdonell RA, et al. Magnetic stimulation of the brain in generalized epilepsy: reversal of cortical hyperexcitability by anticonvulsants. *Ann Neurol* 1993;34:351–355.

9. Kujirai T, Caramia MD, Rothwell JC, et al. Corticocortical inhibition in human motor cortex. *J Physiol (Lond)* 1993;471:501–519.

10. Fong JKY, Werhahn KJ, Rothwell JC, et al. Motor cortex excitability in focal and generalised epilepsy [abstract]. *J Physiol* 1993;459:468P.

11. Chen R, Classen J, Gerloff C, et al. Depression of motor cortex excitability by low-frequency transcranial magnetic stimulation. *Neurology* 1997;48:1398–1403.

12. Linden DJ. Long-term synaptic depression in the mammalian brain. *Neuron* 1994;12:457–472.

13. Weiss SR, Li XL, Rosen JB, et al. Quenching: inhibition of development and statement of amygdala kindled seizures with low frequency stimulation. *Neuroreport* 1995;6:2171–2176.

14. Tergau F, Naumann U, Paulus W, et al. Low-frequency repetitive transcranial magnetic stimulation improves intractable epilepsy [letter]. *Lancet* 1999;353(9171):2209.

PART VI

Oxygen Therapies

CHAPTER 24

Hyperbaric Oxygen Therapy

PETER ROSENBAUM, MD, FRCP(C) AND KASSIA J. JOHNSON, HON. BA, MD

Neurons use oxygen and produce the by-products reactive oxygen species and carbon dioxide (CO_2). Nitric oxide (NO) is also produced by neurons. NO increases cerebral blood flow, which also increases during a seizure (1). Neurons communicate using neurotransmitters, and changes in neurotransmitter activity through neuronal damage or dysfunction can cause a seizure. Every person with epilepsy has a level of disruption that they can tolerate before reaching their seizure threshold.

The average concentration of blood oxygen is over 95%, indicating that most hemoglobin is being used effectively. This amount cannot be much higher, but it can be lower, depending on age and state of health. Although hemoglobin is the most important oxygen carrier, a small amount of free-floating oxygen also is present in the blood. The amount of oxygen that the hemoglobin can carry is steady, but the amount of free-floating oxygen can change. Several processes contribute to the availability of oxygen. When an increase in the free-floating oxygen occurs, more is available to the surrounding body tissues. Changing the barometric pressure in a person's environment can force more oxygen into the blood. This is achieved during deep sea diving and artificially with hyperbaric oxygen (HBO), which has been proposed as an option that can reduce the detrimental effects of seizures and the number of seizures.

Normal Oxygen Conditions

Air is composed of approximately 21% oxygen; the rest consists of nitrogen, carbon dioxide, nitrous oxide, and many other gases. The air pressure (also known as *barometric pressure*) at sea level is 760 mm Hg (referred to as 1 atmosphere, or ATA). Barometric pressure falls as we go higher in the atmosphere (for example, by increasing altitude). A mountain climber who ascends to the top of Mount Everest experiences a barometric pressure of approximately 0.35 ATA. At the other extreme, a deep sea diver experiences a pressure of 2 ATA at 33 feet. As the barometric pressure decreases, the molecules of oxygen in the air are not held as closely together. Therefore, less oxygen is present at a higher altitude and more oxygen is available when the barometric pressure is increased.

Hyperbaric Oxygen

Historically, HBO dates back to Alexander the Great and Aristotle in the fourth century BC. In 1662, the British physician Henshaw used hyperbaric air (not oxygen) to "help digestion … and for the prevention of most afflictions of the lungs" (2). Advances in hyperbaric medicine came with trial and error, and the list of treatable conditions grew with each experience. The list of complications also grew as more experiments were done.

The Undersea and Hyperbaric Medicine Society (3) governs the ethical and scientific certification of HBO in North America and has compiled the official list of indications for HBO, as indicated in Table 24.1. An additional list exists of diseases and conditions for which HBO is used as an experimental treatment, including epilepsy. The treatment of epilepsy with HBO is more popular in Europe than in North America (4).

TABLE 24.1

Various Indications for HBO

Air gas embolism (gas bubble in the bloodstream that can stop blood flow)
Carbon monoxide poisoning
Cyanide poisoning
Clostridial myositis and myonecrosis (a very serious muscle infection)
Crush injuries, compartment syndrome, heart attacks
Decompression sickness (*the bends*, sometimes experienced by scuba and deep sea divers)
Enhancement of healing in certain types of problem wounds
Exceptional blood loss (e.g., after hemorrhage or with severe anemia)
Intracranial abscess (walled-off infection in the head)
Necrotizing soft tissue infections (flesh-eating disease)
Osteomyelitis (bone infection)
Delayed radiation injury (soft tissue and bony necrosis [tissue death])
Skin grafts and flaps (compromised)
Thermal burns

The Basis for Using HBO in Epilepsy

HBO is used by people who believe that it is possible to ameliorate several of the proposed damaging mechanisms of seizures. HBO provides extra, free-floating oxygen in the blood, which—it is argued—increases the cerebral blood oxygen and provides hypoxic neurons with much needed oxygen. Some research indicates that epilepsy and other brain disorders are caused by damaged neurons that can be re-awakened using extra oxygen (5). There is conflicting evidence whether the decrease in cerebral blood flow due to HBO actually helps decrease seizures (6). HBO may also reduce brain swelling, however, by promoting the use of energy by the neurons. It is believed that with all these changes, the poorly functioning parts of the brain recover. HBO is also purported to change cognitive and personality problems caused by seizures (7).

The Administration of HBO

A unit of HBO treatment is known as a dive when it is administered using a chamber, because the artificial change in the barometric pressure is similar to what one would experience during deep sea diving. HBO can be given in a monoplace (one-person) or a multiplace chamber. In a monoplace chamber, the patient is naked or wearing cotton clothing and is often lying down. The oxygen is circulated throughout the chamber. The multiplace chamber can hold anywhere from 2 to 24 people, depending on the model. In these chambers, the patients are seated and each wears a rubber hood or a mask through which they receive oxygen. The multiplace chamber allows children to be accompanied by their parents without their parents also receiving oxygen. The pressure and amount of time in these units depend on the indications and desired treatment outcomes.

Commentary

Hyperbaric oxygen therapy falls within a border zone between standard medical therapy and experimental or alternative therapy. It provides an excellent field from which to view the challenges of linking the "medical" and "alternative" worlds. For example, a quick Internet search finds HBO therapy linked to two broad areas: those that purport to the principles of scientific inquiry (e.g., a PubMed search through the National Library of Medicine at http://www.ncbi.nlm.nih.gov/entrez/) and a search on an Internet search engine, such as Google, that lists many sites promoting the therapy based on subjective experience as well as some that provide more unbiased assessments of our current knowledge about HBO therapy. The rigor of carefully controlled studies and reports of failure is on the scientific side. Failure may be a lack of effectiveness, worsening of the condition one wishes to treat, or harmful side effects. Also found are thoughtful review articles that criticize studies based on their methodology or that combine all the data available in the literature to help better identify the good or bad effects of a treatment. Experience and success in small populations reported by individuals who believe in a therapy—and certainly in the case of HBO therapy—must be critically assessed, especially when there are large fees for treatment.

As discussed by Rosenbaum and Johnson, HBO therapy is definitely effective in treating the variety of disorders listed in Table 24.1. Medicare reimburses for these conditions because good evidence suggests that the benefits are real and outweigh potential dangers. Neurologic disorders such as multiple sclerosis, acute stroke, cerebral palsy, brain trauma, and epilepsy are listed on many Internet sites as conditions that improve with HBO therapy. Scientific data are lacking to clearly support any of these claims, and the evidence varies for each claim.

In multiple sclerosis, a review of published literature by Bennet and Heard of the Department of Hyperbaric Medicine at the University of New South Wales (Sydney, Australia) found "no evidence of significant benefit from the administration of HBO therapy for multiple sclerosis." Yet facilities that offer HBO therapy clearly list multiple sclerosis as one of the disorders for which this therapy is effective. More than 400 cases of human ischemic stroke treated with HBO have been reported. In about half the cases, improvement was claimed on clinical or electroencephalographic grounds (1). Most stroke patients improve unaided, however, and without controls, it remains uncertain whether HBO speeds, slows, or has no effect on recovery. Again, no evidence of clear benefit or harm exists.

A study published in Developmental Medicine and Child Neurology reveals the potential hazards of looking at only one side of a treatment study. This study by researchers at the University of Quebec (2) was a well-designed, double-blind study in which 75 children with cerebral palsy were randomly assigned to a course of HBO therapy. They received 40 sessions of HBO over a 2-month period; each session was 1 hour at 100% oxygen at 1.75 atmospheres absolute (ATA) or a similar course of a sham therapy in the chamber, but at 1.3 ATA, the lowest pressure that can be felt. Thus, the children did not know which group they were in. The pressure was lower than that used in any HBO center because it was considered too low to be effective. On neuropsychologic testing, children in both groups showed better self-control and significant improvements in auditory attention and visual working memory compared with the baseline. Notably, the sham group improved significantly on eight dimensions of the Conners' Parent Rating Scale (a measure of attention deficit disorder), whereas the active treatment group improved only on one dimension. Most of these positive changes persisted for 3 months. Thus, the placebo effect in this study appeared greater than the active treatment effect. Notably, as discussed by Rosenbaum and Johnson, a 2000 study reported on two children with cerebral palsy who were treated with HBO therapy and who developed serious problems that occurred during or immediately after the therapy, suggesting that these were complications of HBO therapy (3). In one case, the child developed aspiration pneumonia, probably from lying flat during therapy. The second child had a stroke that was complicated by seizure activity.

In another well-controlled study of HBO therapy for cerebral palsy that examined motor as well as cognitive functions, 111 children were randomly assigned to active therapy (40 treatments over 2 months at 1.75 ATA) or sham therapy (40 treatments over 2 months at 1.3 ATA) (4). Again, both groups improved very slightly in motor and cognitive areas, but there was no significant difference (e.g., 3.0% in motor function for sham and 2.9% for active therapy). The only statistically significant difference was related to side effects: ear problems were more common in the active treatment group.

A review of the medical literature and more informal lay literature on HBO therapy and epilepsy leads me to strongly endorse the conclusions of Rosenbaum and Johnson, as well as those of the Epilepsy Ontario Web site for alternative medicines (http://epilepsyontario.org/faqs/alternatives.hbot.html): No evidence suggests that HBO therapy reduces seizure frequency or intensity. In contrast, evidence suggests that HBO can cause seizures. Until further studies are done, this is not an alternative therapy that should be endorsed for epilepsy. Rather, physicians should caution individuals with epilepsy to avoid it.

References

1. Nighoghossian N, Trouillas P. Hyperbaric oxygen in the treatment of acute ischemic stroke: an unsettled issue. *J Neurol Sci* 1997;150:27–31.
2. Hardy P, Collet JP, Goldberg J, et al. Neuropsychological effects of hyperbaric oxygen therapy in cerebral palsy. *Dev Med Child Neurol* 2002;44:436–446.
3. Nuthall G, Seear M, Lepawsky M, et al. Hyperbaric oxygen therapy for cerebral palsy: two complications of treatment. *Pediatrics* 2000;106(6):E80.
4. Collet JP, Vanasse M, Marois P, et al. Hyperbaric oxygen for children with cerebral palsy: a randomised multicentre trial. HBO-CP Research Group. *Lancet* 2001;357: 582–586.

Patients experience the pressure changes mainly in their ears—similar to when landing in an airplane—and they are encouraged to swallow to relieve this pressure. The temperature in the chamber also rises as patients dive, but this can be reset to a more comfortable level after the desired pressure is reached (7,8).

Treatment Regimens

HBO is used to treat seizures in varying treatment regimens. One reported regimen listed at the website HBO 4 R KIDS at www.geocities.com (9) requires the treatment to be given at 1.5 to 1.75 ATA for 60 minutes once a day for 40 treatments. This is followed by a break, with 40 subsequent treatments offered if no improvement is seen. Other websites offer a variety of treatment regimens for epilepsy. No standardized treatment approaches for the use of HBO in epilepsy exist because it is still an experimental and unproven treatment for this condition.

Efficacy of HBO in Epilepsy

As with many new and untested therapy ideas, HBO has been applied with good intentions but with little of the careful scientific study that is essential before a good idea becomes an accepted treatment. No clinical trials have assessed whether HBO adds benefit to the drugs and other therapies people with epilepsy are already receiving. We do not know whether HBO does more good than harm, even if it *seems* to be a good idea. This is, of course, essential information, because the golden rule in medicine is "Above all, do no harm." If any treatment is potentially dangerous, expensive, or painful, or if it might interfere with the use of other valuable therapies, we must have strong evidence of benefit that outweighs these risks before we can embrace it.

Much of the excitement surrounding HBO for epilepsy is based on a study done in China in 1987. This study was a report from the Eleventh International Congress on Hyperbaric Medicine; it cited 100 cases of children with epilepsy (10). The children were given a regimen of HBO that lasted for 80 minutes each day for 15 to 30 days. An alleged 82% improvement occurred, reported as a decrease in seizure number and impact. How the improvements were measured, over what period of time, and in what types of epilepsy were all unreported. Therefore, there remains considerable concern that the study was not a methodologically valid assessment of HBO for epilepsy. This study was widely reported on the Internet and was adopted as the foundation for many facilities using HBO to treat epilepsy.

If no scientifically strong evidence exists in favor of HBO for epilepsy, why are people claiming that it works? There are several explanations. Sometimes we see a change in a person's health or function after a treatment is started and assume that it was the treatment that made the difference. Of course, the fact that "B" follows "A" does not mean that "A" and "B" are connected at all, let alone that "B" caused "A" to happen. Anecdotes and individual case reports can be very exciting, but we can never be sure that the report of the success in a single situation happened because of the treatment or for some other reason. Thus, testimonials cannot be the basis for the acceptance of a new treatment. Thus, when an exciting new idea appears, we must control our enthusiasm until unbiased and careful study has taken place. There are simply too many examples in medicine—even in the recent past—where good ideas proved to be bad medicine.

Precautions

Since the 1800s, pure oxygen has been known to cause seizures. Documented research cited this complication in 1945 (11). Animal experiments were developed that identified several dangers in exposing the central nervous system (CNS) to pure oxygen. The damage occurs via several different mechanisms. First, cerebral blood flow increases during seizures. Proponents of HBO feel that the HBO-induced increased cerebral blood flow (CBF) allows more oxygen to reach oxygen-starved neurons, thereby reviving them (12). Several studies looked at this issue and found that HBO initially *decreases* cerebral blood flow by causing vasoconstriction and then causes a sudden increased surge in cerebral blood flow. With this sudden surge come the seizures that can complicate HBO therapy (13–15). The protective mechanism that seems to exist, but which may be overwhelmed, is the production of carbon dioxide (CO_2). Carbon dioxide is the by-product of oxygen metabolism and causes vasoconstriction in the brain. Thus, it seems to lengthen the period of time before the inevitable seizure (16). This leaves open the question as to what brings on seizures: the change in cerebral blood flow, the change in brain chemicals, both of these, or other factors?

The answer may lie in another theoretical cause of seizures: NO. More NO is produced by neurons during HBO therapy (17). Increased NO also increases CBF and may thereby precipitate a seizure. The change in neurotransmitters that is associated with a seizure can also be caused by NO. In particular, NO may increase glutamate, a neurotransmitter that excites the neurons, thereby causing a seizure. New research is examining the protective value of giving patients naturally occurring chemicals that inhibit NO to prevent CNS toxicity (18).

Another finding that raises questions about the safety of HBO concerns the effect of the repeated exposures to HBO advocated by proponents of HBO. This is said to be the only way to receive the benefits of HBO. Some research suggests, however, that repeated exposure sensitizes animals to the detrimental effects of HBO. With each subsequent exposure, they seem to be less able to tolerate the HBO, making them more prone to seizures (18). These seizures also start sooner into the treatment process (19). In addition, increased levels of a precursor to NO, one of the predisposing factors for a seizure, are still found in the system 1 month after HBO exposure (20).

Most of these findings are based on animal studies, but a report by Nuthall et al., in 2000, of a 10-month-old boy with cerebral palsy who had a tonic-clonic seizure following twice daily HBO treatments for 2 days supports these concerns. The child was placed in a monoplace chamber and was not taken above 1.5 ATA. He later had two generalized tonic-clonic seizures and needed IV antiepileptic drug therapy. There was concern that his seizures were caused by oxygen that had not dissolved in his blood, causing a bubble that went to his brain and caused damage and additional seizures (21).

Other complications of the exposure to elevated atmospheric pressure (as happens with HBO) include *barotrauma*, which is pressure manifested by pain in the ears and sinuses, middle ear hemorrhage, and sometimes deafness. Oxygen toxicity can cause convulsions, or water or blood in the lungs, leading to respiratory failure. Decompression sickness can occur with a collapsed lung, nitrogen bubbles in the bloodstream and joints, severe pain, and even death. Other reported complications that may be temporary include near-sightedness, fatigue, headaches, vomiting, and claustrophobia (22). Additionally, in any situation where extra oxygen is present, there is a serious fire hazard because oxygen is so flammable.

Documented Safe Levels of HBO

Proponents of HBO state that 2 ATA of pressure is a safe level below which seizures cannot be induced. This assertion is based on a body of conventional research that observed seizures in animals exposed to 4 or more ATA. Most important research, however, shows the risks of repeated exposures to HBO. Currently, it cannot be said that there is definitely a safe level at which HBO can be applied, especially repeatedly, without any side effects. Side effects are inevitable in any treatment—even with conventional antiepileptic drugs. The differences lie in the large volume of solid clinical research into the effectiveness of most of the drugs currently in use for epilepsy treatment and the predictability of their side effects and long-term outcomes. Such information is largely lacking on the efficacy of HBO therapy, which leads to caution and skepticism about claims of efficacy based on anecdotes and uncontrolled experiences.

Financial Considerations

HBO facilities can be located in regular healthcare facilities, especially in port cities where divers work on ships. An HBO monoplace chamber can also be set up in a house. Several concerns exist regarding the safety of using this therapy in the home, such as fires and explosion (due to pressurized delivery systems). HBO treatment centers have many regulations and controls in place to ensure that all equipment functions properly for the safety of patients and their families.

The cost of equipment used in HBO therapy varies. The following information is quoted in U.S. funds (23). (These amounts do not include patient charges.)

HBOT multiplace chamber	$300,000–2.5 million
Renovation costs to house an HBO therapy facility	$100,000–$450,000
Estimated cost per HBO therapy dive, including physician fees and capital and operating costs	$220 (Canadian funds)

Estimates suggest that one treatment may cost up to $US500. Free services may be provided by companies involved in gathering research evidence on specific diseases. Prices vary depending on the country, state, or province, the equipment operator, and the dive time (24). The high cost of HBO therapy lies partly in the rarity of its use. Some insurance companies have policies regarding HBO, but in Canada, this service is not covered by the provincial government-funded health plans.

Conclusions

HBO is proposed and used as a treatment for childhood epilepsy without scientific evidence to define either its effectiveness or safety. We simply do not know whether it works and, if so, whether it does more good than harm. For this reason, we recommend caution until careful studies have been completed. This may sound overly conservative, but one must accurately estimate the costs and benefits of any novel therapy before trying treatments that might fail to work or that may even cause harm.

References

1. Krings T, et al. Hemodynamic changes in simple partial epilepsy: A functional MRI study. *Neurology* 2000;54(2):524–527.

2. Shah SA. Healing with oxygen: A history of hyperbaric medicine. *The Pharaohs* 2000;3–19.

3. www.uhms.org.

4. Gabb G, Robin ED. Hyperbaric oxygen, a therapy in search of diseases. *Chest* 1987;92(6): 1074–1082.

5. Neubauer RA, Gottlieb SF, Kangan RL. Enhancing "idling" neurons. *Lancet* 1990;335:542.

6. http://www.woundcare.org/newsvol1n3/ar8a.htm.

7. http://www.hbot.com.

8. http://www.sumeria.net/oxy/hot.html.

9. http://www.geocities.com/Heartland/Village/9021/hbo4rkids.html.

10. http://ourworld.compuserve.com/homepages/BazilBrush/hotchina.htm.

11. Bean JW, Siegfried EC. Transient and permanent after-effects of exposure to oxygen at high pressure. *Am J Physiol* 1945;143:656–664.

12. Neubaur RA. Hyperbaric oxygenation for cerebral palsy. *Lancet* 2001;357:2052.

13. Sato T, et al. Changes in nitric oxide production and cerebral blood flow before development of hyperbaric oxygen-induced seizures in rats. *Brain Res* 2001;918:131–140.

14. Chavko M, et al. Role of cerebral blood flow in seizures from hyperbaric oxygen exposure. *Brain Res* 1998;791:75–82.

15. Demchenko IT, et al. Nitric oxide and cerebral blood flow responses to hyperbaric oxygen. *J Appl Physiol* 2000;88:1381–1389.

16. Chavko M, Braisted JC, Outsa NJ, et al. Role of cerebral blood flow in seizures from hyperbaric oxygen exposure. *Brain Res* 1998;791:75–82.

17. Thom SR, et al. Fast track: stimulation of nitric oxide synthase in cerbral cortex due to elevated partial pressures of oxygen: an oxidative stress response. *J Neurobiology* 2002;51(2): 85–100.

18. Chavko M, et al. Increased sensitivity to seizures in repeated exposures to hyperbaric oxygen: role of NOS activation. *Brain Res* 2001;900:227–233.

19. Fenton LH, Robinson MB. Repeated exposure to hyperbaric oxygen sensitizes rats to oxygen-induced seizures. *Brain Res* 1993;632:143–149.

20. Al-Ghoul, WM, Meeker RB, Greenwood RS. Kindling induces a long-lasting increase in brain nitric oxide synthase activity. *NeuroReport* 1995;6:457–460.

21. Nuthall G, et al. Hyperbaric oxygen therapy for cerebral palsy: two complications of treatment. *Pediatrics* 2000;106(6):80.

22. Gabb G, Robin ED. Hyperbaric oxygen, a therapy in search of diseases. *Chest* 1987;92(6): 1074–1082.

23. Mitton C, Hailey D. Health technology assessment and policy decisions on hyperbaric oxygen treatment. *Intl J Tech Assessment Health Care* 1999;15(4):661–670.

24. http://www.facialplasticsurgery.net/HBOT.htm.

CHAPTER 25

The Role of Carbon Dioxide in the Enhancement of Oxygen Delivery to the Brain

CORALEE THOMPSON, MD AND DENISE MALKOWICZ, MD

The human brain is a magnificent organ of great complexity and ability. It requires constant support by a physiologic environment of oxygen, carbon dioxide, glucose, water, and a wealth of nutrients vital to its function. Oxygen is the most vital nutrient and the most frequently threatened component of the brain's environment. The well brain has extensive mechanisms for monitoring and controlling nutrient supplies, but an injured and dysfunctional brain is less able to do this. As a result of brain injury, damage to the respiratory, circulatory, and digestive systems may further impair the delivery of nutrients to the brain.

Carbon dioxide is the main regulator of cerebral blood flow. The physiologic response of the brain to carbon dioxide is vasodilation. In addition, with increased blood levels of carbon dioxide, the respiratory centers of the brain signal an automatic increase in the rate and depth of breathing. A number of scientists became interested in the clinical value of carbon dioxide soon after Schmidt (1928) reported its effect upon respiration and cerebral blood flow (1). Lennox (1929) and Fay (1930) showed that the inhalation of increased carbon dioxide mixtures improved seizure control in some patients (2,3). In 1953, Fay used carbon dioxide mixtures to treat patients with athetoid cerebral palsy resulting in decreased hypertonicity (4). In 1992, Pelligra et al. showed that mixed gases of carbon dioxide and oxygen stimulated neurotransmitter production in children with Rett syndrome, resulting in improved respiratory patterns (5). In the 1950s, Glenn Doman, founder of The Institutes for the Achievement of Human Potential, and other professional pioneers developed a simple procedure of rebreathing exhaled air as a means of increasing carbon dioxide, thereby enhancing oxygen delivery to the brain. This procedure, known as *oxygen enrichment*, is an important part of the comprehensive neurologic programs that staff at The Institutes teach to the parents of brain-injured children.

Over the past half-century, The Institutes have evaluated over 20,000 brain-injured children, many of whom have seizures. The prevalence rate is approximately 450 per 1,000 children evaluated at The Institutes. Of the children with histories of seizures, 55%

were still having seizures at their first visit. The remaining 45% had stopped having seizures by that time. Most of the children with a seizure history met the criteria for symptomatic or secondary epilepsy. (Symptomatic epilepsy is by definition due to a recognized brain injury.) A small number of the children with a positive seizure history met the criteria of primary or idiopathic epilepsy. (Primary epilepsy is a genetically determined lower seizure threshold without other known injury.) Many brain-injured children had syndromes such as infantile spasms or Lennox-Gastaut syndrome. Seizures are one symptom among the plethora of other symptoms of brain injury.

Children with epilepsy have poorly functioning brains and, in that sense, injured brains. The cause of brain injury is usually unknown. It may have occurred at any time during development of the brain or afterward. A number of insults may also provoke seizures in a well brain. Seizures occur when the brain is not getting what it needs, and seizures may occur with very little provocation. Recurrent seizures are a symptom of brain injury. Thus, treatment efforts should be directed toward repairing the underlying cause of the seizures (i.e., the injured and disorganized brain). Fifty years ago, the neuroplastic potential of the brain was not understood as it is today. Yet fifty years ago, The Institutes recognized this potential and understood that the brain grows by use. Treatment programs were built on this principle.

> "In the basic sense, it may be said that all we do at the Institutes is to give the child visual, auditory, and tactile stimulation with increased frequency, intensity, and duration in recognition of the orderly way in which the brain grows."
>
> *Glenn Doman, Founder*

Treatment Principles

The Institutes have five basic treatment principles, which are nonsurgical and nonpharmacological. They are based on the fact that the function of the brain is to relate the organism to its environment. Twenty-six procedures and hundreds of techniques are used within those procedures. The five principles of treatment are:

- Procedures that supply discrete bits of information to the brain for storage.
- Procedures that demand an immediate response from the brain to the discrete bit of information that has just been supplied.
- Procedures that program the brain.
- Procedures that permit the brain to respond to previous programming.
- Procedures that provide an improved physiologic environment in which the brain may function.

Oxygen enrichment is an important part of the fifth treatment principle. The injured brain needs physiologic support to repair itself while it receives the proper visual, auditory, and tactile stimulation.

The brain consumes a high proportion of the body's oxygen supply. Although the brain weighs only about 1% of the body mass, it consumes 20% to 50% of the cardiac output. Without oxygen, neurons die in minutes, because the brain has no way of storing oxygen. Yet giving supplemental oxygen is not an effective way of treating brain injury, nor seizures for that matter. In fact, high concentrations of oxygen can be toxic. In addition, increased levels of oxygen can cause cerebral blood vessels to constrict, thereby decreasing cerebral blood flow.

Cerebral blood vessels respond to levels of carbon dioxide by regulating blood flow. Low levels of carbon dioxide result in vasoconstriction; elevated levels cause vasodilation. Hyperventilation reduces carbon dioxide and thus reduces cerebral blood flow. Hyperventilation is often used during EEG testing to induce slow waves or epileptic spikes. This response is likely due to reduced blood flow to the brain.

A series of physiologic events occurs when carbon dioxide levels in the blood rise. The chemical receptors in the carotid body sense the presence of carbon dioxide. The brain is signaled when levels of carbon dioxide elevate. The respiratory centers of the brain then cause an increase in the rate and depth of breathing. Carbon dioxide acts directly on the cerebral blood vessels to cause vasodilation. Blood flow is increased

Commentary

Drs. Thompson and Malkowicz summarize their experience with masking (rebreathing technique) to increase carbon dioxide levels in the blood, thereby increasing cerebral blood flow and oxygen delivery to the brain. The brain is an enormous consumer of oxygen and glucose, and increased carbon dioxide concentrations open cerebral blood vessels, thus increasing blood flow to brain tissue. Theoretically, increasing oxygen delivery to the brain might help reduce seizure activity or intensity. The program also includes dietary changes and educational-therapeutic interventions.

The overall program includes specific therapies to enhance cortical development and maturation, reduce fluid and salt intake, eliminate sugar and processed foods, and use vitamin supplements. The central component is "oxygen enrichment." The educational and developmental therapies, as well as the oxygen enrichment program, are labor intensive for both the child and parents.

The Institutes for the Achievement of Human Potential has extensive experience treating children and reports remarkable success with its therapeutic program in promoting brain development and maturation, as well as reducing seizures. There are, however, no controls and the results are confounded by numerous factors. For example, improvements in motor, sensory, cognitive, or other functions could result from changes in medication doses, reduction in seizure activity, spontaneous developmental progress (as occurs in all normal and the vast majority of developmentally disabled children when they are viewed over time), other therapies, or the specific therapies in their program. Similarly, the reports of improved seizure control when off antiepileptic drugs is extremely impressive and deserves more careful study in a controlled trial. Seizures were completely controlled in 48% of patients and were reduced in an additional 34% who were taken off all antiepileptic medications. If reproducible in controlled studies, this would represent a treatment that is dramatically more effective than the ketogenic diet or vagus nerve stimulation. Even resective epilepsy surgery is rarely able to fully control seizures in 50% of patients with the elimination of medication. (Some epilepsy surgery centers have seizure control rates of 70% to 90%, but most patients remain on some medication.)

No well documented evidence suggests that directly increasing inspired oxygen concentration or using techniques such as rebreathing reduces seizure activity. If increased oxygen reduces seizure activity, then children and adults could be given nasal prong oxygen to increase the percentage of inspired oxygen. Although high levels of oxygen can be toxic, so too can high levels of carbon dioxide. Similarly, if an area of brain requires more blood flow (and with it, more oxygen and glucose), regulatory processes are well developed to increase circulation to local or more widespread regions. This is very well illustrated by the seizure itself—areas of brain discharge abnormally consume more energy, and the cerebral circulation reflexively delivers more blood to these areas (this is the basis of the ictal SPECT scan to localize seizure activity). Increasing the carbon dioxide level does work differently from simply increasing the percentage of inspired oxygen, but we remain uncertain if either technique has any effect in reducing seizure frequency or severity. Interestingly, hyperventilation just before the administration of the electrical shock at the time of electroconvulsive shock therapy diminishes carbon dioxide levels and increases seizure duration (1). This finding supports a theoretical basis for rebreathing techniques that increase carbon dioxide levels.

Experience with scuba diving provides some cautionary notes. Rebreathing techniques are used to conserve oxygen, but can lead to abnormally high levels of carbon dioxide (carbon dioxide poisoning), which can cause blackouts or impaired consciousness. For scuba divers, high carbon dioxide levels increase the likelihood of tonic-clonic seizures from oxygen toxicity and worsen the severity of nitrogen narcosis. Divers who frequently have headaches after diving may have used air at a low rate and thereby retained carbon dioxide.

We are left with many more questions than answers; however, the remarkable success reported by these physicians challenges both the alternative and traditional medical communities to study the techniques that Drs.

Thompson and Malkowicz have pioneered. We need controlled studies to establish both the safety and efficacy of these therapies. Given the intensive nature of the therapies, it is also important to compare the benefits of the educational therapies against more traditional programs for applied behavioral analysis, speech, occupational, or physical therapies. Similarly, the nutritional and oxygen enrichment programs should be compared with placebo as well as against standard antiepileptic drugs. More data may help to identify which patient populations might benefit from specific therapeutic interventions.

Reference

1. Chater SN, Simpson KH. Effect of passive hyperventilation on seizure duration in patients undergoing electroconvulsive therapy. *Br J Anaesth* 1988;60:70–73.

through vasodilation, and the delivery of oxygen is enhanced. Elevated blood carbon dioxide causes a slight shift toward a more acidic blood pH. This facilitates a release of oxygen from the red blood cell hemoglobin molecule for use at the cellular level of brain tissue. Intermittent rebreathing by the patient of his or her own exhaled air can safely raise levels of blood carbon dioxide.

During oxygen enrichment, a simple mask with a small inlet for air is placed around the nose and mouth. Because exhaled air is higher in carbon dioxide, as the person rebreathes the exhaled air, blood levels of carbon dioxide increase. The mask is kept in place until several seconds of deep breathing occurs. This duration is usually less than 1 minute. No significant decrease in oxygen occurs during this type of intermittent rebreathing. Rather, there is an increase in carbon dioxide, to which the brain is very sensitive. This stimulates increased breathing, vasodilation, and increased oxygen delivery to the brain.

The response to elevated carbon dioxide in the blood is reflexive. In other words, the brain will automatically respond and, thus, the individual does not have to *think* about breathing deeply. This reflex makes deep breathing possible for an individual who is unable to voluntarily take deep breaths. An obvious example of this can be seen in brain-injured children who are physically delayed and as a result have poor respiratory control and lower lung capacity. Poor pulmonary function due to brain injury leads to a number of medical complications, such as frequent respiratory illnesses. By repeatedly inducing brief periods of deep breathing throughout the day, pulmonary function improves, enhancing oxygenation. It has been the experience at The Institutes that all brain-injured children breath inefficiently, some only mildly so, whereas others struggle for every breath. Nearly every brain-injured child benefits from oxygen enrichment through intermittent rebreathing. The oxygen enrichment program directly improves the brain's physiologic environment; the evidence of improved physiology can be measured by clinical improvement.

The following are the major victories achieved by 557 brain-injured children who were seen at The Institutes during the year 2000:

Mobility

- Of the 184 children who were unable to move, 41 (22%) crawled for the first time. In short, they went from being paralyzed to being able to crawl across a room without help. They ranged in age from 8 months to 22 years 7 months.
- Of the 83 children who were unable to creep, 34 (41%) began to do so. This is to say that they defied gravity and moved to the third dimension; they now go all over the house on their hands and knees. They ranged in age from 8 months to 10 years 10 months.
- Of the 90 children who were unable to walk, 19 (21%) began to walk without help for the first time. They ranged in age from 17 months to 7 years 7 months.
- Of the 71 children able to walk but not run, 24 (34%) learned to run for the first time. They ranged in age from 3 years 5 months to 14 years.

Seeing

Of the 48 children who were cortically blind, 34 (71%) saw for the first time. *Cortical blindness* means that the visual apparatus is functioning but the brain cannot process the visual information. Twenty of these children also learned to read. They ranged in age from 8 months to 10 years 6 months. In addition, one 25-year-old regained the ability to see after losing it due to traumatic injury when he was 17 years old.

Hearing

Of the 19 children who were cortically deaf, 17 (89%) heard for the first time. *Cortical deafness* means that the ear functions but the brain cannot process the auditory information. They ranged in age from 14 months to 10 years 6 months.

Understanding

Of the 124 children whose comprehension was not yet equal to that of the average 3-year-old, 102 (82%) were able to understand, as well as a 3-year-old for the first time. They ranged in age from 20 months to 15 years 6 months.

Reading

Of the 126 children who were unable to read, 120 (95%) read for the first time. They ranged in age from 14 months to 13 years 4 months. In addition, one 15-year-old and one 25-year-old regained the ability to read after losing it due to traumatic injury when they were 13 and 17 years old, respectively.

Speech (Language Delay Resulting in No Speech)

Of the 204 children who couldn't speak, 48 (24%) spoke for the first time. They ranged in age from 21 months to 20 years 8 months.

Writing

Of the 135 children who were unable to manually write, 16 (12%) wrote for the first time. They ranged in age from 5 years 6 months to 12 years 8 months. In addition, one 22-year-old regained the ability to write after losing it due to traumatic injury when he was 18 years old.

Health

Of the 370 children eligible to receive a health victory (that is, those who were on the program for at least 1 year), 84 (23%) achieved perfect health for at least 12 consecutive months. Of these, 41 had no illness for more than 24 months, and one has had no illness for 11 years.

Detoxification

Of the 88 children who were on antiepileptic drugs (AEDs), 47 (53%) were completely and successfully detoxified. (They ranged in age from 26 months to 25 years 4 months.) The remaining 41 children are in the process of complete detoxification.

Detoxification is the safe and successful elimination of AEDs, stimulants, antidepressants, or any psychoactive medications. More than 30 years ago, the medical staff of The Institutes began a program of very gradual withdrawal of these drugs from the children who were in the program. In 1971, they brought their concerns about AEDs to the attention of the World Organization for Human Potential (WOHP). Many of their colleagues in other countries shared their concerns. The WOHP issued a cautionary note to the medical world and to the parents of brain-injured children. They expressed concern about the widespread and sometimes indiscriminate use of AEDs in brain-injured children. In our experience, AEDs frequently impair neurologic and cognitive function in brain-injured children.

In 1977, The Institutes did their first statistical look at the results of detoxification from AEDs. Seventy-one children were followed from December 1977 to May 1979. All the children were taken completely off medication while on an active neurologic program designed by the staff at The Institutes. The age limit was 16 years or less. This study documented the change in the number of seizures. Quality of life improved due to the elimination of AED side effects. This was true even for children who were still having seizures. Most children who stopped taking AEDs and continued to have seizures had less intense and shorter seizures than when they were on AEDs.

Results

- The number of children having no seizures was 39 of 71 (55%).
- The number of children having fewer seizures was 22 of 71 (31%).
- Total number of children with an improved seizure picture was 61 or 71 (86%).
- The number of children having the same number of seizures was 2 of 71 (3%).
- The number of children having more seizures was 8 of 71 (11%).

In our experience, these statistics remain quite stable throughout the years. In 1993, of the 132 children who were completely detoxified, similar results were recorded. That year, 48% were having no seizures, and 34% were having fewer seizures, giving a positive outcome of 82%. All these children were under medical supervision during the detoxification program, and they were receiving comprehensive neurologic programs and physiologic support.

Physiologic Environment

The basic programs that improve the physiologic environment of the brain include:

Neurologic Organization Program

Staff at The Institutes evaluate the child and then teach the child's parents neurologic organization programs, including the appropriate visual, tactile, and auditory stimulation. Parents do these intensive neurologic organization programs at home with their child, several hours a day, 7 days a week.

Cortical Maturation

In the *Journal of Pediatrics*, June 2000, Camfield and Camfield state, "Several population-based studies have verified that more than half of the children with epilepsy will outgrow it,… It is now clear that AEDs do not alter the natural history: the epilepsy resolves on its own. AEDs hide the symptoms until brain maturation somehow solves the problem" (6).

This statement agrees with our experience at The Institutes. In addition, The Institutes' programs help accelerate neurologic development and brain maturation. We believe that this is what helps eliminate seizures. The programs include intellectual development in areas such as reading, math, and problem solving. The intelligence programs provide sensory input at a cortical level to promote cortical development and maturation.

Dietary Liquid and Salt Control

A direct correlation exists between seizures and overhydration, which is enhanced by salt intake. Overhydration can result in cerebral edema and brain dysfunction. Brain-injured children who have seizures are particularly sensitive to excessive liquids and salt. At The Institutes, we recommend a limited but safe range of liquid intake. The dietary recommendations include a "no salt added" diet and the elimination of processed foods containing sodium.

Nutrition and Supplemental Support

At The Institutes, we also recommend a balanced diet consisting of unprocessed food and the elimination of sugar, artificial colors, flavors, and sweeteners. In our experience, many brain-injured children have food allergies, especially to milk and wheat products. Any suspected food allergens are eliminated. In addition, we recommend supplements, including healthy fatty acids, probiotics, multivitamins, and minerals: calcium, magnesium, and zinc. Vitamin B6 may also be useful for some children with seizures.

Oxygen Enrichment

The oxygen enrichment program results in improved cerebral circulation and increased oxygen and nutrient supply to the brain. At The Institutes, we have found the oxygen enrichment program to be an effective treatment for seizures. This includes prevention, long-term elimination of seizures, and emergency treatment for prolonged or repeated seizures. The oxygen enrichment program benefits children who have poor mobility, ineffective breathing, and poor circulation. The rate and depth of breathing increases, the lungs are expanded, lung congestion and mucous plugs are reduced, and systemic and brain oxygenation improves.

This procedure of oxygen enrichment should not be done without proper instruction. Parents are taught the oxygen enrichment program only after they attend the "What to do about your brain-injured child" (WTD) course and their child has been evaluated at The Institutes. Alternatively, parents can attend the WTD course and the information can be given to the child's primary doctor, to start the oxygen enrichment program. Oxygen enrichment is not appropriate for some children with cardiac defects. It should not be used in children with respiratory diseases in which carbon dioxide is abnormally retained, such as uncontrolled asthma or obstructive pulmonary disease. Rebreathing should never be done when there is pneumonia, fever, vomiting, or severe upper respiratory infections.

In summary, over the past half-century, The Institutes has treated a great number of children with brain injury, with and without epilepsy. The goal of complete wellness is accomplished by our neurologic organization programs, implemented through teaching the parents to do comprehensive, home-based neurologic organization treatment. The physiologic programs are directed toward improving the environment in which the brain functions. A key program is the oxygen enrichment program, which takes advantage of the powerful effect of carbon dioxide on the brain and respiratory system to enhance oxygen delivery to the brain.

References

1. Schmidt, CF. The influence of cerebral blood flow on respiration. I. The respiratory responses to change in cerebral blood flow. II. The gaseous metabolism of the brain. III. The interplay of factors concerned in the regulation of respiration. *Amer J Physiol* 1928;84:202, 223, 242.
2. Lennox, WG, Cobb S. Relation of certain physio-chemical processes to epileptiform seizures. *Amer J Psychiat* 1929;8:837–847.
3. Fay T. Epilepsy. *J Nerv Ment Dis* 1930;71(5).
4. Fay T. Effects of carbon dioxide (20 percent) and oxygen (80 percent) inhalations on movements and muscular hypertonus in athetoids. *Amer J Phy Med* 1953;32(6).
5. Pelligra R, et al. Rett syndrome: stimulation of endogenous biogenic amines. *Neuropediatrics* 1992;23:131–137.
6. Camfield P, Camfield C. Advances in the diagnosis and management of pediatric seizure disorders in the twentieth century. *J Pediatr* 2000;136:847–849.

PART VII

Manipulation and Osteopathic Therapies

CHAPTER 26

A Chiropractic Perspective on Complementary and Alternative Therapies

BRIAN J. GLEBERZON, DC

Most patients with epilepsy are now managed with prescription medications; however, more than 30% of epilepsy patients either have inadequate seizure control or experience significant adverse drug reactions (1). For example, patients with idiopathic generalized epilepsy may experience an increase in seizure frequency or intensity using medications such as carbamazepine and phenytoin (2). Thus, many individuals with epilepsy may also pursue other types of treatments (2,3). From a chiropractic perspective, this chapter briefly reviews treatment options provided by complementary and alternative (CAM) healthcare providers, utilization rates of CAM, and medical attitudes toward CAM approaches; and then reviews the therapeutic efficacy and safety of chiropractic care, particularly cervical manipulation.

Utilization of Complementary and Alternative Medicines

The term CAM generally refers to the healthcare practices and professions that do not fit into the culturally dominant medical, educational, and financial paradigms (4). Contrary to popular opinion, patients are generally satisfied with the care they receive from medical physicians, and dissatisfaction with conventional medicine does not predict CAM use (4). Thus, many patients combine both allopathic and CAM therapeutic approaches, deriving benefits from both.

A demographic study by Eisenberg revealed that almost 50% of respondents saw a CAM provider, an almost 50% increase from his original study about seven years earlier (5,6). The researchers calculated that this represented an increase from 427 million total visits in 1990, to 639 million visits (by 22 million people) in 1997, a number that exceeds the total visits to all United States primary care physicians (5). The total cost for CAM providers was conservatively estimated at $21.2 billion in 1997, with $12.2 billion paid for by the patient out-of-pocket. The total out-of-pocket expenditures of alternative therapies of all kinds were conservatively estimated to be $27 billion (5).

Although certain therapies, such as herbal medicines, massage, megavitamin therapy, self-help groups, folk medicine, energy healing, and homeopathy increased most in the years between Eisenberg's two studies, visits to chiropractors and massage therapists accounted for nearly half of all visits to CAM providers in 1997 (5,6). Roughly 11% of respondents in the study sought out chiropractic care, and visits to chiropractors accounted for 30% of CAM total visits. Notably, less than 50% of the respondents told their medical doctor they were under the care of a CAM provider (5).

The average demographic profile of a CAM user was Caucasian, aged 25 to 45 years, and of higher education and higher income than nonusers of CAM services. The largest age group of CAM users were the baby boomers (5).

The most common chief complaints prompting patients to consult a CAM provider were, in descending order, chronic low back and neck pain, anxiety, depression, headache, fatigue, insomnia, arthritis, and sprains and strains (6). Patients with back problems, neck problems, headaches, and sprains and strains were most likely to seek chiropractic care. In addition, a study by Hawk (7) reported that nonmusculoskeletal complaints accounted for 10.3% of chief complaints presented to chiropractors. The percentage of patients with epilepsy seeking chiropractic or other CAM approaches is unknown, and it is also unknown what percentage of patients under the care of a CAM provider have epilepsy.

The Appeal of CAM Therapies

Chiropractors and other CAM providers purport to be primarily concerned with the health of the entire person. This sentiment is embraced by the concept of *holism*, considered a basic tenet of chiropractic principles (8). Coulter (9) described the shift in healthcare away from the compartmental, disease-based approach often attributed to allopathic medicine, which sees patients as no more than the sum of their parts, toward a holistic model of health care. The current literature favors a healthcare approach that considers the entire person's health of physiologic abilities, psychosocial interactions, and emotional well-being (9–12). In chiropractic practice (and within some CAM circles), these factors are often grouped together under the umbrella term *wellness*. Hawk (13) recently said that this approach resonates well with the contemporary emphasis on the prevention and promotion of health.

Mootz (14) contrasted the molecular approach to healthcare with the contextual approach. In its simplest form, *molecular medicine* sees a specific causation at the physiologic level. Although many factors contribute to a disease, the role of molecular medicine is often viewed as sort of a background constant. Molecular methods are systematic and allow sequential experimentation (including therapeutic trials) to produce a manageable accumulation of quantitative data. Thus, a molecular medical approach allows tangible breakthroughs in emergent situations (such as myocardial infarcts), environmental virulence (antibodies, for example), and the development of host defenses to known environmental agents (as in vaccination). Molecular medicine has significantly impacted the evolution of healthcare.

The molecular approach may oversimplify problems and fail to account for the unpredictability of complex systems—or simple systems that behave in a complex manner. This approach may exhibit a robustness that is misleading, and researchers may simply ignore phenomena that do not fall into their models. Moreover, reducing a complex system to its component parts may fragment things artificially and, conversely, the extrapolation of laboratory findings to real-world settings may be inaccurate and ultimately misleading.

Contextual medicine views disease as a process rather than a discrete entity, and this approach emphasizes that disease may be the reaction to a variety of environmental, psychosocial, genetic, and other factors (for example, the belief systems of the patient and doctor). Although intuitively attractive because it deals with the richness of human experience and is often easy to explain to a patient, contextual medicine is difficult to quantify. It is a difficult system around which to build a common knowledge base, and often has an outsider status within the scientific community. Conventional healthcare can benefit from a liberal admixture of both these therapeutic approaches (15).

Commentary

Chiropractic therapy is one of the most commonly used forms of CAM therapies. Spinal manipulation, the primary form of chiropractic care, is used to treat neck and back pain, with many studies establishing its effectiveness for some patients. The effectiveness of chiropractic therapy for other disorders, such as headache, fibromyalgia, and other chronic pain disorders, is supported by some data, but the evidence is less robust. As Dr. Gleberzon highlights, no controlled studies support the use of chiropractic therapy in epilepsy. He accurately reviews the essential elements of chiropractic therapy and the lack of any solid evidence that this therapy improves seizure control.

The only data to support chiropractic therapy for epilepsy are individual case studies suggesting that in selected patients, seizure frequency or severity may be reduced by chiropractic therapy directed at the neck (cervical) region; however, as Dr. Gleberzon notes, these are individual case reports and many factors may be responsible. For example, in the one patient reported by Alcantara (1), chiropractic manipulation administered during a seizure led to the abrupt resolution of seizure activity. There are many possible mechanisms. First, the manipulation may have altered some physiologic parameter that stopped the seizure. In the nineteenth century, massage of the neck over the carotid region was sometimes reported to abort seizures (we do not recommend this as it can potentially be dangerous, especially in older individuals). Vagus nerve stimulation may work through a similar mechanism. Cervical manipulation may also send signals to the brainstem that help inhibit seizure activity; however, in this case, the seizure may have also stopped spontaneously, with the timing of the therapy and the cessation of seizure activity as a coincidence. Alternatively, the seizure may not have been epileptic in nature, but may have been psychologically based. These nonepileptic psychogenic seizures are very common and difficult for epilepsy experts to identify without simultaneous video-EEG monitoring. For example, one study in a general neurology clinic found that among patients diagnosed with epilepsy, 37% had psychogenic seizures provoked by suggestive techniques (2). Nonepileptic psychogenic seizures can be aborted by a large variety of suggestive techniques and can potentially complicate all studies of epilepsy patients in both traditional and CAM areas. The potential complications are especially important in considering individual case reports.

It is possible that chiropractic manipulation can improve seizure control. For example in the 17 cases reviewed from the literature by Pistolese (3), 14 improved using upper cervical manipulation to correct misalignments in the cervical vertebrae. These patients may have experienced a reduction in pain or stress that led to a secondary reduction in seizures. Alternatively, controlled investigations in these individual cases could have demonstrated that sham therapy was equally or more effective. We simply don't know.

No established mechanism exists by which chiropractic therapy could improve seizure control. Theories regarding input from spinal receptors to the brain and changes in blood flow to the brain are intriguing, but lack any substantive support.

Finally, therapy is always about risk versus benefit. The benefits of cervical manipulation for epilepsy remain completely unproven. The risk of serious injury is very small, with approximately 1 in 1,000,000 individuals experiencing a stroke. There is a much higher risk of local discomfort, which improves rapidly in the majority of patients.

References

1. Alcantara J, Heschong R, Plaugher G, et al. Chiropractic management of a patient with subluxation, low back pain and epileptic seizures. *J Manip Physiol Ther* 1998;21:410–418.
2. Bazil CW, Kothari M, Luciano D, et al. Provocation of nonepileptic seizures by suggestion in a general seizure population. *Epilepsia*. 1994;35:768–770.
3. Pistolese RA. Epilepsy and seizure disorders: a review of the literature relative to chiropractic care of children. *J Manip Ther Physiol* 2001;24:199–205.

The Chiropractic Profession

Chiropractic is a profession and not a treatment modality. It is the third largest health profession in North America, behind medicine and dentistry, with approximately 60,000 practitioners in the United States (15). In general, chiropractic is a drugless, conservative approach to healthcare. Case management protocols reflect approaches standard to all healthcare disciplines, including history taking, diagnostic evaluation, and care planning. Therapeutic interventions commonly include spinal manipulation (or adjustment) and other manual therapies, exercise and rehabilitation methods, physiotherapeutic modalities, and advice on lifestyle, nutrition, ergonomics, hygiene, and health promotion, as well as other complementary and alternative procedures (15). Spinal manipulation is a high-velocity, low-amplitude thrust, usually delivered onto a specific spinal structure to correct its aberrant function or motion (sometimes referred to as *subluxation*). This motion is often accompanied by a popping or cracking sound, thought to be the result of the release of gas from the joint space; however, several therapeutic approaches in chiropractic use forms of spinal adjustments that do not result in audible joint cavitations. Over 100 different technique systems are used in chiropractic, and thus the interchangeable use of the terms "spinal manipulation" and "spinal adjustment" is only accurate outside a chiropractic context (16).

Chiropractic does not represent a unified clinical approach, although most practitioners use spinal adjusting as a central focus of therapy. Similar to conventional medicine, chiropractic also represents a spectrum of perspectives toward clinical interventions and philosophical principles. For example, most chiropractors maintain that spinal manipulation enhances joint mobility and resolves symptoms, whereas other chiropractors also believe that the chiropractic adjustment has significant and far-reaching neurophysiologic effects (16–19).

Chiropractic Efficacy and the Safety of Spinal Manipulation

Meeker and Haldeman reviewed and reported on the impressive accrual of evidence supporting spinal manipulative therapy (SMT) for acute and chronic neck and low back pain (20). Similarly, clinical trials support the use of SMT for tension and migraine headaches (21–24), fibromyalgia (25), and cervical vertigo (26).

Bronfort (27) recently compiled evidence for SMT for acute and chronic neck and low back pain, and reviewed clinical guidelines from the United States, United Kingdom, Australia, and Sweden. Taken as a whole, the clinical guidelines from these countries advocate the use of SMT for acute and chronic low back pain, and chronic neck pain. The evidence also supports the use of SMT for chronic headaches. At this time, however, the evidence supporting the use of chiropractic care for nonmusculoskeletal conditions is much less robust compared with the evidence for musculoskeletal conditions. No clinical trials or studies specifically examine the efficacy of chiropractic care for epilepsy.

Adverse Reactions to Spinal Manipulation

The reported incidence of adverse reactions to spinal manipulation is high, with a frequency as high as one of every two patients, but these reactions are generally reported to be mild and self-resolving. In one of the largest studies examining the incidence of side effects from SMT, Senstead (28) reported that the most common side effect was local discomfort (53%) of mild or moderate intensity (85%) that resolved within 24 hours (74%). No serious injuries or complications were reported during the study (28). Similarly,

Haldeman et al. (29,30) reported that stroke, often associated with cervical manipulation, is a rare, remote, and unpredictable risk, with causes that include both minor and major traumas. Haldeman found examples of stroke following minor trauma, such as those experienced during yoga, archery, and getting one's hair washed, as well as after major trauma, such as a car accident. Currently accepted estimates of the frequency of a stroke resulting in serious neurologic complications or death following manipulation are between 1 and 3 per million adjustments, and one in 400,000 patients (20,30,31). The most commonly accepted estimate of the risk of stroke (with or without serious neurologic complications) following manipulation is 1 in 1,000,000 patients (20,31).

Medical Acceptance of CAM Approaches

Studies indicate an increased interest in and acceptance of CAM within the medical community. For example, of the 117 (of 125) medical schools in the United States that responded to a survey documenting information about CAM education within their curricula, 64% offered some kind of CAM instruction (3). Most classes offered were electives, although some institutions provided information within required courses. Common topics included chiropractic, acupuncture, homeopathy, herbal therapies, and mind-body techniques. In another study, when asked, 39% of medical physicians described chiropractic as a legitimate medical practice (3). In addition, a growing number of prestigious journals, including the *New England Journal of Medicine*, the *Journal of the American Medical Association*, and the *Archives of Internal Medicine* are devoting more and more space to CAM.

Treatment by CAM Providers

An eclectic approach to the treatment of epilepsy is not a phenomenon unique to the modern era. For example, the first known documented case of epilepsy in China appeared in *The Yellow Emperor's Classic of Internal Medicine*, written by a group of physicians around 770 B.C. (32). At that time, the treatment of epilepsy, based on the principles of Ying Yang Wu Xing, consisted of herbs, acupuncture, and massage (32). Centuries later, accounts of epilepsy were reported in pre-Columbian America (33). Both the Aztecs and Incas associated epilepsy with magic and religion. Both these ancient cultures used magical therapies, as well as botanical medicines that may have had an empirical benefit.

In additional to a plethora of antiepileptic drugs (AEDs) commonly used today, a number of nonpharmacological options are available. Two of these approaches, the ketogenic diet (high-fat, low-protein, and low-carbohydrate) and vagal nerve stimulation (implantation of a stimulating device in the chest wall), are well supported by the literature. In addition, after chiropractic adjustments (often directed to the upper cervical region), several case studies (2,34–38) have documented improvements in patients with epileptic seizures. The use of acupuncture, yoga, and a host of supplements has been met with much more limited success.

Chiropractic Treatment in Epilepsy

Over the past 40 years, numerous case studies documenting the successful resolution of epileptic seizures following chiropractic care were published in peer- and non-peer-reviewed journals (2,34–38). Pistolese (2) recently reviewed the literature regarding chiropractic care in patients with epilepsy. His paper reviewed 17 documented case reports since 1966. A recent history of trauma was reported in 10 of 16 cases. Fourteen of the 17 patients were receiving AEDs, which were unsuccessful in controlling the epilepsy of these patients. Upper cervical adjustments were administered to correct vertebral subluxations (joint dysfunction) in 15 patients, and all patients reported positive outcomes as a result of chiropractic care (2).

Pistolese wrote that many of the patients who benefited from chiropractic care experienced the onset of epileptic seizures early in childhood (2). Moreover, careful examination of the cases reviewed showed that none of the patients experienced a sudden miracle cure. Instead, they demonstrated a steady decline in the frequency and duration of seizure activity during therapy that spanned months to more than a year. Several of the treating chiropractors reported that patients often required fewer AEDs after chiropractic care began, and some patients did not require any further AED therapy.

Alcantara described a 21-year-old woman who presented with low back pain after a fall and a history of grand and petit mal seizures (34). Before treatment, the patient reportedly experienced a seizure every 3 hours, with a duration of 10 seconds to 30 minutes per episode. Treatment consisted of spinal manipulative therapy directed to the cervical, thoracic, and lumbar regions. During one seizure, the chiropractor administered a cervical adjustment. On administration of the adjustment, the seizure stopped abruptly. This is the only published report of such a phenomenon. At the 18-month follow-up, the patient reported that her low back complaint had resolved, and her seizures had reduced in frequency to as little as one every 2 months (34).

Amalu (35) described a 5-year-old boy with tonic-clonic and absence seizures, as well as other impairments, who experienced 30 or more seizures a day. The boy was treated with phenobarbital and phenytoin. Amalu administered two upper cervical adjustment during the first week, reducing the number of seizures to 10 per day. By the third week of care, all generalized tonic-clonic seizure activity ceased. Between treatment weeks 7 and 12, all seizure activity had abated. Over the next 10 months of care, the child's neurologist reduced his medication levels. After additional testing, the neurologist concluded that the boy no longer had epilepsy and withdrew all medications (2,35).

No well-defined mechanisms explain these clinical observations. Many theories exist, however, as to how cervical adjustments may positively influence seizure activity. Alcantara (34) suggested that cervical adjustments may activate spinal receptors to send impulses to appropriate pathways and sites in the brain, resulting in a decrease or cessation of seizure activity. Similarly, Hymann (2) theorized that the correction of vertebral subluxations in the upper cervical spine by chiropractic adjustments may reduce aberrant nerve impulses to the brain.

Amalu (35) has provided two theories of neurophysiologic mechanisms that may account for the relationship of epilepsy and spinal adjustments. These are (i) central nervous system facilitation, possibly from a trauma (e.g., birth, falling) resulting in entrapment of intra-articular meniscoids and segmental hypomobility of some areas of the spine and compensatory hypermobility of other areas of the spine; or (ii) cerebral penumbra or brain cell hibernation. In Amalu's cerebral penumbra model, a state of neural hibernation occurs when a threshold of ischemia is reached. In this theory, cells remain alive but cease to perform their designated function. Note that case reports such as those described cannot distinguish the effects of therapy from the placebo effect or natural history.

Spinal Dysfunction and the Nervous System

Most authors (18,19,39) suggest that poor or aberrant biomechanical motions of the cervical spine, coupled with its high concentration of mechanoreceptors and the position of the cervical sympathetic ganglia, may account for the clinical observations of improvements in different neurophysiologic symptoms (such as seizure activities) after cervical adjustments; however, the proof of these relationships and their underlying mechanisms are still under investigation.

Other CAM Approaches

Several studies have investigated the benefits of acupuncture, yoga, and various supplements in epilepsy patients. In general, these studies show minimal, if any, clinical benefits derived from any of these approaches.

The Cochrane Collaboration reviewed the evidence of the effects of yoga in epilepsy patients (40). Only one study met the reviewers' selection criteria, and they felt that no reliable conclusions could be drawn regarding the efficacy of yoga as an epilepsy treatment (40).

One study investigating the effects of acupuncture in chronic intractable epilepsy reported that patients receiving true acupuncture and patients receiving sham acupuncture both had a reduction in seizure activity, as well as an increase in the number of seizure-free weeks (41). A more recent study monitoring changes in quality of life found no benefit from acupuncture (42). A few studies, however, reported reduced seizure activity in dogs after acupuncture (43,44).

Several studies report the improvement of seizures using Chinese traditional medicines (45), taurine (an amino acid) (46), and the pineal hormone melatonin (47). In addition, a case study documented the successful resolution of epileptic seizures following osteopathic manipulation (48). Osteopathic manipulation differs from chiropractic manipulation, in that osteopathic manipulation is more of a mobilization, a procedure that moves a joint within a patient's passive range of motion.

Conclusions

There is an expectation by healthcare stakeholders (patients, third-party payers, and healthcare professionals) of an evidentiary foundation on which healthcare decisions are based. According to Sackett, evidence-based medicine is the "conscientious, explicit, and judicious use of the current best evidence in making decisions about the care of individual patients" (49). He goes on to say that "evidence-based medicine means integrating individual clinical expertise with the best available external clinical evidence from systematic research ... especially from patient-centered clinical research" (49). Thus, the current best evidence is not limited to randomized clinical trials, but also includes anecdotal evidence, case studies, practitioner experience, and practice-based studies, as described in this chapter.

At this time, some evidence supports the use of some CAM therapies to augment the medical case management of a patient with epilepsy. Evidence supports the use of the vagal nerve stimulator and the ketogenic diet. In the case of SMT directed at the cervical spine, some anecdotal evidence suggests that this approach may have significantly positive benefits in a person with epilepsy, and that this treatment approach is safe.

Patients currently on prescription medications should not discontinue them. Insufficient evidence suggests a patient abandon an allopathic model of management altogether. An individual with epilepsy may consider combining medical and CAM approaches after consultation with his medical physician. This coordination of healthcare services resonates well with the current impetus toward an interdisciplinary healthcare team; however, patients should be advised to exercise caution before self-prescribing a CAM approach, particularly with respect to the use of botanical medicines, herbs, or other supplements that may potentially adversely react with a prescription medication (50).

Although some CAM therapeutic approaches do not have any scientific evidence to support their use at this time, physicians should bear in mind the adage that "absence of evidence is not evidence of absence" (51). Although most chiropractic evidence is in the form of case studies, such evidence should not be disregarded out-of-hand. Several experts in the evidence-based practice arena have emphasized the importance of the clinician's experience, having felt that the pendulum has swung too far towards the over-reliance on randomized clinical trials as the final arbiter of clinical practice activities. This is because, as Haynes et al. opined, "evidence does not make decision ... people do" (52). Thus, an individual may benefit from one or more of the therapeutic approaches described in this chapter, even with the absence of supporting evidence. Clinical practice is an art, science, and philosophy. As O'Malley said, "there are many instances of a seemingly capricious patient whose response varies from the textbook outcome" (53). If some preliminary precautions are taken, a person with epilepsy can consider including a CAM approach in his healthcare plan, and should do so on a trial basis.

References

1. Herman ST, Pedley TA. New options for the treatment of epilepsy. *JAMA* 1998;280:693–694.
2. Pistolese RA. Epilepsy and seizure disorders: a review of the literature relative to chiropractic care of children. *J Manip Physiol Ther* 2001;24:199–205.
3. Meeker WC. Public demand and the integration of complementary and alternative medicine in the U.S. Health care system. *J Manip Physiol Ther* 2000;23:123–126.

4. Rapin I. Autism. *N Engl J Med* 1997;337:97–104.
5. Eisenberg D, Davis R, Ettner S, et al. Trends in alternative medicine use in the United States, 1990-1997. *JAMA* 1998;280:1569–1575.
6. Eisenberg D, Kessler R, Foster C, et al. Unconventional medicine use in the United States. *N Engl J Med* 1993;328:246–252.
7. Hawk C, Long CR, Boulanger KT. Prevalence of nonmusculoskeletal complaints in chiropractic practice: report from a practice-based research program. *J Manip Physiol Ther* 2001;24:157–169.
8. Gatterman M: *Chiropractic Management of Spinal-Related Disorders*. Baltimore: Williams & Wilkins, 1990.
9. Coulter I. Alternative philosophical and investigatory paradigms in chiropractic. *J Manip Physiol Ther* 1993;16:419–425.
10. Gerin P, Dazord A, Boissel J, Chifflet R. Quality of life assessment in therapeutic trials: rationale for and presentation of a more appropriate instrument. *Fundam Clin Pharmacol* 1992;6:263–276.
11. Coulter ID. *Chiropractic. A Philosophy for Alternative Health Care*. First Printing. Oxford, UK: Butterworth-Heinemann, 1999.
12. Wilson I, Cleary P. Linking clinical variables with health-related quality of life. *JAMA* 1995;273:59–65.
13. Hawk C. Should chiropractic be a "wellness" profession? *Top Clin Chiro* 2000;7:23–26.
14. Mootz RD. The contextual medicine of manual methods: challenges of the paradigm. *J Chiro Humanities* 1995;5:28–40.
15. Gleberzon BJ, Mootz RD. Different health care strategies for the older person. In: Gleberzon BJ, (ed.) *Chiropractic Care of the Older Person*. Oxford, UK: Butterworth-Heinemann, 2001.
16. Cooperstein R, Gleberzon BJ. *Technique Systems in Chiropractic*. Edinburgh, UK: Churchill-Livingston, 2004.
17. Owens EF. Theoretical constructs of vertebral subluxation as applied to chiropractic practitioners and researchers. *Top Clin Chiropr* 2000;7:74–79.
18. Haldeman S. Neurologic effects of the adjustment. *J Manip Physiol Ther* 2000;23:112–114.
19. Budgell BS. Reflex Effects of subluxation: the autonomic nervous system. *J Manip Physiol Ther* 2000;23:104–106.
20. Meeker WC, Haldeman S. Chiropractic: a profession at the crossroads of mainstream and alternative medicine. *Ann Intern Med* 2002;136:216–227.
21. Boline PD, Kassak K, Bronford G, Nelson C, Anderson AV. Spinal manipulation vs. amitriptyline for the treatment of chronic tension-type headaches: a randomized clinical trial. *J Manip Physiol Ther* 1995;1:148–154.
22. Nelson CF, Bronfort G, Evans R, et al. The efficacy of spinal manipulation, amitriptyline and the combination of both therapies for the prophylaxis of migraine headache. *J Manip Physiol Ther* 1998;21:511–519.
23. Nilsson N, Christensen HW, Hartvigsen J. The effects of spinal manipulation in the treatment of cervicogenic headaches. *J Manip Physiol Ther* 1997;20:326–330.
24. Nelson C. Principles of effective headache management. *Top in Clin Chirop* 1998;5:55–61.
25. Blunt KL, Rajwani MH, Guerriero RC. The effectiveness of chiropractic management of fibromyalgia patients. A pilot study. *J Manip Physiol Ther* 1997;29:389–399.
26. Bracher ESB, Almeida CIR, Almeida RR, Duprat AC, Bracher CBB. A combined approach for the treatment of cervical vertigo. *J Manip Physiol Ther* 2000;23:96–100.
27. Bronfort G. Spinal manipulation and the scientific evidence. Presentation at the CMCC Sixth Annual Conference on Advancements in Chiropractic. Oct. 23, 2000.
28. Senstead O, Leboueuf-Yde C, Borchgrevink C. Frequency and characteristics of side effects of spinal manipulative therapy. *Spine* 1997;22:435–441.

29. Haldeman S, Kohlbeck FJ, McGregor M. Risk factors and precipitating neck movements causing vertebrobasilar artery dissection after cervical trauma and spinal manipulation. *Spine* 1999;24:785–794.

30. Haldeman S., Kohlbeck FJ, McGregor M. Unpredictability of cerebrovascular ischemia associated with cervical spine manipulation therapy. *Spine* 2002;27(1):49–55.

31. Terrett A. Vertebrobasilar stroke following manipulation. National Chiropractic Mutual Insurance Company. West Des Moines, Iowa. 1996.

32. Lai CW, Lai YH. History of epilepsy in Chinese traditional medicine. *Epilepsia* 1991;32:299–302.

33. Elferink JG. Epilepsy and its treatment in the ancient cultures of America. *Epilepsia* 1999;40:1041–1046.

34. Alcantara J, Heschong R, Plaugher G, Alcantara J. Chiropractic management of a patient with subluxation, low back pain and epileptic seizures. *J Manip Physiol Ther* 1998;21:410–418.

35. Amalu W. Cortical blindness, cerebral palsy, epilepsy and recurring otitis media: a case study in chiropractic management. *Today's Chiropractic* 1998;27:16–25.

36. Hospers LA, Sweat RW, Hus L, et al. Response of a three-year-old epileptic child to upper cervical adjustments. *Today's Chiropractic* 1987(Dec/Jan);69.

37. Goodman RJ, Mosby JS. Cessation of a seizure disorder: correction of the atlas subluxation complex. *J Chiropr Res Clin Invest* 1990;6:43–46.

38. Converse ML, Converse TA, Dall LD. Cervicocranial adjustments in seizure management: a case report. *Dig Chiropr Econ* 1991(Jan/Feb);27–28.

39. Morgan LG. Psychoneuroimmunology, the placebo effect and chiropractic. *J Manip Physiol Ther* 1998;21:484–491 [Commentary].

40. Ramaratnam S, Sridharan K. Yoga for epilepsy. *Cochrane Database Syst Rev* 2000;2:CD001524.

41. Kloster R, Larsson PG, Lossius R, et al. The effect of acupuncture in chronic intractable epilepsy. *Seizure* 1999;8:170–174.

42. Stavem K, Kloster R, Rossberg E, et al. Acupuncture in intractable epilepsy: lack of effect on health-related quality of life. *Seizure* 2000;9:422–426.

43. Klide AM, Farnbach GC, Gallagher SM. Acupuncture therapy for the treatment of intractable, idiopathic epilepsy in five dogs. *Acupunct Electrother Res* 1987;12:71–74.

44. Panzer RB, Chrisman CL. An auricular acupuncture treatment for idiopathic canine epilepsy: a preliminary report. *Am J Chin Med* 1994;22:11–17.

45. Chen LC, Chen YF, Yang LL, et al. Drug utilization pattern of antiepileptic drugs and traditional Chinese medicines in a general hospital in Taiwan—a pharmaco-epidemiologic study. *J Clin Pharm Ther* 2000;25:125–129.

46. Birdsall TC. Therapeutic application of taurine. *Alt Med Review* 1998;3:128–136.

47. Birdsall TC. Biological effects and clinical use of the pineal hormone melatonin. *Alt Med Review* 1996;1:94–102.

48. Patel F, Holt S. Osteopathy cured my daughter's epilepsy. *Proof! What works in alternative medicine.* 1999;3:10.

49. Sackett D. Evidence-based medicine [Editorial]. *Spine* 1998;23:1085–1086.

50. Miller LG. Herbal medicines. Selected clinical considerations focusing on known or potential drug-herb interactions. *Arch Intern Med* 1998;158:2200–2211.

51. Altman DG, Bland M. Absence of evidence is not evidence of absence. *BMJ* 1995;311:485.

52. Haynes RB, Devereaux PJ, Guyatt GH. Physician's and patient's choices in evidence-based practice. *BMJ* 2002;324:1350.

53. Malley J. Towards a reconstruction of the philosophy of chiropractic. *J Manip Physiol Ther* 1995;18:285–292.

CHAPTER 27

The Osteopathic Approach to Children with Seizure Disorders

Viola M. Frymann, DO, FAAO, FCA

The osteopathic approach to healthcare originated in the work of Andrew Taylor Still, M.D. (1), who founded the American School of Osteopathy in Kirksville, Missouri in 1884. A student of that school, William Garner Sutherland, D.O. (2), through sudden inspiration and diligent research, extended the osteopathic principles and practice to the head region. Osteopathy in the cranial field was first published in a book by Sutherland called *The Cranial Bowl* in 1938 (3). The fundamental principles, practice, and concepts of osteopathic medicine are as sound in their therapeutic efficacy now as they were in the very beginning, but the profession has grown, as has the medical profession, and it now includes all the standard diagnostic and therapeutic procedures in medicine. Therefore, osteopathic physicians treating a child with epilepsy will refer the child for an electroencephalogram (EEG), magnetic resonance imaging (MRI), and the appropriate blood or urinary tests, as needed.

The osteopathic approach has distinguishing features. First, the osteopathic physician examines the presenting problem of seizure disorder and the patient suffering from it as *a dynamic unit of function*, not as a case of epilepsy. The whole history, from the moment of conception to the present, is explored. The history covers events in the lives of the parents before birth, including during pregnancy as well as the duration, conduct, difficulty or ease of labor, and delivery. Trauma after birth, such as falls down stairs, off counters, scooters, or bicycles, out of trees, in sports, and any other untoward events are recorded. We are not only concerned with the major trauma, loss of consciousness, or fractures that parents rarely forget, but also with minor head injuries, a field that has received more and more attention in the last decade. A history of immunizations, the dates, and any reactions that followed are important and may contribute to the analysis of this problem. A high fever, disturbed sleep, irritability, inconsolable crying, and even encephalitis following immunization are relevant examples.

Second, any child is a delicately designed and superbly integrated structural-functional unit. Each part is interrelated with every other. The structures are designed to move together and might be compared to a clock in which every wheel, every part must move efficiently with every other or the clock fails to correctly tell time. Every bone is designed to move, whether in the spine, pelvis, arm, leg, hand, foot, and even the head.

The ribs of the chest cage and the bones of the head move rhythmically and perpetually without conscious effort, activated by a force from within the patient. These are respiratory motions. If a decision is made to inhale deeply and hold the breath, one can consciously override the usual inherent rhythm. Yet a moment may come when it can no longer be held and either a deep gasp of air will be inhaled or consciousness will be lost and the patient will fall to the floor. The movement of the bones of the head—that motion within the cranial mechanism—would nevertheless continue, for this is the *primary respiratory mechanism* (PRM) that controls every function of every organ in the body (4). Any trauma that interferes with the inherent motion of the PRM will impair central nervous system (CNS) function. Thus, the neurologic performance and development of the child can be impaired by disturbances in the circulation of arterial and venous blood, or the motion of the cerebrospinal fluid nourishing the brain.

Third, these concepts lead to the realization that diseases are *effects* (5), the manifestations of impairments of function due to disturbances of the delicate structural integration of some part of the total patient.

Osteopathic Treatment and Its Physiologic Effect

Osteopathic manipulative treatment may be performed using various techniques depending on the age and state of well-being of the patient, the region of the body to be treated, the experience of the practitioner, and the particular issues being addressed at the time. The whole patient must be considered. The initial evaluation includes a general physical examination. If possible, the patient's structure will be evaluated in the standing and sitting position, and then lying comfortably on the back. The examination progresses from the feet to the pelvis, the sacrum, the spinal column, the breathing motion of the ribs and the diaphragm, and the head. Scars, in any location, may be of great importance. If they are surgical scars, attention is addressed to the scar tissue deep beneath the visible scars. Structural and functional abnormalities are correlated with events described in the history.

Asymmetry of structure may be immediately obvious. For example, the head may have a parallelogram form; the forehead may be more prominent on one side; the occipital region may be long, narrow, and especially hard to the touch; one eye may be larger or higher than the other; or the chin may have shifted to the right or the left of the vertical line of the midface. Our primary concern, however, is always *motion.* Distorted, reduced, or impaired motion helps to identify the problem within. The palpating hands of the practitioner on the head follow the moving cranial bones—movement is possible because there are developing sutures or joints between the bones. The motion may not be functioning in a healthy physiologic pattern. It may be distorted because some injury is compressing one or more sutures. The motion is caused by the cerebrovascular system—the blood flow through arteries and veins—and the cerebrospinal fluid system—the fluid that occupies the cavities within the brain, surrounds the brain deep to the membranes, and provides the water-cushion under the brain (6). Further, the brain has an inherent rhythm that is analogous to the inherent pulse rhythm of the heart or the breathing rhythm in the lungs. The osteopathic physician evaluates the competency of the PRM with gentle sensitive palpation and then applies appropriate techniques to restore its optimal function. The cerebrospinal fluid is one of the most important known elements contained within the human body, and unless the brain furnishes this fluid in abundance, a disabling condition of the body will result (7).

A distortion in the flow of energy occurs during an epileptic seizure. No disease causes the muscle to jerk as if recurrently startled or thrash uncontrollably like a fish pulled out of the water; no ocular disease causes the eyes to become blind momentarily; nor is there a pathology in the lungs that produces apneic spells. Rather, the problem is at the source, and that source is within the brain, despite the absence of organic pathology visible to the naked eye on autopsy or even ultramicroscopic cellular abnormality sought by the histopathologist. Nevertheless, despite the absence of structural errors in the CNS, one can monitor the production and distribution of life energy within the brain. The EEG can penetrate into the operation of the system and can sometimes identify the cause of the malfunction or localize a breakdown in the complex electrical system of the brain, despite the absence of structural abnormalities.

The development of the fetal nervous system may be distorted or impaired by drugs taken by the mother during pregnancy. The dangers of street drugs, such as marijuana and cocaine, are widely recognized. But the dangers of legitimate medication are too often ignored under the delusion that "it cannot happen to me." Many of the prescription drugs approved by the FDA, however, can adversely affect a growing baby. For example, antiepileptic drugs (AEDs) may adversely affect the child. The mother is then faced with a painful dilemma: stop the drug and risk seizures during her pregnancy or take medication that can potentially affect the child.

Commentary

Osteopathy is a system of diagnosis and therapy that focuses on the structural and functional integrity of the body. Osteopathy has expanded enormously since its early emphasis on bones. Whereas traditional medicine often looks most closely at "disease," osteopathic medicine carefully examines the ways in which abnormalities in the function of body structure cause pain and disability. The most common problems treated by osteopathy include back pain, postural changes related to pregnancy or work, sports injuries, repetitive strain injuries, arthritis pain, and colic and sleep problems in babies. Currently, doctors of osteopathy undergo training analogous to medical training, and many of them are vital elements in academic medical centers and private practices of neurology. In such instances, their approach to diagnosis and care often closely parallels that of medical doctors. In many cases, the diagnostic evaluation and recommended therapies for epilepsy patients (and other patients) by physicians with osteopathic degrees and those with medical degrees is identical.

Dr. Viola Frymann and her colleagues provide a different approach to the care of children with epilepsy from that of medical physicians and also many other osteopathic physicians. They first focus on a detailed history from conception through pregnancy, often closely examining pieces of information considered irrelevant by traditional medicine. Next, they examine the whole patient, including the motion of the body. Dr. Frymann formulates a therapeutic strategy from her diagnostic evaluation and applies "appropriate techniques to restore optimal functioning." We are unfortunately told little about the specifics of these techniques. For example, how does one translate the history of a minor trauma or fever after immunization into a specific therapy?

Dr. Frymann is a figure of enormous character, purpose, and clinical strength. One suspects her hands and her mind possess an intuitive brilliance. Her experience and the numbers she reports suggest her approach can help where standard medical/surgical or dietary approaches have not. Yet the content of her chapter leaves us asking for more substance. Exactly what did she do? How long was the follow-up in patients whose seizures were fully controlled or improved?

How do subtle movements of cranial bones alter the electrical activity in the brain? Dr. Fryman discusses potential injury to cranial nerves at birth, although evidence is lacking. Problems with sucking or breastfeeding are attributed to isolated cranial nerve disorders. Such problems are often not a result of neurologic disorders, and when they are neurologic, most problems result from brain or muscle abnormalities, not cranial nerve abnormalities. Similarly, a relationship between difficulty passing through the birth canal and trauma to the foramen magnun is postulated as leading to excessive crying and sleep problems. What is the evidence for this?

Medical physicians must remain humble about the leap from identifying effective therapies to understanding how they work. Aspirin has been long recognized as an effective therapy for fever and pain, although its mechanism of action—inhibiting prostaglandins—was discovered relatively recently. Francis Gall, the father of phrenology, correctly localized speech to the left frontal lobe by correlating skull bumps and language skills. His theory was wrong; his localization of speech was correct. The mechanisms of disease suggested in this chapter come into sharp conflict with many scientific facts. The therapy may be quite effective, however, if still unproven.

Dr. Frymann's interpretation of other data also differs from traditional scientific views. Two topics are the definitive linking of minor head injury and minor immunization reactions to the cause of subsequent epilepsy. Post-traumatic epilepsy is the most frequently delayed sequelae of head injury, occurring in approximately 5% of patients hospitalized after a nonmissile head injury (1). The risk for developing post-traumatic epilepsy is related to the severity of the injury (brain trauma dose) (1–3). Previous epidemiologic studies on large patient samples using careful definitions and powerful statistical analyses found that patients with mild head injury (i.e., loss of consciousness or amnesia lasting up to 30 minutes but without skull fracture) do not have a significantly greater incidence of seizures or epilepsy than the general population (2). In clinical practice, epilepsy is observed in minor head injury (e.g., cases with significant trauma causing a loss of consciousness for 20 minutes). Such cases may represent a coincidence of frequent minor head injuries in the general population and new-onset epilepsy, as suggested by the epidemiologic studies. Alternatively, mild head injury may occasionally cause sufficient brain trauma to cause subsequent seizures and epilepsy.

In 1996, one of us reported a dozen cases of medically mild head injury as a potential contributing factor in epilepsy (4). These cases included what most lay individuals would consider severe head injury (e.g., a policeman punched repeatedly by multiple assailants; he was badly bruised, required emergency room care, and developed his first seizure within a week of this trauma). The association found in these cases and others with clinically significant but medically mild head trauma and epilepsy remains unproven. Clinical common sense supports such a causal relation in some cases. Scientifically, the association remains uncertain and, even if proven, evidence for cause and effect remains a speculation (despite our "clinical belief.") Minor head injury is ubiquitous in children. As one child neurologist said, one can often find a minor head injury in each month of a perfectly healthy boy's life; it is just a question of looking carefully.

Defining immunization as a possible cause of seizures and its relationship to epilepsy is complex and controversial. Multiple immunizations are given annually to tens of millions of children. Febrile seizures occur in 2% to 3% of children between the ages of 6 months and 6 years; these are also the peak ages for immunization. Single seizures and epilepsy are common in children. The opportunity for coincidence of two common childhood events: immunization and seizures/epilepsy is great. Extensive and carefully controlled scientific studies have examined this issue in large pediatric populations. The findings consistently find no evidence that immunizations cause epilepsy; however, a seizure may occur within several days of an immunization, especially if it is followed by a fever. In such cases, the child probably had a 'benign' febrile seizure. When the child receives subsequent immunizations, the parents should ask the doctor about using acetaminophen (Tylenol®) or ibuprofen (Advil®, Motrin®) before a fever develops. Children who have a single seizure following an immunization can usually receive further immunizations. Rarely, a child develops seizures within 24 hours after an immunization and then develops epilepsy and often cognitive and behavioral problems.

Was the immunization contributory? Available scientific studies say "no." Common sense says "yes." As with the cases of "medically mild" but "actually severe" head injury, it is hard to discount a causal relationship when the seizures follow so soon after the seemingly provocative cause. Our own clinical sense is that in both "medically mild" injuries (although these are, in reality, severe with significant trauma) and immunizations followed by severe reactions and seizures that occur very soon after the immunization and continue, there may well be a causal relationship. There may not, however, and it may truly be coincidence, despite the power of our common sense.

Finally, the finding that osteopathy can lead to changes in cerebral blood flow is highlighted in Dr. Frymann's research section. This provides little evidence that osteopathy has any direct effect on seizures or brain function. Cerebral blood flow can be modified by many forms of relaxation (deep breathing, massage), muscle activity in the limbs, and mental activity, such as thinking of words that begin with a specific letter of the alphabet. It is, therefore, a leap from observing changes in blood flow during an osteopathic manipulation to correlating these changes to a mechanism of antagonizing seizure activity.

Can osteopathy improve seizure control in some children and adults? Anecdotal reports suggest that it can. The jury remains out; no scientific data support this. We anxiously await more information on both the specifics of techniques and studies to carefully evaluate the effectiveness of the osteopathic approach in treating people with epilepsy.

References

1. Jennett B, Teasdale G. *Management of Head Injuries.* Philadelphia: FA Davis, 1981;281–287.
2. Annegers JF, Grabow JD, Groover RV, et al. Seizures after head trauma: A population study. *Neurology* 1980;30:683–689.
3. Weiss GH, Feeney DM, Caveness WF, et al. Prognostic factors for the occurrence of post-traumatic epilepsy. *Arch Neurol* 1983;40:7–10.
4. Devinsky O. Epilepsy after minor head trauma. *J Epilepsy* 1996;9:94–97.

The delivery of the baby may be long and traumatic, and associated with hypoxic or anoxic periods. Lack of oxygen during delivery can injure critical areas of the brain. Compression of the delicate infant head impairs the vital, inherent motion of the PRM.

Certain immunizations can precipitate encephalitis, injuring part or all of the brain to various degrees. The manifestation of a seizure within hours or days of receiving immunizations suggests a cause and effect relationship (8).

Sports, car accidents, bicycle and scooter mishaps, and skiing and skating injuries are examples of events that can inflict brain injury that may sooner or later precipitate seizures. Regrettably, we now recognize that many children are abused by a relative, shaken by a frustrated babysitter, or traumatized in other ways. The list goes on; many different forms of trauma can eventually lead to seizure disorders.

Genetic studies revealing perverted chromosome organization and structure provide an understanding of some of the other factors that deform or impair brain development and may eventually manifest as seizures.

The mystery is that a far greater number of children who have suffered an accident or other trauma do not develop seizures. It is rare for two children in the same family to have one of these problems and develop epilepsy.

The Story of Jerome

Clues can help explain this apparent inconsistency of individual variability, which the story of Jerome illustrates. He was his mother's second pregnancy. She developed bronchitis and was treated with erythromycin during the first trimester. She was happy, healthy, and active for the rest of the pregnancy. Jerome was delivered on his due date by an easy nine-hour labor. He was a beautiful baby, nursed well, and grew fast. He never crawled, but he sat up at 6 months and crept on his hands and knees at 10 months. As a 6-month-old baby, he would become terrified if thrown into the air; he held his left hand in a fist; and his arms and back were weak. These observations were noted but received no medical intervention. He flopped forward when sitting at 8 months, and he would suddenly jerk into a hyperextension position when he was in the swimming pool. His knees would give way when standing at 10 months. Seizures caused him to fall sideways when learning to walk. Then he experienced a tonic-clonic seizure with apnea and bulging of his eyes that sent him to the hospital. A diversity of frequent seizures led to the diagnosis of Lennox-Gestault syndrome, defined as "generalized myoclonic astatic epilepsy in children with mental retardation resulting from various cerebral afflictions, such as perinatal hypoxia, cerebral hemorrhage, encephalitides, maldevelopment, or metabolic disorders of the brain characterized by generalized tonic seizures or kinetic attacks and mental deterioration with diffuse slow spike and wave patterns on EEG" (9).

Various drugs were prescribed, and he started the ketogenic diet at 16 months. For 36 hours he had no seizures while fasting in the hospital. But within 6 weeks, a tonic-clonic seizure occurred that was followed by another at 7 weeks. Drop seizures began and increased to 80 to 100 a day. By the time he arrived at the Osteopathic Center for Children (OCC), his count was 100 to 120 drop seizures per day. This was in August 1997; Jerome was 2 years 10 months old.

At the OCC, we search the history for critical and sometimes previously unrecognized events. Jerome's third DPT was given in April 1995, and his first seizure occurred in July of that year. This interval of 3 months decreases the likelihood of a causative relationship; however, after the MMR in May,1996, he had a high fever and many seizures. To me, this indicates a significant relationship. He fell down the stairs in November of 1995. He had suffered many falls, fracturing his feet four times before August 1997. He had received all the traditional immunizations through May 1996. He received 35 osteopathic treatments in 8 months and had his last seizure in April 1998, following an accident and a fall on the back of his head.

Summary of Jerome's History

- During early pregnancy, mother had a respiratory infection treated with an antibiotic. I have observed that respiratory or influenzal illnesses during the early weeks of pregnancy may adversely affect the fetal brain, which is undergoing very rapid development at this time.
- His delivery was uneventful, and his immediate neonatal history was satisfactory.
- His neurologic development was mildly impaired; he never crawled; his arms and upper back were described as weak; and his left hand was held in a fist. Opisthotonic (infantile) spasms developed by 9 months, a sign of brain injury.
- At 13 months, he fell down the stairs. It was not regarded as worthy of medical attention but from an osteopathic point of view, it probably added a mild degree of structural impairment that disturbed the important, delicate, inherent motion of the PRM.
- His early immunizations were not followed by any recognized problems, but his first tonic-clonic seizure occurred within 3 months of his third DPT and polio immunization at 14 months; however, after the MMR at 21 months, he developed a high fever and the number of seizures increased.

Thus, a sequence of minor events interfered with Jerome's neurologic function, eventually culminating in major seizures. His seizures were not controlled by AEDs or by the ketogenic diet. Ultimately, he had no further seizures after 9 months of osteopathic treatment.

Traditional Approaches to Seizure Disorders

I am not a neurologist, neurosurgeon, or epileptologist. When the first child with a major seizure disorder was brought to me many years ago, I had no idea what osteopathic principles and practice could accomplish concerning the seizures, but I knew that their application would enable the child to function closer to the optimum of his potential. Since that early challenge, I have treated approximately 90 children, whose records were retrospectively studied. Every type of seizure was observed. The various therapeutic measures these children received included ACTH in early infancy, the whole spectrum of AEDs, the ketogenic diet, the vagus nerve stimulator, and brain surgery. A search of the literature reveals that all these modalities help many children, but many still remain who live with the insecurity and uncertainty of unpredictable seizures. These children find their way to the OCC. We know the children whose neurologic development was arrested—never to get back on track—after ACTH was administered. We meet the children—once happy, fun-loving, and outgoing—who became mean, aggressive, vindictive, grouchy, and angry as a direct effect of various AEDs. For the child who reacts in this way to one therapy, all are a psychologic hazard. The ketogenic diet can make some children virtually seizure-free and it has, in certain instances, made them happier and friendlier, probably in part because AEDs are reduced. However, many children cannot tolerate this diet of overwhelming fat without fresh fruits, vegetables, and whole grains, or their seizures are not sufficiently controlled to permit reduction of AEDs. The diet is often abandoned for these reasons. The vagus nerve stimulator—whose mode of action is unknown—disturbs the sensitive and delicate balance between the sympathetic and parasympathetic aspects of the autonomic nervous system. However, modest seizure reduction is reported in about 20% to 50% of children with its use. Brain surgery can be dramatically therapeutic if a circumscribed epileptogenic focus is localized that can be removed with minimal trauma to the surrounding brain. These conditions, however, cannot always be fully met. The result is a patient with additional brain injury, persistent seizures, heavy scar tissue (both externally and internally), probable mental delays, and disturbance in other areas of brain function. Conversely, Wilson et al. (10) observed that surgical alleviation of seizures in chronic epilepsy can bring with it the "burden of normality." The successful alleviation of seizures through temporal lobectomy does not necessarily provide psychosocial benefits for the patient. Occasionally, patients decline in functioning as they adjust to life without epilepsy. Patients may spontaneously report problems adjusting to normality up to 10 years post surgery.

The Trauma of Birth

The osteopathic physician looks at the interrelationship of structure and function. Is there evidence of trauma during delivery? Plagiocephaly (a crooked head) may be evident to the untrained naked eye in 10% of newborn babies (11). The other 90% of newborns may look symmetrical and without deformity, but when the trained physician puts experienced hands on the head, impairment or distortion of the inherent motion is apparent in 80% of newborns. Perhaps 10% of the babies were delivered by an easy labor without delays or the need for stimulating intervention (Pitocin®), or instrumental assistance for extraction (forceps or vacuum extraction), or epidural analgesia. They not only look beautiful, alert, responsive, and of good color, but they feel good on palpatory examination. The focus of concern is the inherent motion within the body, including the head. The baby may show you in his inimitable fashion soon after birth that there was some stress as he negotiated the birth canal. For example:

- He does not immediately latch on to the nipple and suck effectively (12th cranial nerve).
- He spits up or vomits after many of his feedings (10th cranial nerve).
- He cries excessively and does not sleep well (foraman magnum).

The occiput leads the way out of the birth canal. The 10th and 12th cranial nerves may be compromised if the occiput is compressed by the forces of labor. The brainstem passes through the developmental parts of the occiput and may be compromised if delay or difficulty occurs during birth. The physician looks for rapid, irregular, shallow breathing or whether the skin is cyanotic or a little dusky. This may indicate that the temporal bones that articulate bilaterally with the occiput were stressed as the fetus passed down the birth canal and are not freely and symmetrically in motion. While the baby lies on a bed or firm surface on his back, note whether his head and feet are in the same vertical line, or whether there is a lateral curve to one side. This suggests some stress in the vertebral area, but trained hands are required to find and release the area of somatic dysfunction (i.e., a structural change that distorts function).

The physician may ask whether the baby begins to move her legs alternately, as if getting ready to crawl when you place her prone on her belly. As the weeks go, parents should watch to see if she responds to this opportunity to develop mobility in her body and lifts her head to survey the world.

When the first immunizations are scheduled, make sure that the baby has no fever or a cold. Ask the parents to carefully observe how he responds after the shot. Look for fever, irritability, excessive crying, or excessive sleeping. Adverse reactions to immunizations are more likely to occur if you noticed some of the factors listed above. Is the baby well integrated in his movements? Is he efficient as he crawls, lies flat on his belly, and then creeps on hands and knees? Learning to walk is often the beginning of falls. If he becomes irritable after a fall, the delicate mechanisms may have sustained strain, impairing the vital and inherent rhythmic respiratory motion. Osteopathic treatment can correct these traumatic events from the time of birth through the growing years, thus enabling the child to function at the optimum of his potential.

For the child with epilepsy, the osteopathic physician explores the history and physical examination for all the problems enumerated above. Dietary habits are studied and constructive changes may be recommended. No changes in the neurologist's protocol will be considered until the following are apparent: (i) a new level of well-being; (ii) a distinct change in seizure occurrence; and (iii) an improved EEG.

Research Concerning Osteopathy in the Cranial Field

Intensive research into the PRM is an ongoing commitment of Yuri Moskalenko (12) and his colleagues at the Russian Academy of Science in St. Petersburg. Transcranial Dopplerography is a physiologic noninvasive method that evaluates the volume and velocity of blood flow through a specific major artery. Bioelectric impedance records the change of electrical conductivity between plate electrodes placed on the human head to monitor for high frequency electric current. Because the electrical conductivity of blood and cerebrospinal fluid are different, their comparative volume changes alter electrical conductivity. Measurable changes occur in the middle cerebral artery following specific cranial technique. Also, one can visualize the proportional cerebrospinal fluid compensatory mobility by analyzing the simultaneous recordings of transcranial Dopplerography and bioelectric impedance.

Clinical Results

Clinical results after osteopathic manipulative treatment in children with seizure disorders include: out of 65 children we cared for at OCC, 19 achieved full seizure control without medication (30%). Eleven achieved reduced frequency and intensity (17%). Sixteen reported improved general well-being, even though seizures persisted (24%). Three patients (4.5%) did not observe significant changes during the course of eight treatments. One patient with a long and intensive history of various types of seizures, and who had received all modalities of AED therapies, died in his sleep several months after his last treatment.

Not every child with epilepsy becomes seizure-free, but some do; some have reduced episodes; many live successfully on less medication; and, with osteopathy, *all enjoy an improved level of well-being.*

References

1. Hildreth AG. *The Lengthening Shadow of Dr. Andrew Taylor Still.* Hildreth and Vleck, p.xi.
2. Sutherland AS. *With Thinking Fingers.* Cranial Academy, 1962;10.
3. Sutherland AS. *The Cranial Bowl.* Published by author, 1939. Reprinted by Cranial Academy, 1948.
4. Magoun HI. *Osteopathy in the Cranial Field.* Published by author, 1966;23.
5. Truhlar RE. *Doctor A.T. Still in the Living.* Published by author, 1950;36.
6. Hilton J. Walls S, Philipp EE, Atkins HJB, (eds.) *Rest and Pain.* (Originally published in 1863 as *On the Influence of Mechanical and Physiological Rest in The Treatment of Accidents and Surgical Diseases and the Diagnostic Value of Pain.*) JB Lippincott Co., 2nd ed., 1950;24.
7. Truhlar RE. *Doctor A.T. Still in the Living.* Published by author, 1950;43.
8. Drug Bulletin. FDA, October 1990;8.
9. *Stedman's Medical Dictionary*, 25th ed. New York: Williams and Wilkins, 1990.
10. Wilson, et al. The longitudinal course of adjustment after seizure surgery. *Seizure* 2001;10:165–172.
11. Frymann VM. Relation of disturbances of craniosacral mechanism to symptomology of the newborn. Study of 1250 infants. *JAOA* 1966;1059–1075.
12. Moskalenko Y, Frymann VM, Kravchenk T, et al. Fundamental background of the cranial rhythmic impulse and primary respiratory mechanism. Sechenov Institute of Evolutionary Physiology and Biochemistry, Russian Academy of Science, St. Petersburg, Russia.

CHAPTER 28

Craniosacral Therapy

GINGER NASH, ND

Craniosacral therapy is difficult to define because it is experientially oriented. As a craniosacral practitioner, it is easier to put my hands on somebody and feel what is happening than to describe what I feel with words. With this caveat, I will attempt to provide a basic understanding of craniosacral work and how it may help individuals with epilepsy.

The cranial bones and sacrum, and the membrane structures that connect these areas, form an anatomic and physiologic system. A distinct rhythm is present within this system (the craniosacral rhythm), created by the flow of cerebrospinal fluid (CSF) through the membrane complex. A craniosacral practitioner assesses this rhythm and uses it to treat subtle imbalances in the nervous and musculoskeletal systems. Even subtle imbalances can profoundly affect a person's health and well-being because the nervous system controls the entire body.

The craniosacral system was discovered by Dr. William Sutherland in the early part of the twentieth century. Dr. Sutherland was an osteopathic physician who, for 20 years, contemplated and conducted limited research into the idea that the bones of the skull were movable. By applying different pressures and constraints on different cranial bones, he described problems with coordination and corresponding areas of pain, as well as different mental and emotional reactions. Dr. Sutherland developed a system to examine and assess the movements of the skull bones. He also developed methods to adjust, or more accurately, to help his patients self-correct the movements of these bones. Thus, he developed methods to treat these imbalances, a discipline now referred to as cranial osteopathy.

The healing approach of cranial osteopathy was initially practiced by a small number of physicians who studied with Sutherland. In the 1970s, the osteopathic physician and surgeon Dr. John Upledger directly observed the rhythmic movements within the membranes that surround the brain and spinal cord. He researched these movements and coined the term *craniosacral system*. In 1975, Upledger joined the faculty at Michigan State University as a clinician-researcher, focusing his work on the craniosacral system.

The brain and spinal cord, essentially the core of our being, are encased in both bone and connective tissue. The brain is housed in the skull bones and the spinal cord in the vertebral column, with the sacral bone forming its base. The connective tissue consists of the *meninges*, three specialized membranes that are wrapped tightly around the brain and spinal cord, much like a stocking. The *pia mater* closely follows the contours of the central nervous system; the *arachnoid membrane* lies on top of the pia; and the thickest *dura mater* forms the outer layer. The entire body is encased in the *fascia*, the connective tissue that forms a sheath around various bodily structures, including the bones, muscles, and internal organs. These membranes surrounding the spinal cord and brain and those surrounding the skull and vertebral bones comprise the craniosacral system. The proper alignment of this connective tissue system is essential for the optimal transmission of nerve impulses. It can also affect blood and lymph circulation to different tissues.

The craniosacral system also includes the bones of skull, mouth and face, and the sacrum. The brain and spinal cord are lubricated with CSF, which is pumped out by specialized cells lining the ventricles of the brain. The CSF system is a semi-closed hydraulic system, with the fluid moving up and down the spinal cord as pressures build from increased output. Just as the pumping action of the heart can be determined by palpation of the pulse at the wrist or neck, the cranial rhythm can be palpated very easily at certain points on the body (i.e., certain locations in the skull bones and the sacrum, because that is where the meninges attach to bone.) Experienced practitioners can palpate this rhythm anywhere on the body.

Normally, the human body continually regulates this physiologic process. When an individual fails to self-regulate (e.g., because of trauma, poor circulation, or poor anatomic alignment), areas of restriction and diminished function are created. This results in certain body parts not responding rhythmically to the gentle CSF pulsations. This pathologic process can affect a person's health in various ways and in different clinical scenarios; however, the bulk of cranial work is performed on patients with neurologic problems, chronic pain, and long-standing psychological issues, such as depression and anxiety. I also commonly treat endocrine or hormonal imbalance. Craniosacral work can affect hormone secretions due to the connection with pituitary and pineal glands, located deep inside the skull and in close contact with the meningeal system.

Other common reasons for the inhibition of proper functioning of the craniosacral system are scarring or adhesions, inflammation, and vascular accidents. Any abnormalities in the structure or function of the nervous system, the musculoskeletal system, endocrine, or respiratory system may alter functioning in the craniosacral system. Conversely, an imbalance in the craniosacral system can impair normal functioning in these physiologic systems.

The craniosacral technique uses gentle, light-force manipulation of the aforementioned bodily structures, including the cranial bones. The technique relies largely on the body's inherent ability for self-correction and is noninvasive. It does not cause side effects, in any traditional sense. The skilled practitioner detects any weakened cranial rhythm, asymmetry in the rhythm, and areas of restriction, and then employs particular techniques, always gently, to accommodate proper movement of the structures involved.

Patients often ask me how so little force can change the positioning of the bones or other structures. It makes sense from the perspective of pure physics. The craniosacral

Commentary

Craniosacral therapy is a growing field with expanding numbers of practitioners, centers, and potential applications; however, the growth in clinical activity is not paralleled by the growth in clinical or basic research. Fundamental issues underlying this therapy remain uncertain. Do cranial bones move? If so, can such minor motion of these bones result from craniosacral treatment? Can minor movements in cranial bones improve certain disorders? Can craniosacral practitioners reliably palpate a craniosacral rhythm (CSR)? Does craniosacral therapy work for any disorder? No adequately controlled studies support the use of craniosacral therapy for any disorder; however, some websites for craniosacral treatment centers list more than 60 disorders that might benefit from this therapy. The use of craniosacral therapy in epilepsy remains unproven.

Rogers and Witt (1) reviewed the literature on cranial bone motion and found the published research scant and inconclusive. Although animal and human studies demonstrate a potential for small-magnitude motion, they found no evidence to link such potential motion with therapeutic outcomes. Also, one study on human cadavers that found changes in the length of the *falx cerebri* (a prominent membrane within the skull) was uncontrolled and unblinded (2).

The British Columbia Office of Health Technology Assessment reviewed the objective data regarding craniosacral therapy and found the evidence to be insufficient to support this therapeutic modality for any disorder (3). They used a three-dimensional evaluative framework: (i) craniosacral interventions and health outcomes; (ii) validity of craniosacral assessment; and (iii) pathophysiology of the craniosacral system. They reviewed all published data in Medline, Embase, Healthstar, Mantis, Allied and Alternative Medicine, Scisearch, and Biosis from their start date to February 1999. Notably, one study reported mild negative side effects in 5% of outpatients with traumatic brain injury who received craniosacral therapy (4).

Several studies found that the reliability of palpating a craniosacral rhythm is poor between practitioners (5,6). Palpating the CSR is a fundamental clinical diagnostic skill and forms the basis of therapy. In one study (6), two registered osteopaths with postgraduate training in craniosacral techniques simultaneously palpated the head and the sacrum of 11 normal healthy subjects. They did not know each other's findings (i.e., they were blinded). Intrarater reliability (repeated measures for the *same examiner* in the same patient) at either the head or the sacrum was fair to good (correlation coefficients from 0.52 to 0.73). Interexaminer reliability (simultaneous measures for *different examiners* in the same patient; one at the cranium and one at the sacrum) for simultaneous palpation at the head and the sacrum was poor to nonexistent (correlation coefficients from -0.09 to 0.31). The results failed to support the construct validity of the CSR hypothesis as traditionally held by craniosacral therapists.

Much uncertainty remains regarding the theoretical basis of craniosacral therapy, the ability of different practitioners to palpate an actual CSR, and the role of this therapy in treating various disorders. No evidence suggests that it benefits individuals with epilepsy; however, craniosacral therapy may work through the relaxation response, or it may work in other ways that could potentially benefit individuals with epilepsy. Thus, we are left with many more questions than answers.

References

1. Rogers JS, Witt PL. The controversy of cranial bone motion. *J Orthop Sports Phys Ther* 1997;26:95–103.
2. Kostopoulos DC, Keramidas G. Changes in elongation of *falx cerebri* during craniosacral therapy techniques applied on the skull of an embalmed cadaver. *Cranio* 1992;10:9–12.
3. Green C, Martin CW, Bassett K, et al. A systematic review of craniosacral therapy: biological plausibility, assessment reliability and clinical effectiveness. *Complement Ther Med* 1999;7:201–207.
4. Greenman PE, McPartland JM. Cranial findings and iatrogenesis from craniosacral manipulation in patients with traumatic brain syndrome. *J Am Osteopath Assoc* 1995;95:182–188; 191–192.
5. Hanten WP, Dawson DD, Iwata M, et al. Craniosacral rhythm: reliability and relationships with cardiac and respiratory rates. *J Orthop Sports Phys Ther* 1998;27:213–218.
6. Moran RW, Gibbons P. Intraexaminer and interexaminer reliability for palpation of the cranial rhythmic impulse at the head and sacrum. *J Manip Physiol Ther* 2001;24:183–190.

practitioner uses a minimal amount of force (approximately the weight of a nickel) over a long period of time (anywhere from 30 seconds to several minutes depending on individual circumstances and how quickly the person's body responds). A more forceful manipulation may exert many times more pressure on the system in just a second, or fraction of a second. During craniosacral therapy, the amount of energy put into the body is approximately the same as some chiropractic adjustments, just over a longer period of time.

Craniosacral practitioners are more interested in larger areas, indeed the entire body, including all the soft tissue structures, not simply the bones. They are trained to follow the body's self-correcting processes and use their intention to help foster balance. During a craniosacral treatment, many patients experience different sensations in their bodies—strong images may come into the patient's mind; others feel the release of emotion or tension; some simply fall asleep. Individual perception and response to therapy can vary. In many cases, patients report that after two or three treatments they can feel their own cranial rhythm, either during the treatment or spontaneously during times when their bodies are still.

Most patients require a series of three to six treatments for lasting results, and maintenance visits are encouraged once every few months, although a single treatment may dramatically benefit the patient in some cases. Treatments last approximately 45 minutes to one hour in length.

Precautions

The most effective craniosacral work is achieved when the practitioner taps into the body's self-corrective abilities, and when obstacles are removed or areas of restriction are reintegrated into the entire system. Patients rarely experience any side effects. Infrequently, patients may feel worse after a treatment for a short period of time before they feel better or notice benefits. This may be due to areas of the body "waking up," so to speak, and therefore being more sensitive than previously. Also, the rebalancing process can sometimes take longer than the duration of the treatment, and the body needs extra time to adjust to the new energy flowing through it.

Craniosacral therapy is not recommended in a few special circumstances. These include conditions where a slight alteration in cranial pressure could be injurious. Examples include an acute aneurysm, severe bleeding disorders, or cerebral hemorrhage.

Therapeutic Approaches

Three schools of craniosacral work exist. They are similar but have slightly different therapeutic approaches. The sutural approach, popularized by Dr. Sutherland, focuses on the mobility of the cranial bones. The meningeal approach incorporates the membrane system into its work. The reflex approach was developed by Dr. De Jarnette, a student of Dr. Sutherland's, in the 1920s. This school uses sacro-occipital techniques to turn off stress signals affecting different organs in the body.

Osteopathic physicians are trained in osteopathic medicine, which incorporates many of these concepts. Other practitioners—such as naturopathic physicians, medical doctors, physical therapists, dentists, nurses, occupational therapists, psychiatric specialists, psychologists, acupuncturists, massage therapists, and other professional body-workers—can receive training from the organizations created by the pioneers and leaders in this field. No standardized credentialing requirements exist, except as determined by each educational organization.

Craniosacral Therapy in Epilepsy

Unfortunately, no controlled trials using craniosacral therapy to treat epilepsy have been undertaken; however, some studies provide clinical evidence that craniosacral therapy can improve several neurologic disorders. When treating patients with seizure disorder, as with any other complaint, the functional integrity of the entire system should be addressed from the scalp down or the feet up. Common findings in the skeletal system for people with epilepsy are rotation in the temporal bones. Often one is internally rotated and one externally rotated; these corrections can usually be made in one session. The parietal bones are always assessed, and some resistance also often is present in the mobility of those bones. Advanced cranial work also assesses the brain lobes. Normally, one feels a smooth alternating rhythm from side to side in corresponding lobes. Typically, the lobes cycle through this alternating movement 5 to 6 times per minute. The brain lobes often feel sluggish in patients with epilepsy. Often the temporal lobe is involved, meaning the mobility or motility of the lobes is palpably different. Sometimes the movements are out of synch or barely palpable, there may be a racheting quality, or the presence of scar tissue can be identified by very sensitive hands. The quality of this movement can greatly improve over the course of a session, or several sessions, and can hold for many days, or even weeks, depending on the individual.

Craniosacral treatments range in cost from approximately $40 to $200 per session. Costs are largely determined by geographical area and the practitioner's credentials and experience. Most health insurance plans cover the treatment as a soft tissue manipulation, for those craniosacral practitioners who accept health insurance.

Conclusion

Craniosacral work is difficult to explain succinctly and is therefore challenging to discuss with practitioners who are unfamiliar with this therapy. The therapy is very gentle and safe; little or no risk is involved in receiving treatment. Most patients find it an extremely relaxing experience and, on this basis alone, its clinical implications are enormous. Craniosacral work is truly holistic medicine, integrating all aspects of one's self and working with the body instead of against it.

Resources

The Upledger Institute: http://www.upledger.com/
The International Association of Healthcare Practitioners: http://www.iahp.com/
The American Academy of Osteopathy: http://www.ohwi.org/
Sacro Occipital Technique Organization: http://www.sorsi.com/

PART VIII

Music, Art, and Pet Therapies

CHAPTER 29

Music Therapy

Concetta M. Tomaino, DA, MT-BC

Music affects us in many ways. It can help us relax, reminisce, and generally feel better. This is because music affects the brain on many levels, and it can be used in therapy to alleviate or help improve certain physical, psychologic, and cognitive conditions. Music can also be a powerful stimulus that may trigger seizure activity in some individuals; however, research into how certain tones and rhythmic patterns influence brain activity indicates that specific types of music may provide a therapeutic benefit for people with epilepsy. In addition, specific uses of music to affect emotional well-being may be applied within the context of therapy through a trained music therapist. This chapter provides an overview of the clinical application of music therapy.

Definition

Music therapy is the systematic use of music within a developing relationship between a therapist and patient to restore, maintain, and/or improve physical, emotional, psychosocial, and neurologic function. Not only songs are used, but the various components of music, such as a specific tone or frequency of sound, certain patterns of beat or rhythm, harmony, and melody can be used independently to provide a clinical effect. The music therapist works with the patient to select the type of music that provides the most benefit.

History

The general public is becoming more familiar with the use of music therapy for a variety of medical and psychologic benefits, but many people are unaware that the therapeutic properties of music have been documented since the time of Socrates and Plato. An interest in the potential of music therapy and developing a professional practice arose in the United States after both World Wars, when musicians provided entertainment programs for the veterans who were being treated for the physical and emotional traumas of war. Medical staff took notice that the most withdrawn, and even some of the catatonic patients, exhibited a response when music was playing. The need to investigate the therapeutic aspects of music and train professionals to apply music for special populations led to the establishment of college curricula. The first was at Michigan State University, in 1944. The American Music Therapy Association, representing over 5,000 music therapists, was founded in 1998, as a union of the National Association for Music Therapy (established in 1950) and the American Association for Music Therapy (established in 1971).

Length of Treatment

The effects of certain types of rhythmic patterns or songs can be almost immediate. The sessions may range from 30 minutes to 1 hour if the individual is attempting to overcome anxiety related to his epilepsy or trying to learn self-help or behavior modifying techniques. The therapist will estimate how often sessions should take place and work out a treatment plan.

Treatment Protocols

The use of music as therapy, and its potential for abating seizure activity, is still a subject for research and clinical investigation. For this reason, no standard exists for what type of music may work or how long the treatments may take. A trained music therapist who is helping an individual build self-help techniques or develop techniques for reducing stress, anxiety, or other emotional triggers that may set off their seizures may schedule weekly sessions until the individual's goals are met.

Other Conditions

Music therapy has been used in many different medical, educational, and psychologic treatments include the following:

- To help people with Alzheimer's disease and other types of cognitive impairments to improve memory.
- In medical treatments, to alleviate or minimize the experience of pain.
- During physical rehabilitation, to assist in the recovery of motor function and speech following a stroke or other traumatic brain injury.
- In psychiatric cases, to help individuals express and deal with their fears, anxieties, mental blocks, and resistances so that they can gain more control over their personal health and well-being.

Treatment Plans

Treatment may involve listening to music with or without verbal guidance by the therapist, improvising music, or actively making music with the therapist. After the music-making experience, there is usually time to discuss the experience with the therapist. In treatments in which music has been specifically programmed to produce a therapeutic

Commentary

Many people with epilepsy, particularly those whose seizures are not under complete control, experience increased levels of stress because of psychosocial difficulties. Stressful problems can arise at school or work, or may result from conflicts with family members, friends, or other people, often leading to anxiety, depressed mood, and trouble sleeping. Unfortunately, increased stress can make seizures worse, creating even more stress.

Several methods for reducing stress levels are described in this book that do not involve medications, including music therapy. These therapies and techniques can be quite helpful.

Although scientific studies of music therapy for people with epilepsy have not been conducted, it is reasonable to believe that the potential beneficial effects would be similar to those derived by people without epilepsy. Even so, studies would be helpful to know which people with epilepsy are most likely to benefit from music therapy, how much their stress and anxiety levels may improve, and whether other possible effects may occur, such as improved concentration and memory.

We concur with the precautions Ms. Tomaino highlights. Patients whose seizures are triggered by music, strong beats, or tones should probably not undergo music therapy. Interested patients should seek out music therapists who are knowledgeable about epilepsy and know how to respond in the event of a seizure during treatment.

effect, the treatment may be simply listening to recorded sounds while the doctor or therapist performs an EEG test to see how the music affects brain waves and seizure activity.

Precautions

Music can induce seizure activity in some individuals. This is due to either the emotional aspects of the music or the specific areas of the brain that are stimulated when a specific type of music is heard. This varies with each individual. Sometimes the rhythm of the music will trigger physical ticks or jerks; sometimes it is the meaning or emotion associated with a particular sound that will trigger a seizure. Musicogenic epilepsy is the term applied when an individual has a seizure due to a specific type of music being played. This is well documented in the medical journals, although rare.

Training and Credentials

A music therapist is a professional who has undergone rigorous education and training at an approved academic program and completed a 1,000-hour clinical internship under the supervision of a trained music therapist. Individuals are eligible to sit for the national exam offered by the Certification Board for Music Therapists upon completion of training. Music therapists who successfully complete the independently administered examination hold the music therapist-board certified credential (MT-BC). The National Music Therapy Registry (NMTR) serves qualified music therapy professionals with the following designations: RMT, CMT, ACMT. These individuals have met the accepted educational and clinical training standards and are qualified to practice music therapy.

Effectiveness of Music Therapy in Epilepsy

Although the research in the field of music therapy in epilepsy is limited, hundreds of peer-reviewed articles are available on the applications of music therapy to improve psychologic well-being. Several published clinical studies have shown that certain types of music can decrease seizure activity. Increased research into specifically how music is processed in the brain will soon help explain the anecdotal reports of this therapeutic effect in the treatment of epilepsy. Using various measurement tools, such as electroencephalogram (EEG) and functional magnetic resonance imaging (fMRI), scientists are beginning to see precisely how this happens. Of particular note is a review of the research by John Hughes (1) that explored the "Mozart Effect" in persons with epilepsy. His article examined the patterning of the melodic line of Mozart's music and EEG measurements of epileptiform patterns. He suggested that the superorganization of the cerebral cortex resonates with the great organization found in Mozart's music. In one study, John Hughes et al. (2) studied 29 epilepsy patients (3–47 years of age), all of whom had frequent seizures either in the waking or comatose state. They carefully monitored the occurrence and duration of abnormal brain wave episodes during five conditions: (i) baseline silence; (ii) Mozart's Sonata for Two Pianos (K.448); (iii) following a period of silence; (iv) old-time pop tunes; and (v) a final period of silence. The investigators found a statistically significant reduction in discharges in 23 of 29 cases. Moreover, the effect was confined to Mozart's music, and the degree of effect was not small. The average amount of time these patients had seizures was reduced from 62% to 21%. Old-time pop tunes had no effect.

Lubar and Bahler (3) found that training individuals with severe seizure activity to use an EEG biofeedback of the sensorimotor rhythm could decrease seizure intensity and duration when the subjects learned to increase the 12- to 14-Hz EEG activity from the regions overlying the Rolandic area in the brain. This sensorimotor rhythm was hypothesized by Sterman (4) to be related to motor inhibitory processes.

Music is not processed in one specific region of the brain, but rather is processed in many cerebral and subcortical areas. Rhythm—the actual pulse or beat pattern of music—does have a therapeutic affect. Rhythm can serve as an entrainment device, driving cortical rhythms as a result of auditory stimulation. Certain rhythmic patterns can drive or excite the motor cortex to coordinate movement. In diseases such as Parkinson's or stroke, where the internal initiation or sequential patterning of movement may be damaged, the cueing of specific patterns through an outside source can allow for such a function to be initiated and executed.

Melodic perception differs from rhythmic perception and is processed primarily in the right temporal lobe. There it excites a tonotopic map indicative of specific pitches or tones. In temporal lobe epilepsy, the spontaneous stimulation of this region during a seizure can result in the hearing of tones or specific melodies.

Music also has strong emotional components and associations. The auditory nerve has an almost immediate connection to the limbic area of the brain, including the thalamus, making it easy to have an emotional response even before the title of the song is recognized or recalled. Because of the strong associations attributed to songs or particular harmonies, music can be used to affect mood states. In a study by Blood and Zatorre (5) using position emission tomography (PET) to study the neural mechanisms underlying intensely pleasant emotional responses to music, the researchers found that increases were found in brain structures that are known to be active in response to other euphoria-inducing stimuli, such as food, sex, and drugs of abuse.

The following aspects of music therapy—developed during clinical work with individuals having seizure disorders—have been documented:

- Music can produce a generalizing relaxation affect; however, music that is relaxing to one person may not be relaxing to another. An individual can keep a journal noting the music that affects his mood and/or activity level to learn what types of music provide a specific response. By using music to provide relaxation or to promote sleep, the need for sedative drugs or other substances, some of which may exacerbate seizure activity, may be decreased.

- When emotional or social integration issues arise, especially with young children, participation in a formal music therapy group is beneficial. The therapist is trained to use music both in improvisations and songs to build self-esteem and provide group cohesion and integration. Music can be used to promote movement, relaxation, self-awareness, learning, communication, self-expression, creativity, social interaction, and personal development. These skills may help children gain important social skills, decrease their feelings of isolation, increase their self-esteem, and gain control over their lives.

- If music can stimulate, it can also relax by providing rhythmic patterns that can entrain brain waves to a slower pattern. Techniques similar to the relaxation exercises used in meditation and yoga can be facilitated by music to cue slower breathing and entrain slower brain wave patterns.

Precautions

Many case studies reported that music can induce seizure activity. Norman Weinberger, a cognitive neuroscientist at the University of Irvine in California, wrote:

Musically induced seizures can occur in epileptic patients for whom there are other triggers for seizures (e.g., blinking lights). In some cases, music is the only trigger. There are no specific epileptogenic features of music; seizures can be induced by the type of music, type of instrument, type of emotional content, and even by a certain composer. But actual music need not be present; seizures can occur while thinking or even dreaming of music. The seizures are not immediately "reflexive" but many take tens of seconds to several minutes to develop. They appear to originate most commonly in the right temporal lobe, which houses the right auditory cortex, an area implicated in the processing of melody. Exactly how music induces epileptic episodes is unknown (6).

Some musicogenic seizures are a reflex epilepsy triggered by certain types of music or even specific frequencies of pitch for which the person's brain has a low threshold or tolerance. These sounds trigger focal epileptiform EEG discharges in a very specific part of the brain. This may result in a complex partial seizure, but may also induce other seizures, such as tonic-clonic seizures.

Musicogenic seizures usually involve a degree of cognitive or emotional appreciation of stimulus.

Vizioli (7) suggested that music is too complex to limit it to just rhythm or melody. He considers that three levels of integration involve music: a sensory level (lowest), an emotional level and waking level (second), and an aesthetic level (highest). Vizioli noted that musicogenic epilepsy may be related to limbic brain function, which is associated with the second level of integration.

Weiser et al. (8) studied 83 patients with musicogenic epilepsy according to musical triggers, type of epilepsy, presumed location of seizure onset, and demographic data. Their results showed that 14 of the 83 seizures (17%) were triggered exclusively by music. They noticed that the characteristics of the music that were significant included musical category, familiarity, and instrumentation. They concluded that musicogenic epilepsy is a particular form of epilepsy with a strong correlation to the temporal lobe and right-sided preponderance. The majority of seizures did not fall into the strictly "reflex epilepsy" category but appeared to depend on certain emotional reactions mediated through the limbic temporal lobe structures.

A case study by Sutherling et al. (9) described a 67-year-old organist minister with diabetes mellitis who had stereotypic focal seizures of the left lower face, jaw, and neck. Attacks occurred spontaneously or were induced when he played a specific hymn on the organ. The seizures did not happen by reading, singing, hearing, or playing the hymn silently. In this case, the seizures were caused by playing a specific sound in a specific hymn on the organ. Right temporofrontal seizures were recorded on an EEG.

Information about the types of sounds or rhythms that induce seizures is extremely useful for the physician because it may indicate a specific location of seizure activity as well as provide a basis for desensitizing the individual to the particular stimulus.

Sometimes seizure activity triggers the "sound of music." In his book *The Man Who Mistook His Wife for a Hat*, Dr. Oliver Sacks (10) discussed a few cases where people have actually experienced "musical epilepsy." One woman, Mrs. O'C, woke up one night hearing Irish music playing loudly. For weeks, she thought someone had left the radio on. When she reported this, she discovered that she was the only one who heard the music. She was first referred to a psychiatrist, who then referred her to a neurologist. When she went to see Dr. Sacks, he had difficulty speaking with her because the music playing in her head overpowered all other sounds in the room. She could hear him only during the quieter songs. After an EEG, it was evident that Mrs. O'C was having temporal lobe seizures, and this was causing the *reminiscence* or *experiential hallucination*. Dr. Sacks soon discovered that Mrs. O'C had suffered a stroke, and as the local damage in the stroke area resolved, the music in her head diminished.

Certain drugs can also "turn on the music." For example, aspirin can cause tinnitus or ringing in the ears. These noises can take many forms, with descriptions ranging from whistling and humming to paper rustling. Some people hear noises as tunes and melodies. The common factor with all these sounds is that they do not originate from an external source.

Likewise, certain drugs used in treating epilepsy can change the perception of sound. One 18-year-old woman being treated with carbamazepine (CBZ) developed an auditory disturbance (flat tone). She was placed on CBZ 400 mg/day because she had tonic-clonic seizures during sleep. She stated that the musical instrument she normally played sounded a half tone lower immediately after taking the medication. All exams and magnetic resonance images were normal. Given that this particular subject was a well-trained musician who could identify pitch changes, the authors questioned whether or not the subtle side effect of CBZ in pitch perception was common and needed further investigation (11).

Financial Considerations

The cost of an individual session of music therapy is based on geographic area, and may range from $40 to $100 per hour.

At present, some insurance companies reimburse for prescribed music therapy if the procedure or service is covered under standard Current Procedural Terminology (CPT) and the service provider has received prior approval by the insurance company's case manager to bill for music therapy services for the specific procedure or treatment. Some individuals who are unable to receive insurance coverage may choose to pay privately to participate in music therapy.

Assessing the Standards and Methods of a Music Therapist

Music therapists must maintain their credentials on a regular basis through continuing education. Not all music therapists are knowledgeable about the effects of music on epilepsy. For this reason, it is always important to know what types of patients a therapist typically works with. This allows potential patients to understand their ability to work with the issues related to seizure disorders. Patients can contact the National Music Therapy Registry or the Certification Board for Music Therapists to check whether a music therapist is credentialed.

Conclusion

Music therapy may help some people with epilepsy decrease the number of seizures they experience and promote a general sense of well-being and self-control. It may also help with the emotional issues related to having a diagnosis of epilepsy. People interested in pursuing music therapy as a treatment option should find a trained therapist who has experience in this area. In using any of the new specialized "brain rhythm entrainment" music programs, it is important to be aware of any significant change in seizure activity—either an increase or decrease—and any other lasting effects. Music can have a powerful effect on some seizure activity, so treatment should not be taken lightly or without discussing the program with your primary healthcare professional.

References

1. Hughes J. The Mozart Effect. *Epilepsy and Behavior* 2001;2(5):396–417.
2. Hughes JR, Daaboul Y, Fino JJ, et al. The "Mozart effect" on epileptiform activity. *Clinical Electroencephalography* 1998;29:109–119.
3. Lubar JF, Bahler WW. Behavioral management of epileptic seizures following EEG biofeedback training of the sensorimotor rhythm. *Biofeedback Self Regulation* 1976;1(1):77–104.
4. Sterman MB, Macdonald LR, Stone RK. Biofeedback training of the sensorimotor electroencephalogram rhythm in man: Effects on epilepsy. *Epilepsia* 1974;15(3):395–416.
5. Blood, Zatorre. Intensely pleasurable responses to music correlate with activity in brain regions implicated in reward and emotion. *Proc. Natl Acad Sci USA* 2001;98(20):11818–11823.
6. Weinberger N. Music and epilepsy as treatment. *Musica Notes* 1998;5(3):5–6.
7. Vizioli R. Musicogenic epilepsy. *Intl J Neuroscience* 1989;47(1–2):159–164.
8. Wieser HG, Hungerbuhler H, Siegel AM, et al. Musicogenic Epilepsy: Review of the literature and case report with ictal single photon emission computed tomography. *Epilepsia* 1997;38:200–207.
9. Sutherling WW, Hershman LM, Miller JQ, et al. Seizures induced by playing music. *Neurology* 1980;30(9):1001–1004.
10. Sacks OW. *The Man Who Mistook His Wife for a Hat.* Summit Books: New York, 1985; 125–142.
11. Mabuchi K, Hayashi S, Nitta E, et al. Auditory disturbances induced by carbamazepine administration in a patient with secondary generalized seizure. *Rinsho Shinkeigak.* May 1885;35(5):553–555.

Bibliography

Adrian ED, Matthews BC. The Berger Rhythm: potential changes from occipital lobes in man. *Brain* 1934;57:355–384.

Birbaumer N, Lutzenberger W, Rau H, et al. *Perception of Music and Dimensional Complexity of Brain Activity.* Technical Report CCSR-95-4, Center for Complex Systems Research, The Beckman Institute, Univ. of Illinois at Urbana-Champaign, 1995.

Bregman AS. *Auditory Scene Analysis: The Perceptual Organization of Sound.* Cambridge, MA: The MIT Press, 1994.

Buser P, Imbert M. *Audition* translated by R.H. Kay. Cambridge, MA: MIT Press, 1992.

Crichtley M. Musicogenic epilepsy, I. The beginnings. In: Critchley M, Henson RA, (eds.) *Music and the Brain.* Heinemann Medical: London, 1977;344–353.

Deutsch D. *The Psychology of Music.* San Diego: Academic Press, Inc., 1982.

Evan JR, Clynes M. *Rhythm in Psychological, Linguistic and Musical Processes.* Springfield, IL: Charles C. Thomas, 1986.

Fraisse F. (Deutsch). *The Psychology of Music.* Orlando, FL: Academic Press, 1982;149–180.

Glass L. Synchronization and rhythmic processes in physiology. *Nature* 2001;410:277–294.

Hart M, Lieberman F. *Planet Drum.* Grateful Dead Books, 1991.

Lane JD, Kasian SJ, Owens JE, et al. Binaural auditory beats affect vigilance performance and mood. *Physiology Behav* 1998;(2):249–252.

Neher A. Auditory driving observed with scalp electrodes in normal subjects. *Electroencephalography Neurophysiology* 1961;13:449–451.

Penhume, VB, Zatorre, RJ, Evans AC. Cerebellar contributions to motor timing: a PET study of auditory and visual rhythm reproduction. *J Neuroscience* 1998;29(6):752–765

Reisberg D, (ed.) *Auditory Imagery.* Hillsdale, NJ: Lawrence Erlbaum Associates, 1982.

Simpson GV, Pflieger ME, Foxe JJ, et al. Dynamic neuroimaging of brain function. *J Clin Neurophysiology* 1995;12(5):432–449.

Straum M. Music and rhythmic stimuli in the rehabilitation of gait disorders and clinical applications. *J Music Ther* 1983;23:56–122.

Taylor D. *Biomedical Foundations of Musical Therapy.* St. Louis: MMB Inc., 1997.

Thaut M, Brown S, Benjamin J, et al. Rhythmic facilitation of movement sequencing: effects on spatial-temporal control and sensory modality dependence. In: R.R. Pratt & Spintge (eds.) *Music Medicine.* St. Louis: MMB Music, Inc., 1994;2:104–109.

Thaut MH, Kenyon GP, Schauer ML, et al. The connection between rhythmicity and brain function. *IEEE English Medical Biolog Mag* 1999;18(2):101–108.

Tomaino (ed.) *Clinical Applications of Music in Neurologic Rehabilitation.* St. Louis: MMB Music, 1998.

Zifkin BG, Zatorre RJ. Musicogenic epilepsy. In: Zifkin G Z, Andermann F, Beaumanoir A, Rowan AJ, (eds.) *Reflex Epilepsies and Reflex Seizures: Advances in Neurology.* Philadelphia, PA: Lippincott-Raven, 1998;75:273–281.

Resources

The following websites provide useful information about music therapy, how to find a music therapist, music brain research, and applied sound research:

The American Music Therapy Association; www.musictherapy.org

The Certification Board for Music Therapists: www.cbmt.org

The World Music Therapy Federation: www.musictherapyworld.de

The Institute for Music and Neurologic Function: www.musicaspower.org

Information on Specialized Sound Recordings and Other Helpful Information

Advanced Brain Technologies: www.advancedbrain.com

The Relaxation Company: www.therelaxationcompany.com

Medical Music Resonance Therapy: www.scientificmusictherapy.com

www.epilepsyontario.org

www.epilepsy.org.uk/info/mozart.html

www.appliedmusic.com

CHAPTER 30

Art Therapy

Elizabeth Coss, MA, ATR-BC and Steven C. Schachter, MD

Art therapy is about giving form to feelings. Our culture and society mainly rely on words to communicate our thoughts, feelings, and intentions to each other. Often we are defensive when verbally communicating to one another. At other times, what we say is not really what we feel, and this may be hurtful. Some people find it difficult to communicate or talk about circumstances and feelings that are painful or unconscious.

Art therapy is a creative process that can recreate the space where a child or adult learns to be creative and authentic (1,2), making it difficult to disguise true feelings. In addition, because the creative process keeps one closer to authentic feelings, unconscious and repressed feelings surface with greater ease.

Art therapy can be especially helpful to people with epilepsy who isolate themselves and have difficulty engaging with others and feeling comfortable in social settings. Because parents and people with epilepsy are often concerned with safety and the possibility of embarrassment, their lives can become further limited in terms of interaction—socially, educationally, or in the workplace. For these reasons, children with epilepsy may not make a confident transition to a more autonomous lifestyle as they become adults. Therefore, art therapy can be very helpful in the processes of engagement, transition, and socialization.

Art therapy helps a patient become more interactive because the art therapist provides a safe space wherein the patient can communicate in a fun and subtle way without using words. According to Deri, "creativity refers to the innumerable ongoing actions, reactions, decisions, and choices—unconscious, preconscious, and conscious—that give form and texture to an individual life" (3). In the art room, the patient can test out "life-shaping activities" (3) with the art therapist through symbolism or imagery.

Winnicott (2) talks about development in terms of an infant transitioning from being merged and dependent upon the mother (parent) through the capacity to symbolize. The capacity to symbolize starts with the baby's first found object: the transitional object. This object is a symbol of the baby's union with the parent, whether it be a blanket or another object that the baby holds onto when the parent is not in the baby's presence. The object becomes a symbol for the parent. Because the baby can now symbolize the parent, the baby can also be separate from the parent. By contrast, the person with epilepsy may not fully separate from her family. Consequently, she may not have practiced the behaviors that lead to a sense of independence. Art therapy can create an environment in which the patient creates a transitional object, which may help the patient find words or images that help her transition to more independence.

In most cases, art therapists are well trained artists and psychotherapists with additional skills in interpreting artwork. Art therapists work in settings as varied as schools, hospitals, or their own private practices. A clinically trained art therapist has a master's degree in art therapy from an accredited university or a program approved by the American Art Therapy Association. An art therapist with the title "ATR" is a registered art therapist who has had at least 1,000 hours of patient contact time after graduation, including 100 hours of clinical supervision. An art therapist who is an ATR-BC is also board certified, meaning he has passed a lengthy test that evaluates his theoretical and clinical knowledge of the field.

Case Study

Here is an example of how one particular patient with epilepsy benefited from art therapy. He became engaged in the art making process and made a transition from being anxious and withdrawn to a more socially fulfilling life.

Kevin is a 20-year-old African American man who participated in an art therapy group for people with epilepsy. Kevin was struggling with adolescent issues of transition to autonomy and independence. He experienced his first seizure at 15 months of age. In addition to art therapy, Kevin was involved in a support group and saw an individual therapist. Kevin still lived at home, and when he started traveling to see an individual therapist, it was the longest trip he had ever made on his own using public transportation.

Commentary

Coss and Schachter provide an overview of art therapy that is focused on the care of individuals with epilepsy. Unlike many of the therapies in this volume, art therapy is not intended to directly reduce seizure frequency, although that may be an added benefit for some individuals. Rather, art therapy is a tool, quite different from the instruments that a parent, friend, doctor, or nurse is likely to use, that can creatively allow an individual to discover and process feelings.

We all fall into ruts, paths that take us to one spot but exclude other options. Medicine is no different. Physicians recognize the critical role of a person's emotional well-being. In quality-of-life studies of epilepsy patients, emotional well-being strongly correlates and is the largest single factor in predicting quality of life (1). Physicians are adept at prescribing antidepressant drugs for sadness, antianxiety drugs for anxiety, and hypnotic agents for insomnia. Referrals to psychologists and other therapists may, however, be the critical step in improving emotional well-being for many individuals. Their problems are not due to deficient serotonin, even if that deficiency and the resultant depression is a by-product of their underlying disorder. An antidepressant may be indicated and improve some symptoms, but such medications alone rarely restore self-esteem or resolve the personal demons that can sap an individuals' vitality and verve. "Talk therapy" has fallen somewhat out of favor with the explosion of biologic psychiatry and the downfall of Freudian psychology. Yet there is enormous value in psychotherapy, and for many individuals, it is *the* therapy they need.

Art therapy is an especially valuable tool for children in communicating their feelings; it is psychotherapy that begins without words. In many cases, the feelings may be those that the child is unaware of and that the parents might consider impossible. Those feelings and issues can be the key to finding the path towards a better quality of life, greater self-esteem, and the resolution of negative emotions that fester and can destroy a child's spirit.

There are no risks in the conventional sense. As with any therapy, "chemistry" must exist between therapist and patient for the interaction to succeed. Finding the right art therapist may be challenging, especially for children whose feelings lie under many protective layers, and those who distrust adults or members of a certain gender or other groups. Yet this is true for all therapies, and the rewards of finding the right therapist can be enormous.

References

1. Devinsky O, Vickrey BG, Cramer J, et al. Development of the quality of life in epilepsy (QOLIE) inventory. *Epilepsia* 1995;36(11):1089–1104.

First Group

Initially, Kevin was quiet and had a shy demeanor. He seemed anxious and conscientious and had difficulty expressing himself verbally and with confidence. He seemed very excited about making art. During the first group, members were asked to draw a picture of how they would introduce themselves to others in the group. The group members had a choice of many different materials, including pencils, pastels, crayons, and markers.

Kevin chose to work in pencil, and made a very detailed drawing of himself doing chores at home, such as washing dishes and cleaning the floor (Figure 30.1). Kevin included the room where he watches television in the drawing, which is possibly a place where he experiences pleasure and some engagement with the outside world, albeit from the security of his home. It was, however, still a reference to staying in his home, where he felt safe and where most of his life was centered.

At the end of this group, Kevin drew another picture (Figure 30.1a) and spoke about being quiet, hardworking, smart, and fast. He said his needs included his television and bed. He wished he was stronger, had money and a car, and worked outside his home. Kevin seemed to be most expressive about what he needed and wished for, giving money the most color.

Although Kevin worked and spoke in extraordinary detail, he had difficulty creating a bigger, more colorful picture of the world or himself. He was holding onto the safety of his home, not venturing out into the world to pursue his dreams.

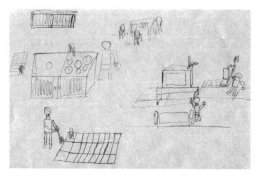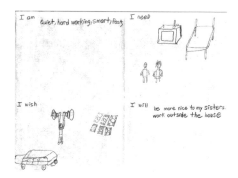

FIGURES 30.1 AND 30.1A

Second Group

In the second group, participants were given paint and large pieces of cardboard. They were asked to paint a landscape that reflected who they are. Kevin had expressed a strong interest in painting, and he worked in a focused manner over the next few weeks on a painting of his room (Figure 30.2). (This painting remains unfinished.) Kevin experimented with where he put colors and with mixing colors, which was daring and expansive for him. He appeared freer and more comfortable in the group.

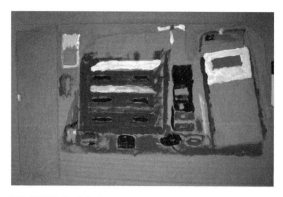

FIGURE 30.2

Kevin spoke in exacting detail about all of his belongings: his football, book bag, slippers, dustpan, and broom. He shared a very personal part of himself, and it became apparent that he was becoming more comfortable in the group by showing the members his belongings (transitional objects), which were extremely familiar to him and reassuring in his day-to-day life.

Third and Fourth Groups

The next group utilized an art therapy exercise designed to increase Kevin's level of comfort with being a little looser and freer in his work, and then possibly in his own life. The group members were asked to make a squiggle on a large piece of paper in a color of their own choosing. They were then asked to look at the squiggle from different angles and turn it into a drawing.

Kevin had difficulty with the spontaneity of the squiggle exercise. After thinking about it, he eventually made several rather tight squiggles in bright colors. Kevin turned his squiggles into brightly colored flowers, and what appeared to be an outdoor scene (Figure 30.3). This was a breakthrough for Kevin because his drawing was of something outside of his house and room. Kevin talked in a fairly animated manner about the places he was visiting that he had never seen before.

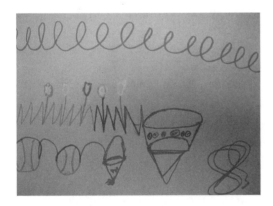

FIGURE 30.3

In the next session, group members made two masks—one with the face they usually show the world and one that showed an internal face that they hid from the world. Kevin's response was amazing. He described his first mask (Figure 30.4, left) as a "Tom and Jerry" mask, saying he identified with the cat, who was "shy and quiet." Kevin was able to put this mask on while describing the mask, projecting a fairly high level of comfort with himself, the group, and his feelings.

Kevin initially appeared frustrated with the second mask (Figure 30.4, right), but after some discussion, he was able to talk about his feelings of sadness and loss, and how he was trying to convey these feelings with the second mask but did not know how. It was explained to Kevin that sadness can be a lack of expression, color, and activity, so that he was probably accurately depicting the feelings he keeps inside.

Kevin made some big gains after this group. He worried less, was more comfortable reaching out to others, and expressed a genuine need to have contact with others.

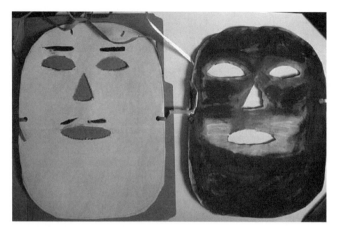

FIGURE 30.4

Other Groups

A form of sculpting clay in different colors was used for the next group. The group was asked to make objects that they liked and some that they didn't, and to then have the objects interact with each other. The objects Kevin made were related to activities he enjoyed and to chores. Kevin may have been trying to balance and integrate the difficulties in his life with the fun and pleasure. This was possibly a metaphor for his own difficulty of balancing the limitations of his illness with his desire for more participation in the outside world. Kevin had difficulty organizing the pieces into a structure or order, indicating he was still struggling with integrating the feelings this project evoked.

During the next group, members were asked to use their imaginations and an assortment of materials to turn empty shoe boxes into whatever they liked, with the option to use both the inside or outside of the box. Kevin painted the Statue of Liberty with a smile on her face and surrounded by water on the inside of the box. The Statue of Liberty seemed to correlate with Kevin's newfound freedom of expression as well as the incorporation of more independence and adventure into his life. For the outside of the box, Kevin returned to the safe objects of his home—mainly the room where he watches television. When describing the outside of the box, Kevin said he retreats to this room to watch television when he is sad. This seemed to express his loneliness about the insular life he was living.

At this point, it seemed that Kevin started to make a transition to the outside world. He engaged with art with more ease, as well as with the art therapist and the other art therapy students. Over the following months, Kevin continued to develop this engagement, seeming less anxious and making art with much more confidence. He has recently attended more activities on his own, such as a Christmas party and a large fun-filled gathering for people with epilepsy, where he did not know anyone. He is also in a job-training program that he is quite excited about. Kevin is more expressive, happy, and confident each week.

The Benefits of Art Therapy

Kevin's experience in art therapy illustrates how the combination of art and therapy can be a powerful tool for helping people with epilepsy. Art therapy can be a slow and subtle process. At the beginning, there is usually encouragement to create, with little emphasis on talking until the patient feels comfortable. This allows the patient to develop and discover their own symbols or transitional objects that will assist them in communicating comfortably. It also helps to ensure that the person is communicating authentically and with little pressure to please anyone other than himself. Working on how to relate to others is slowly and carefully integrated into the therapeutic process.

Kevin appeared to be comfortable being quiet and alone, but he had difficulty talking about feelings that are not easy to share, such as fear of being rejected by others. It took time for Kevin to see that he could express himself through the art making process. It also took time for him to develop trust and confidence in the art therapist. Only then did Kevin seem to feel comfortable verbalizing his feelings. Kevin first became comfortable testing out "life shaping activities" (3) in his art, then with the art therapist, and then more actively with the world at-large.

The process of engagement, transition, and socialization through art therapy—although it is at times slow and arduous—is usually rewarding and fun, and its effects are long lasting. Winnicott, in discussing the need for authenticity and creative living in development, says that, "The infant's ego is building up strength" (1). People with epilepsy have different levels of need in terms of engagement, transition, and socialization. This depends on the severity of the seizures, the age of onset, the degree of protectiveness they have experienced in their families, and other factors. Art therapy can effectively develop creativity and authenticity, giving (ego) strength to the person with epilepsy. With the support of the art therapist, the person with epilepsy can create transitional objects that increase his ability to be more confident socially. Therefore, people with epilepsy may live more fully and creatively within their given circumstances, through utilizing this form of therapy that assists with engagement, transition, and socialization.

References

1. Winnicott DW. *Ego Distortion in Terms of True and False Self*, 1960. *The Maturational Processes and the Facilitating Environment, Studies in the Theory of Emotional Development.* International Universities Press, Inc., 1965.
2. Winnicott DW. *The Location of Cultural Experience. Playing and Reality.* Tavistock Publications Ltd., 1971.
3. Deri SK. *Symbolism and Creativity.* International Universities Press, Inc., 1994.

CHAPTER 31

Pet Therapy

STEPHEN W. BROWN, FRC PSYCH

Employees experience lower stress levels when they are allowed to bring their pets into the workplace. The presence of pets has a positive effect on employee health and on the workplace in general. In one study by Wells et al., the authors noted that "participants who brought their pets to work experienced greater benefits than participants who did not bring their pets to work and participants who did not own pets" (1). The presence of a dog in a room can lower the blood pressure of children, both while resting and while reading, and reduce the stress associated with a demanding experimental situation. In this case, the presence of the dog appears to modify the children's perception of the situation so that they find it less threatening and friendlier (2). Having a dog present in the room reduces the behavioral features of distress exhibited by young children undergoing a physical examination (3). Children with a disability who are accompanied by a dog receive more social acknowledgment than those without a dog (4), and the presence of a dog acts as a social catalyst for adults (5). Dog ownership by older people is associated with an increase in the activities of daily living and positively effects on mood (6).

Companion Animals and Human Health

Studies of Alzheimer's disease patients showed that animal-assisted therapy (especially with dogs) is associated with less aggression, agitation, and wandering, and more social interaction (7–10). Companion animals also have benefits for caregivers (11). Although people with Alzheimer's disease may have seizures as a consequence of the condition, studies of the effect of this therapy present little comment on seizure frequency. Work with people who have spinal cord injury suggests that animal-assisted therapy may provide sensory stimulation, reduce stress, increase self-esteem, and help the patient express feelings (12). At least one report documents the benefits of pet ownership for people living with HIV infection—pet ownership is said to promote self-esteem—although the evidence for this and for the use in spinal cord injury rehabilitation is mainly anecdotal (13).

Other Zootherapies

The relationship between other nondomestic animals and humans has been studied for therapeutic potential, including hippotherapy (using horses) and dolphin-assisted therapy. Programs aimed at assisting people with disabilities to ride horses are popular in a number of countries, and potential benefits are said to come from a variety of aspects of horse–human interaction. Dolphin therapy has been used with children with learning disabilities, autism, and motor developmental delay, as well as with adults with chronic pain. These groups presumably would have included children with difficult-to-control epilepsy, but the specific impact on seizures has hardly been studied. Working with dolphins requires special preparation and circumstances, and it is unlikely to develop into a mainstream therapeutic option. Nevertheless, some positive long-term follow-up studies suggest that the dolphin's echolocation system may play a role in some cases, possibly by the emission of high frequency sound waves that affect human tissues (14–16). Although the patient groups described in these reports often have a high incidence of seizure disorders, little is reported on the outcome of this type of therapy on epilepsy.

Dog-Assisted Therapy

The use of assistance dogs for people with visual impairment is well known and has a long history, and is not further described here. The therapeutic use of dogs in reacting to human situations falls into two main categories: *response* and *alert*. Response dogs assist humans by behaving in a specific, useful way when a particular event occurs, such as drawing the hearing-impaired human's attention to the presence of a visitor at the door. Alert dogs are said to anticipate certain kinds of impending events and provide a useful warning to humans. In psychiatry, dog therapy has been advocated for the anticipation of panic attacks (alert type), for desensitizing people to phobias, and for reducing social anxiety (mainly response type). Little research data support such claims, and these topics require further investigation.

The use of support dogs in human epilepsy has a number of particular issues.

Dogs and Human Seizures

Many of us who work in clinical epileptology are aware of anecdotal reports of pet dogs developing a premonition of human seizures. Probably up to two-thirds of adults with epilepsy lack a useful warning method for their seizures. Occasionally, we hear that other family or household members may recognize premonitory signs of seizures before the person with epilepsy does. That household member with a premonition may be the pet dog. When we look more closely, however, we see hazards associated with ordinary pet dogs who lack special training. During or after a seizure (or if the dog spontaneously anticipates a human seizure), the dog may attack the person with epilepsy or anyone else in the vicinity. This reaction may generalize to the exhibition of aggression to other similar humans, such as children. The dog may show a flight, fright, freeze, or appeasement reaction. We know of at least one dog that choked on a leash as a result.

It is important to know how common this problem is. We reported 36 cases known to us (17), and hope we will be able to set up a survey in a geographically defined area.

Commentary

Pets can be "just what the doctor ordered" for people with epilepsy. Nonjudgmental and full of unconditional love, pets can provide a boost to a person's self-esteem, provide a sense of security, and help lower stress levels.

Dr. Brown reviews the medical evidence that pets have positive health benefits in people with a variety of medical conditions. He then discusses seizure-alert dogs, a subject that interests many people. Dr. Brown emphasizes the importance of the training process for these dogs and discusses his own research in which he measured seizure frequency in people who were given seizure-alert dogs. These results are very interesting and warrant additional studies.

The question arises: Can dogs be properly trained to react to human seizures? I suggest the answer is "yes."

Seizure Alert Dogs

My colleague, Val Strong, of the not-for-profit charity Support Dogs, based in Sheffield, United Kingdom, developed a specific program to train seizure alert dogs, who are especially chosen for their suitability for this work. They are socialized by working with a trainer and the person with epilepsy, and have no contact with the person with epilepsy before being introduced under controlled conditions by the trainer. The dogs undergo an intensive reward-based operant conditioning regime, beginning in a special setting and generalizing later. The trainer rewards the dog when the person with epilepsy has a seizure. More than 20 dogs have been trained by Support Dogs, and one scientific paper has described six of the dogs (18). Dogs trained in this way can anticipate a seizure in the significant human and warn the person from 15 to 45 minutes beforehand by attracting the person's attention and then giving a particular signal. Dogs will not be stressed by seizure events if they have been properly trained.

The original purpose of our work was to assist people with epilepsy who did not have a useful warning of their seizures, so that they could take appropriate action for their own protection when they knew a seizure was approaching. An unexpected finding from the early work was that people reported a reduced seizure rate; therefore, we began investigating whether this was a useful effect by using seizure frequency as an outcome measure, which we had not done before. Initially, we followed 10 people with epilepsy who all had tonic-clonic seizures. They kept seizure diaries for 12 weeks after enrollment, but before being assigned to a dog. Each person was then introduced to a specially selected dog and a 12-week training period began. The people entering the study were followed for 24 weeks after the 12-week training period. Seizure rates fell, on average, during the training period (Figure 31.1), and this improvement continued during 24 weeks of follow-up. Nine of the 10 subjects had some reduction in seizure frequency (Figure 31.2), with only one showing no improvement. These reductions in seizure frequency are statistically significant.

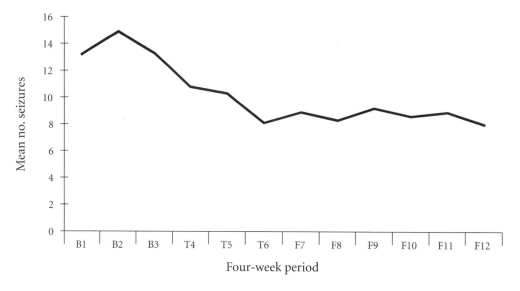

B1 – B3 = Baseline; T4 – T6 = Training; F7 – F12 = Follow-up

FIGURE 31.1

Change in mean seizure frequency of 10 people with tonic-clonic seizures after training with a selected dog.

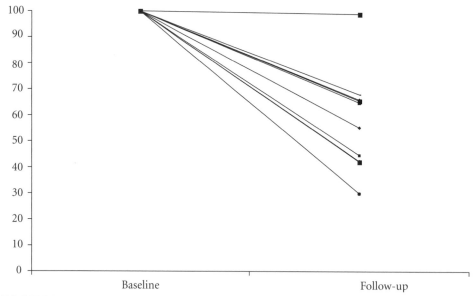

FIGURE 31.2

Percentage change in seizure frequency in the same persons after seizure-alert dog training. Outcomes for each of 10 persons.

Seizure Precipitation

If we are training people to recognize that when their dog behaves in a certain way they are about to have a seizure *and* the dog has learned this by being rewarded for it, the possibility exists that the seizure may be a consequence of the dog's alert, rather than the dog's alert being a result of the impending seizure. The best evidence against this possibility, however, as we have shown in small numbers so far, is that in most cases, the person with epilepsy reports a reduction in overall seizure frequency.

Harm or Stress on the Dogs

Dogs that spontaneously react to human seizures may show serious stress reactions that have adverse consequences for the health and well-being of the dogs themselves, the people with epilepsy, and other humans. The dogs trained in the way described here, however, are not affected by such consequences and, indeed, the training is specifically designed to avoid such an outcome.

Efficacy of Dog-Assisted Therapy in Epilepsy

In the cases reported so far, we were careful to solicit the opinion of the neurologists caring for the person with epilepsy, and we excluded any people with the possibility of nonepileptic attack disorder (pseudoseizures). In our ongoing study of 30 people, we have built in more safeguards to be certain of the diagnosis and outcome. We acknowledge that the issue needs to be addressed further. It is possible that this may be a treatment that can be applied to both epileptic and nonepileptic seizures. We have more evidence for efficacy in epilepsy than in nonepileptic attack disorder, however.

Having a greater degree of predictability for seizures means being able to take more control over one's activities, leading to increased self-confidence. There has been much interest in the relationship between well-being in epilepsy and its relationship to whether people perceive themselves as acting effectively in the world and directing their own behavior, or whether they see themselves as passive recipients of events around them (19–22). Being able to go out more may allow people to engage in more activities and may reduce some of the fear previously associated with epilepsy. Whether this increased self-confidence alone is sufficient to alter seizure frequency is not clear, but increased levels of activity and engagement in tasks may possibly have an effect (23).

Conclusion

Our opinion—based on observation and bearing in mind the training method that has been developed—is that the dogs detect subtle changes in the behavior of the human subject that characteristically precede a clinical seizure. The dogs may be using other cues such as smell; this is difficult to investigate further and remains an interesting speculation.

Acknowledgment

I thank my colleague, Val Strong, of Support Dogs (Sheffield, UK), who developed the technique described in this chapter.

References

1. Wells M, Perrine R. Critters in the cube farm: perceived psychological and organizational effects of pets in the workplace. *J Occup Health Psychol* 2001;6:81–87.
2. Friedmann E, Katcher AH, Thomas SA, et al. Social interaction and blood pressure. Influence of animal companions. *J Nerv Ment Disease* 1983;171:461–465.
3. Hansen KM, Messinger CJ, Baun MM, et al. Companion animals alleviating distress in children *Anthrozoos* 1999;12:142–148.
4. Mader B, Hart LA, Bergin B. Social acknowledgements for children with disabilities: effects of service dogs. *Child Dev* 1989;60:1529–1534.
5. McNicholas J, Collis GM. Dogs as catalysts for social interactions: robustness of the effect. *Br J Psychol* 2000;91:61–70.
6. Raina P, Waltner-Toews D, Bonnett B, et al. Influence of companion animals on the physical and psychological health of older people: an analysis of a one-year longitudinal study. *J Am Geriatr Soc* 1999;47:323–329.
7. Kongable LG, Buckwalter KC, Stolley JM. The effects of pet therapy on the social behavior of institutionalized Alzheimer's clients. *Arch Psychiatr Nurs* 1989;3:191–198.
8. Forbes DA. Strategies for managing behavioural symptomatology associated with dementia of the Alzheimer type: a systematic overview. *Can J Nursing Research* 1998;30:67–86.
9. Bernstein P-L, Friedmann E, Malaspina A. Animal-assisted therapy enhances resident social interaction and initiation in long-term care facilities. *Anthrozoos* 2000;13:213–224.
10. Kanamori M, Suzuki M, Yamamoto K, et al. A daycare program and evaluation of animal-assisted therapy (AAT) for the elderly with senile dementia. *Am J Alzheimer's Dis Other Demen* 2001;16:234–239.
11. Fritz CL, Farver TB, Hart LA, et al. Companion animals and the psychological health of Alzheimer patients' caregivers. *Psychol Rep* 1996;78:467–481.
12. Counsell CM, Abram J, Gilbert M. Animal-assisted therapy and the individual with spinal cord injury. *Sci Nurs* 1997;14:52–55.
13. Allen JM, Kellegrew DH, Jaffe D. The experience of pet ownership as a meaningful occupation. *Can J Occup Ther—Revue Canadienne d'Ergotherapie* 2000;67:271–278.
14. Lukina LN. Influence of dolphin-assisted therapy sessions on the functional state of children with psychoneurologic symptoms of diseases. *Hum Physiol* 1999;25:676–679.
15. Servais V. Some comments on context embodiment in zootherapy: the case of the autidolfin project. *Anthrozoos* 1999;2:5–15.
16. Nathanson D. Long-term effectiveness of dolphin-assisted therapy for children with severe disabilities. *Anthrozoos* 1998;11:22–32.
17. Strong V, Brown S. Should people with epilepsy have untrained dogs as pets? *Seizure* 2000;9:427–430.
18. Strong V, Brown SW, Walker R. Seizure alert dogs—fact or fiction? *Seizure* 1999;8:62–65.
19. Gehlert S. Perceptions of control in adults with epilepsy. *Epilepsia* 1994;35:81–88.
20. DiIorio C, Faherty B, Manteuffel B. Epilepsy self-management: partial replication and extension. *Res Nurs Health* 1994;17:167–174.
21. Amir M, Roziner I, Knoll A, et al. Self-efficacy and social support as mediators in the relation between disease severity and quality of life in patients with epilepsy. *Epilepsia* 1999;40:216–224.

22. Hermann BP, Wyler AR. Depression, locus of control, and the effects of epilepsy surgery. *Epilepsia* 1989;30:332–338.
23. Jenkins L, Owen L. Work and epileptiform activity. *Seizure* 1992;1(suppl A):P14/18.

Index

NOTE: Boldface numbers indicate illustrations; *t* indicates a table.